ABL

$77-00

Department of Renal Medicine

—

Do Not Remove

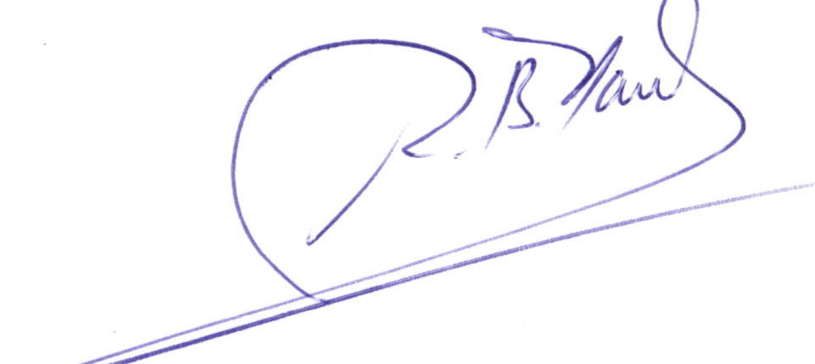

Advances in Nephrology®
Volume 21

Advances in Nephrology®

Volumes 1 through 15 (Out of Print)

Volume 16

Vasopressin Antagonists, *by Serge Jard*
From the Renin Gene to Renin Inhibitors, *by Pierre Corvol and Joël Ménard*
Cardiovascular and Renal Effects of Atrial Natriuretic Factor, *by Friedrich C. Luft, Rudolf E. Lang, Heikki Ruskoaho, R. Bernd Sterzel, Thomas Unger, and Detlev Ganten*
Do Glucocorticosteroids Play a Role in the Regulation of Blood Pressure? A Study Performed With a Glucocorticosteroid Antagonist, *by Jean-Pierre Grünfeld, Laure Eloy, Blanca Ramos-Frendo, Augusto Araujo, Eugène Rothschild, and Françoise Russo-Marie*
Thick Ascending Limb—Anatomy and Function: Role in Urine Concentrating Mechanisms, *by Lise Bankir, Nadine Bouby, Marie-Marcelle Trinh-Trang-Tan, and Brigitte Kaissling*
Hormonal Control of Renal Medullary Functions, *by Christian de Rouffignac, Jean-Marc Elalouf, and Nicole Roinel*
Multiple Hormonal Control of the Thick Ascending Limb, *by Claude Amiel, Claire Bailly, and Gerard Friedlander*
Pharmacology of Loop Diuretics: State of the Art, *by Jean-Louis Imbs, Mariette Schmidt, and Eva Giesen-Crouse*
Acute Renal Failure: A Disease of the Elderly? *by Joseph Rosenfeld, Joseph Shohat, Itamar Grosskopf, and Geoffrey Boner*
Glomerular Cells in Vitro, *by Gary E. Striker, Mary Ann Lange, Karen MacKay, Kenneth Bernstein, and Liliane J. Striker*
Endourology, *by Joseph W. Segura*
Treatment of Idiopathic Membranous Nephropathy, *by Claudio Ponticelli, Pietro Zucchelli, Patrizia Passerini, Leonardo Gagnoli, and Enrico Imbasciati*
Drug-Induced Autoimmune Disease, *by C. J. Spears and J. R. Batchelor*
Physiopathologic Aspects of Tamm-Horsfall Protein: A Phylogenetically Conserved Marker of the Thick Ascending Limb of Henle's Loop, *by Pierre Ronco, Michel Brunisholz, Monique Geniteau-Legendre, Francoise Chatelet, Pierre Verroust, and Gabriel Richet*
Antireceptor or Antihormone Autoimmunity and Its Relationship With the Idiotype Network, *by Jean-François Bach*
Berger's Disease: Recent Advances in Immunology and Genetics, *by Marie-Christine Bene and Gilbert Faure*
Autoimmunity and Glomerulonephritis, *by Christopher Martin Lockwood, Christine Bowman, D. Bakes, A. Pressey, and A. Dash*
Kidney Transplantation in Children: Results of 383 Grafts Performed at Enfants Malades Hospital From 1973 to 1984, *by Michel Broyer, Marie-*

France Gagnadoux, Genevieve Guest, Daniel Buerton, Patrick Niaudet, Renee Habib, and M. Busson

Cyclosporine in Pediatric Kidney Transplantation, *by Johannes Brodehl, Gisela Offner, and Peter F. Hoyer*

Cardiovascular Stability on Hemodialysis, *by Thierry Petitclerc, Tilman Drüeke, Nguyen-Khoa Man, and Jean-Louis Funck-Brentano*

Erythropoietin: Structure, Function, Origin, *by Armin Kurtz*

Erythropoietin: Origin, Bone Marrow Receptors, and Relation to Renin Substate (Angiotensinogen), *by Frej Fyhrquist, Katarine Rosenlöf, Matti Autero, and Tytti Kärkkäinen*

Volume 17

Glomerular Hemodynamics in Experimental Glomerulonephritis, *by Roland C. Blantz, Francis B. Gabbai, and Curtis B. Wilson*

Glomerular Adaptations to Renal Injury: The Role of Capillary Hypertension in the Pathogenesis of Focal and Segmental Glomerulosclerosis, *by Helmut G. Rennke*

Glomerular Hemostasis in Normal and Pathologic Conditions, *by Jean-Daniel Sraer, Alain Kanfer, Eric Rondeau, and Roger Lacave*

Recent Immunologic Data on Human Glomerulonephritis, *by Philippe Lesavre, Renato C. Monteiro, Alain Chevailler, Jean Berger, Lise Halbwachs-Mecarelli, and Laure-Hélène Noël*

Update, on Immunosuppressive Therapy in Human and Experimental Glomerulonephritis, *by Christian Jacquot, Dana Baran, Benoît Vendeville, Lucette Pelletier, and Philippe Druet*

Early Diabetic Nephropathy: Detection and Prevention, *by GianCarlo Viberti and Jeremy J. Bending*

The Nephropathy Related to Acquired Immune Deficiency Syndrome, *by Jacques J. Bougoignie, Ruth Meneses, and Victoriano Pardo*

Treatment of Corticoresistant Idiopathic Nephrotic Syndrome in the Adult: Minimal Change Disease and Focal Segmental Glomerulosclerosis, *by Alain Meyrier and Pierre Simon*

Treatment of Severe Childhood Nephrosis, *by P. Niaudet, R. Habib, M. F. Gagnadoux, M. J. Tete, and M. Broyer*

Nephrotoxicity of Antitumoral Agents, *by J. P. Fillastre, G. Viotte, J. P. Morin, and B. Moulin*

Renal Involvement in Essential Mixed Cryoglobulinemia: A Peculiar Type of Immune-Mediated Renal Disease, *by G. D'Amico, G. Colasanti, F. Ferrario, A. R. Sinico, A. Bucci, and A. Fornasier*

Lead and the Kidney, *by Eberhard Ritz, Johannes Mann, and Markus Stoeppler*

Recent Developments in Pheochromocytoma Diagnosis and Imaging, *by P.-F. Plouin, G. Chatellier, M.-A. Rougeot, J. M. Duclos, J.-Y. Pagny, P. Corvol, and J. Menard*

Volume 18 **(Out of Print)**

Volume 19 **(Out of Print)**

Volume 20

Advances in Nephrology® From the Necker Hospital

French Editors

Jean-Pierre Grünfeld, M.D.

Corresponding Editor-in-Chief, Department of Nephrology, Necker Hospital, Paris, France

Jean François Bach, M.D., D.Sc.

Department of Clinical Immunology, Necker Hospital, Paris, France

Henri Kreis, M.D.

Department of Nephrology, Necker Hospital, Paris, France

American Editor

Morton H. Maxwell, M.D.

Director of Hypertension Service, Cedars-Sinai Medical Center, Los Angeles, California

Volume 21 • 1992

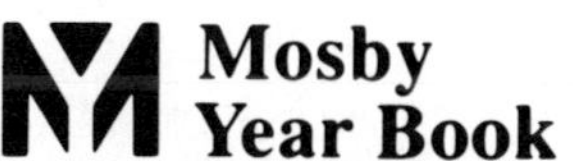

St. Louis Baltimore Boston Chicago London Philadelphia Sydney Toronto

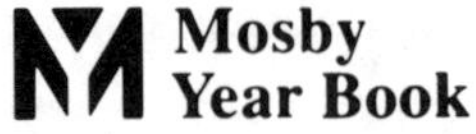

Dedicated to Publishing Excellence

Sponsoring Editor: Amy L. Reynaldo
Associate Managing Editor, Manuscript Services: Denise Dungey
Assistant Director, Manuscript Services: Frances M. Perveiler
Production Coordinator: Max Perez
Proofroom Manager: Barbara M. Kelly

Mosby–Year Book, Inc.
11830 Westline Industrial Drive
St. Louis, MO 63146

Editorial Office:
Mosby–Year Book, Inc.
200 North LaSalle St.
Chicago, IL 60601

International Standard Serial Number: 0084-5957
International Standard Book Number: 0-8151-3590-4

Contributors

Jean Michel Achard

Chef de Clinique, Service de Néphrologie du Centre Hospitalier Régional et Universitaire d'Amiens, France

Elisabetta Baldi, Ph.D.

Department of Pathophysiology, University of Florence, Florence, Italy

Jean-Pierre Benhamou, M.D.

Service d'Hépatologie and Unité de Recherches de Physiopathologie Hépatique (INSERM), Hôpital Beaujon, Clichy, France

Henri Bernardi

Institut de Pharmacologie Moléculaire et Cellulaire de Centre National de la Recherche Scientifique, Sophia Antipolis, Valbonne, France

Virginia M. Black, B.S.

Life Science Research Assistant, Division of Nephrology, Department of Medicine, Stanford University School of Medicine, Stanford University Medical Center, Stanford, California

Odile Blanchet, M.D.

INSERM U93, Hôpital Saint-Louis, Paris, France

Christian Boitard, M.D.

Department of Clinical Immunology, INSERM U25, Hôpital Necker, Paris, France

Bernard Boudailliez

Practician Hospitalier, Service de Pédiatrie I du Centre Hospitalier Regional et Universitaire, d'Amiens, France

Liesbeth Breslau-Siderius

Department of Clinical Genetics, Academic Hospital Maastricht, Maastricht, The Netherlands

Martijn H. Breuning, M.D., Ph.D.

Department of Human Genetics, State University Leiden, Sylvius Laboratories, Leiden, The Netherlands

Christopher R. Burrow, M.D.

Assistant Professor, Division of Nephrology, The Johns Hopkins University School of Medicine, Baltimore, Maryland

Johannes G. Dauwerse

Department of Human Genetics, State University Leiden, Sylvius Laboratories, Leiden, The Netherlands

William M. Deen, Ph.D.
Professor of Chemical Engineering, Department of Chemical Engineering, Massachusetts Institute of Technology, Cambridge, Massachusetts

Françoise Degos, M.D.
Service d'Hépatologie and Unité de Recherches de Physiopathologie Hépatique (INSERM), Hôpital Beaujon, Clichy, France

Laurent Degos, M.D., Ph.D.
INSERM U93, Hôpital Saint-Louis, Paris, France

Jan R. de Weille, Ph.D.
Institut de Pharmacologie Moléculaire et Cellulaire de Centre National de la Recherche Scientifique, Sophia Antipolis, Valbonne, France

Gilles Dietrich, M.B.
INSERM U28 and Service d'Immunologie, Hôpital Broussais, Paris, France

Tilman B. Drüeke, M.D.
Director, Associate Professor, INSERM U90, Department of Nephrology, Necker Hospital, Paris, France

Jean-Louis Dufier, M.D.
Department of Ophthalmology, Hôpital Necker, Hôpital des Enfants-Malades, Paris, France

Michael J. Dunn, M.D.
Hanna Payne Professor of Medicine, Director, Division of Nephrology, Departments of Medicine and Physiology/Biophysics, Case Western Reserve University School of Medicine, Cleveland, Ohio

Kai-Uwe Eckardt, M.D.
Assistant, Physiologisches Institut der Universität Regensburg, Germany

Michel Fosset, Ph.D.
Institut de Pharmacologie Moléculaire et Cellulaire de Centre National de la Recherche Scientifique, Sophia Antipolis, Valbonne, France

Albert Fournier, M.D.
Professor of Medicine, Service de Néphrologie, Centre Hospitalier Régional et Universitaire d'Ameins, France

Dominique Ganeval, M.D.
Department of Nephrology, Necker Hospital, Paris, France

Henri-Jean Garchon, M.D.
Department of Clinical Immunology, INSERM U25, Hôpital Necker, Paris, France

Violaine Guérin, M.D.
Department of Nephrology, Necker Hospital, Paris, France

Claus Hammer, M.D., Ph.D.
Professor, Institute for Surgical Research, University of Munich, Klinikum Grosshadern, Munich, Germany

Jacques Hors, M.D.
INSERM U93, Groupe d'études des Oligonucléotides de Diagnostic, Hôpital Saint-Louis, Paris, France

Denise Jobin, M.D.
INSERM U28 and Service d'Immunologie, Hôpital Broussais, Paris, France

Paul Jungers, M.D.
Department of Nephrology, Necker Hospital, Paris, France

Claudine Junien, Pharm.D., Ph.D.
Professor of Genetics, INSERM U73, University of Paris V, Paris, France

Srinivas V. Kaveri, Ph.D.
INSERM U28 and Service d'Immunologie, Hôpital Broussais, Paris, France

Michel D. Kazatchkine, M.D.
INSERM U28 and Service d'Immunologie, Hôpital Broussais, Paris, France

Mark Kester, Ph.D.
Departments of Medicine and Physiology/Biophysics, Case Western Reserve University School of Medicine, Cleveland, Ohio

Iman Khalil
Groupe d'Etudes des Oligonucléotides de Diagnostic, Hôpital Saint-Louis, Paris, France

Andrzej S. Krolewski, M.D., Ph.D.
Chief, Section on Epidemiology and Genetics, Research Division, Joslin Diabetes Center; Assistant Professor, Department of Medicine, Harvard Medical School, Boston, Massachusetts

Armin Kurtz, M.D.
Professor, Physiologisches Institut der Universität Regensburg, Germany

Lori M.B. Laffel, M.D., McPott.
Investigator, Section on Epidemiology & Genetics, Research Division, Joslin Diabetes Center; Instructor, Department of Pediatrics, Harvard Medical School, Boston, Massachusetts

Paul Landais, M.D.
Department of Nephrology, Necker Hospital, Paris, France

Michel Lazdunski, Ph.D.
Institut de Pharmacologie Moléculaire et Cellulaire du Centre National de la Recherche Scientifique, Sophia Antipolis, Valbonne, France

Gérard Lefranc, M.S., Ph.D.

Professor, Laboratoire d'Immunogénétique Moléculaire, Unité de Recherche Associée 1191, Centre National de la Recherche Scientifique, Université Montpellier II, Sciences et Techniques du Languedoc, Montpellier, France

Marie-Paule Lefranc, M.S., Ph.D.

Professor, Laboratoire d'Immunogénétique Moléculaire, Unité de Recherche Associée 1191, Centre National de la Recherche Scientifique, Université Montpellier II, Sciences et Techniques du Languedoc, Montpellier, France

Virginia Lepage, M.D.

Laboratoire Universitaire, Groupe d'Etudes des Oligonucléotides de Diagnostic, Hôpital Saint-Louis, Paris, France

Philippe Lesavre, M.D., Ph.D.

Department of Nephrology, INSERM U90, Necker Hospital, Paris, France

Micheline Lévy, M.D.

INSERM U155, Château de Longchamp, Bois de Boulogne, Paris, France

C. Martin Lockwood, M.D.

Department of Medicine, School of Clinical Medicine, Addenbrooke's Hospital, Cambridge, United Kingdom

Patrick Marcellin, M.D.

Service d'Hépatologie and Unité de Recherches de Physiopathologie Hépatique (INSERM), Hôpital Beaujon, Clichy, France

Paolo Mené, M.D.

Cattedra di Ne Frologia Medica, University of Rome, Rome, Italy

Philippe Morinière, M.D.

Service de Néphrologie du Centre Hospitalier Régional et Universitaire d'Amiens, France

Christiane Mourre, Ph.D.

Institut de Pharmacologie Moléculaire et Cellulaire du Centre National de la Recherche Scientifique, Sophia Antipolis, Valbonne, France

Bryan D. Myers, M.D.

Professor of Medicine, Division of Nephrology, Department of Medicine, Stanford University School of Medicine, Stanford University Medical Center, Stanford, California

Tomohiro Osanai, M.D.

Department of Internal Medicine, Hirosaki University, Hirosaki City, Japan

Pascale Paul, Ph.D.

INSERM U93, Hôpital Saint-Louis, Paris, France

Nathalie Pertuiset, M.D.
Department of Nephrology, Necker Hospital, Paris, France

Cécile Rabian, M.D.
Department of Nephrology, Necker Hospital, Paris, France

Françoise Rossi, M.D.
INSERM U28 and Service d'Immunologie, Hôpital Broussais, Paris, France

Stephen G. Rostand, M.D.
Professor of Medicine, Nephrology Research and Training Center, Division of Nephrology, Department of Medicine, University of Alabama School of Medicine, University of Alabama at Birmingham, Birmingham, Alabama

Jasper J. Saris
Department of Human Genetics, State University Leiden, Sylvius Laboratories, Leiden, The Netherlands

John D. Scandling, M.D.
Associate Professor of Medicine, Division of Nephrology, Department of Medicine, University of Rochester School of Medicine and Dentistry, Rochester, New York

Michael S. Simonson, B.S.
Department of Medicine, Case Western Reserve University School of Medicine, Cleveland, Ohio

Jean Paul Soulillou, M.D
University Hospital, INSERM U211, Nantes, France

Yvette Sultan, M.D.
Laboratoire d'Hemostase, Hôpital Cochin, Paris, France

Christie P. Thomas, M.D.
Department of Medicine, Case Western Reserve University School of Medicine, Cleveland, Ohio

Gert-Jan B. van Ommen, Ph.D.
Department of Human Genetics, State University Leiden, Sylvius Laboratories, Leiden, The Netherlands

Martin C. Wapenaar
Department of Human Genetics, State University Leiden, Sylvius Laboratories, Leiden, The Netherlands

James H. Warram, M.D., Sc.D.
Investigator, Section on Epidemiology & Genetics, Research Division, Joslin Diabetes Center, Boston, Massachusetts

Patricia D. Wilson, Ph.D.

Associate Professor, Department of Physiology and Biophysics, University of Medicine and Dentistry of New Jersey, Robert Wood Johnson Medical School at Rutgers, Piscataway, New Jersey

Johanna Zingraff, M.D.

Department of Nephrology, Necker Hospital, Paris, France

Preface

In recent years, the concept has emerged that genetic predisposition to disease plays an essential role in medicine. This idea is not new, but the tools necessary to test it were developed only through recent progress in molecular biology. Several papers in the first part of this volume point out how this genetic susceptibility can be analyzed (and, in some cases, predicted) in renal medicine, such as in glomerulonephritis, autoimmune diseases, diabetic nephropathy, malignant renal tumors, nephrosclerosis and, obviously, in inherited kidney diseases. These advances have raised further questions that are discussed in some of these papers: how such information can be used in families for early detection of disease and with what precautions, how these data shed light on the pathogenesis of the diseases, and how this genetic predisposition interplays with environmental factors.

This volume also contains information on advances in therapy in renal patients. Some of them are already applicable. The prevention of bone disease in dialysis patients remains a main concern for nephrologists. This volume contains an extensive review of new modalities of treatment in secondary hyperparathyroidism. Attention is focused on some therapeutic issues in renal patients that are often discussed with consulting physicians: e.g., treatment of chronic viral hepatitis in dialysis or transplant patients, indications of intravenous immunoglobulins in some autoimmune diseases, and management of patients with multiple myeloma. Some other therapeutic advances are heralded by recent progress in pharmacology and immunology: how to analyze and later to antagonize the renal effects of endothelin, the future for potassium channel agonists in cardiovascular medicine, and how to better understand the effect of erythropoietin on target cells and subsequently to better use it in renal patients. Recent therapeutic advances in kidney transplantation are presented in the last part of the book. Bioreagents comprise a growing family of monoclonal antibodies, modified monoclonal antibodies, and artificial molecules aimed at target immunocompetent cells. This family includes, among others, anti-interleukin 2 receptor monoclonal antibody, the use of which in human kidney transplantation has afforded promising results. Finally, xenografting, which is a formidable challenge in future organ transplantation, is considered in the last chapter of this volume.

The title of this series, *Advances in Nephrology,* is once again fully justified; the present volume brings together some major advances in concepts and understanding of renal diseases, and in the treatment of renal patients.

Jean-Pierre Grünfeld, M.D.

Contents

Part I

Genetic Factors in Renal Diseases

The Constant Region Genes of the Immunoglobulin Heavy Chains

Marie-Paule Lefranc, M.S., Ph.D.

Professor, Laboratoire d'Immunogénétique Moléculaire, Unité de Recherche Associée 1191, Centre National de la Recherche Scientifique, Université Montpellier II, Sciences et Techniques du Languedoc, Montpellier, France

Gérard Lefranc, M.S., Ph.D.

Professor, Laboratoire d'Immunogénétique Moléculaire, Unité de Recherche Associée 1191, Centre National de la Recherche Scientifique, Université Montpellier II, Sciences et Techniques du Languedoc, Montpellier, France

The human immunoglobulins (Ig) are the products of three unlinked sets of genes: the heavy (IGH) chain genes, and the κ (IGK) and λ (IGL) light chain genes.

The Ig heavy chain locus (IGH) is mapped on chromosome 14[1] at band q32[2]; the κ and the λ chain loci are mapped respectively on chromosomes 2 (2p12)[3, 4] and 22 (22q11).[5, 6] In this paper, we shall review the synthesis of the Ig chains and the organization of the constant region genes (Ig CH) of the human Ig heavy chains.

Synthesis of the Ig Chains

In the germ line state, the κ and λ loci consist of variable (V), joining (J), and constant (C) region genes. The synthesis of, for instance, a κ chain involves the joining of a Vκ gene[7, 8] with one of the five Jκ segments located about 2.5 kb upstream of the Cκ gene[9, 10] and the transcription of the rearranged Vκ-Jκ gene and of the Cκ gene. The synthesis of a λ chain involves the joining of a Vλ gene[11] with a joining segment Jλ located 1.5 kb upstream of one of the functional Cλ genes.[12–16]

The human heavy-chain locus consists of four linked families of variable (VH),[17-19] diversity (D),[20–23] joining (JH), and constant (CH)[24–27] genes. The synthesis of a heavy chain involves two joining events, first between D and JH, then between VH and D-JH.[28, 29] The Vκ-Jκ, Vλ-Jλ, and VH-D-JH joinings require the presence of characteristic heptamer-nonamer sequences separated by 12 or 23 base pairs and located at the 3′ end of the V genes, at the 5′ end of the J segments, and on both sides of the D segments.[30, 31] The V-J and V-D-J joinings result in the deletion of the intermediate sequences by a loop excision mechanism.[32–34] To express a complete and functional light or heavy chain, the corresponding genes must be correctly recombined at the DNA level in B cells.[35, 36] There is a chronology of the rearrangements observed in B cells with rearrangement of the heavy chain locus occurring first. A functional heavy chain μ appears to be required to initiate a κ gene rearrangement, and a λ gene rearrangement only occurs if κ genes are aberrantly rearranged or deleted.[37, 38] Once rearranged, the genes are transcribed into a nuclear RNA precursor that contains the fused V-J (or V-D-J) rearranged gene and the constant region exon(s) and which, like virtually every eukaryotic messenger RNA, must be processed by RNA splicing. Characteristic nucleotides 5′/GT-intron-AG/3′ at the junctions between introns and exons are required for correct splicing.

The Ig Class Switch

In humans, there are five classes of antibodies (IgM, IgD, IgG, IgE, and IgA) that are characterized by the isotypic antigenic determinants, physicochemical properties, and biologic activities of their heavy chains (μ, δ, γ, ϵ, and α, respectively). Furthermore, subclasses are known for IgG and IgA which are IgG1, IgG2, IgG3, and IgG4 (containing γ1, γ2, γ3, or γ4 heavy chains, respectively) and IgA1 and IgA2 (containing α1 or α2 chains). The heavy chains are defined by their CH region (for instance Cμ, Cδ, Cγ, and so on). The commitment of a human B-cell starts with the production of an IgM antibody of a given specificity which implies the synthesis of a μ chain and that of a κ or a λ chain. For the expression of IgG, IgA, or IgE antibodies, the H-chain genes have to undergo the so-called class switch. The switch from IgM to IgG, for example, requires no further light chain gene rearrangement but involves the recombination (or switch) of the previous expressed VH gene from Cμ to one of the Cγ subclass genes. This process involves the mediation of switch or S sequences that contain short tandemly repeated motifs and which are located about 2.0 kb upstream of all CH genes except Cδ.[39–41] The switch results in the deletion of the CH genes located between Sμ and the switch sequence of the new active CH gene,[42–44] by a loop excision mechanism.[32, 45, 46]

Organization of the Human Ig CH Locus

In human DNA, there are differences with the mouse locus shown first by the existence of two Cα genes (A1 and A2),[24, 26] second by the presence of a pseudo-γ gene GP,[47] and third, by the existence of three ϵ genes.[48, 49] (Nomenclature of the Ig CH genes is according to the recommendations of the

Human Gene Mapping committee.) Two of the ε genes (the active E gene and the pseudogene EP1) are located in the CH locus on chromosome 14, whereas the third (EP2) is a processed pseudogene located on chromosome 9.[50] The human M and D genes are linked[51] 8 kb apart.[52]

Two groups of cosmid clones (covering about 83 kb and 72 kb of the genome) were isolated, which encompassed G3-G1-EP1-A1 (region A) and G2-G4-E-A2 (region B)[24] (Fig 1). These results confirmed the linkage of the G2 and G4 genes previously established from phage library clones[47, 53] and showed that the human CH locus evolved by duplication of a large segment of DNA containing γ-ε-α or γ-γ-ε-α.[54]

The pattern of a large Ig CH gene deletion in individuals lacking IgG1, IgG2, IgG4, and IgA1 immunoglobulins[55] enabled the ordering of the two groups of cosmid clones with region A in the 5′ of region B, as the deletion starts downstream of G3 (region A) and ends upstream of the active E gene (region B) (deletion I, Fig 1).[26]

Moreover, the absence of the GP gene showed that the GP gene was also included in the deletion and therefore must be located between the A1 and G2 genes on chromosome 14.[25, 26] The order of the human Ig CH genes is, therefore, the following[24–26]:

$$5' \text{ M} \overset{8\text{kb}}{\text{——}} \text{D-. . .-G3} \overset{26\text{kb}}{\text{——}} \text{G1} \overset{19\text{kb}}{\text{——}} \text{EP1} \overset{13\text{kb}}{\text{——}} \text{A1-. . .}$$

$$\text{-GP-. . .-G2} \overset{18\text{kb}}{\text{——}} \text{G4} \overset{23\text{kb}}{\text{——}} \text{E} \overset{10\text{ kb}}{\text{——}} \text{A2} - 3'$$

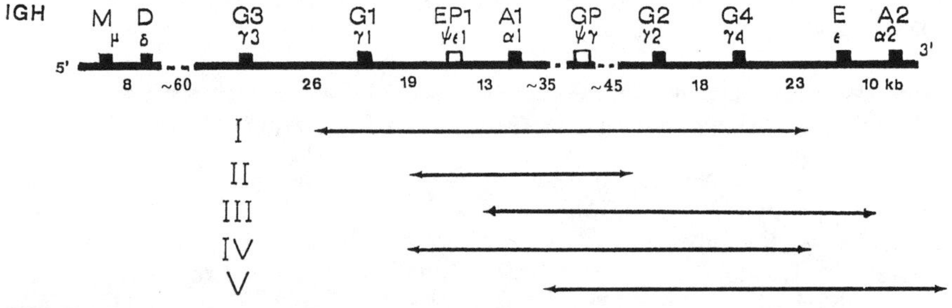

FIG 1.

Organization of the human immunoglobulin heavy chain constant region locus.[24–26, 82] Nomenclature of the Ig CH genes is according to the recommendations of Human Gene Mapping Committee. Multigene deletions in the Ig GH locus have been described in healthy individuals, either homozygous for one type of identical deletion on the two chromosomes 14 or heterozygous for two different deletions.[68, 69] Types of Ig CH multigene deletions are designated I to V according to the chronologic order of their findings.[78] Deletion I and other multigene deletions involve highly homologous regions that are hot spots of recombination, outside the switch sequences.[78] We have estimated with pulsed field gel electrophoresis (PFGE) that deletion I encompasses 160 kb.[78] Given these data[78] and those of Flanagan and Rabbitts,[24] the distance between A1 and G2 may be estimated to be 85 kb. A similar estimation (80 kb) has been obtained with PFGE of normal DNAs.[82] Deletion I = del G1-EP1-A1-GP-G2-G4. Deletion II = del EP1-A1-GP. Deletion III = del A1-GP-G2-G4-E. Deletion IV = del EP1-A1-GP-G2-G4. Deletion V = del GP-G2-G4-E-A2.[82]

Structure of the Ig CH Genes

The human genomic Ig CH genes have been completely sequenced: M,[51] D,[56] G3,[57, 58] G1,[59] EP1,[49] A1,[60] GP,[61] G2,[53] G4,[62] E,[48, 49] A2.[60, 63] The constant region of the μ[51] and ε chains is encoded by four distinct exons corresponding to each domain. The μ chain and the other heavy chains exist as membrane or as secretory forms with a distinct C-terminal region originating from different splicing events.[64–66]

The IGHG genes have a similar organization with each domain of the protein (CH1, CH2, CH3) and the hinge (h) coded on separate exons.[67] However, the hinge coding region of the G3 gene is made of three or four distinct exons separated from each other by short introns.[57, 58] This arrangement is distinct from the other IGHG genes in that these genes possess only one hinge exon.

The pseudogene EP1 has lost the CH1 and CH2 but possesses the CH3 and CH4 exons with the CH3 nucleotide sequence lacking four residues at its 5′ end (including the RNA splicing site).[48, 49] Adjacent to and upstream of the CH3 exon, a nucleotide sequence is found (absent from the active IGHE gene) with strong homology to S sequences. The unexpected location of this sequence implies its involvement in the deletion event.[54]

The A1 and A2 genes contain three exons. The hinge region is encoded at the beginning of the second exon.[60] This organization is different from that of the IGHG genes and from the D gene which have one (G1, G2, G4) or more (two for D, three or four for G3) small separate hinge coding exons.

Identification of the Ig CH Genes on Southern Blots

The Ig CH genes can be detected on Southern blots with Cμ, Cδ, Cγ, Cε, and Cα probes.[25, 26] Hybridization with these different CH probes revealed that the absence of several Ig subclasses observed in several healthy individuals was due to extensive deletions encompassing several heavy chain genes (Fig 1).[68, 69] The Cγ probe detects all the IGHG genes since they cross-hybridize with the genes for the various subclasses.[26] Moreover a restriction fragment length polymorphism (RFLP) exists for the different IGHG genes and, for example, five to ten hybridizing bands can be detected with genomic DNAs cut with the BamHI restriction enzyme.[26, 70–73] However a G3 hinge region probe[74] enabled identification of the G3 gene on Southern blot. This first specific human immunoglobulin subclass probe allowed study of the G3 polymorphism and demonstrated that an IgG3 selective deficiency was not due to a deletion of the G3 gene.[74]

Allele Determination With RFLP

The constant region of the γ1, γ2, γ3, α2, and ε heavy chains can be identified by allotypic antigenic determinants located on one or the other of the CH domains. These antigens, detectable with the classic hemagglutination inhibition technique, provide genetic markers for IgG1, IgG2, IgG3, IgA2, and IgE and are, consequently, called G1m, G2m, G3m, A2m, and Em allotypes, respectively. These allotypes are useful tools for the characterization of populations, disease association and linkage analyses, forensic medicine, and genetics of immunoglobulins.[75] Some of the alleles encoding these allotypes can be determined at the DNA level with RFLP using appropriate restriction enzymes. An example of such a determination is shown at the A2 locus where two allelic forms, $\alpha 2$ $A2m^1$ and $\alpha 2$ $A2m^2$, exist. The amino acid responsible for the A2m(2) allotype is encoded by nucleotides that are part of an EcoRI restriction site. Due to a nucleotide substitution, this site is absent in the $A2m^1$ allele. Thus, whereas the restriction enzyme PstI yields two fragments containing the A1 (1.2 kb) and A2 (2 kb) genes[24, 26] when DNAs are probed with a Cα probe, double digests EcoRI – PstI will show two different patterns: one similar to the PstI one for the $A2m^1$ allele and the other with a new 0.9 kb band for the $A2m^2$ allele due to the existence of the EcoRI site.[76] The determination of alleles with RFLP is particularly useful when reagents are not readily available for the serologic determination of the allotypes.[76, 77] Moreover it is the only way to identify alleles when no serum is available (for instance cell lines).

Conclusion

Extensive polymorphism has been observed with coding probes. Additional information may be obtained by the use of flanking region probes.[78] The vast number of RFLPs for immunoglobulin genes provides markers for genetic analysis of risk factors involved in the development of disease. The relative associations described between diseases and constant as well as switch region RFLPs[79–81] are likely to reflect an association with a given set of VH genes thus determining the repertoire of available antibodies. Such linkage between VH and CH genes has previously been described, but very limited data are available at present both with regard to normal linkage patterns and associations to disease. The recent description of multiple VH and CH genes as well as switch region RFLPs will therefore be of marked importance in the development of this area of research.

References

1. Croce CM, Shander M, Martinis J, et al: Chromosomal location of the genes for human immunoglobulin heavy chains. *Proc Natl Acad Sci USA* 1979; 76:3416–3419.
2. Kirsch IR, Morton CC, Nakahara K, et al: Human immunoglobulin heavy chain genes map to a region of translocations in malignant B lymphocytes. *Science* 1982; 216:301–303.
3. Malcolm S, Barton P, Murphy C, et al: Localisation of human immunoglobulin

kappa light chain variable region genes to the short arm of chromosome 2 by in situ hybridization. *Proc Natl Acad Sci USA* 1982; 79:4957–4961.

4. McBride OW, Hieter PA, Hollis GF, et al: Chromosomal location of human kappa and lambda immunoglobulin light chain constant region genes. *J Exp Med* 1982; 155:1480–1490.
5. Emanuel BS, Cannizzaro LA, Magrath I, et al: Chromosomal orientation of the lambda light chain locus: Vλ is proximal to Cλ in 22q11. *Nucleic Acids Res* 1985; 13:381–387.
6. Erikson J, Martinis J, Croce CM: Assignment of the genes for human λ immunoglobulin chains to chromosome 22. *Nature* 1981; 294:173–175.
7. Bentley DL, Rabbitts TH: Human Vκ immunoglobulin gene number: Implication of the origin of antibody diversity. *Cell* 1981; 24:613–623.
8. Straubinger B, Huber E, Lorenz W, et al: The human Vκ locus. Characterization of a duplicated region encoding 28 different immunoglobulin genes. *J Mol Biol* 1988; 199:23–34.
9. Hieter PA, Maizel JV, Leder P: Evolution of human immunoglobulin κ J region genes. *J Biol Chem* 1982; 257:1516–1522.
10. Hieter PA, Max EE, Seidman JG, et al: Cloned human and mouse kappa immunoglobulin constant and J region genes conserve homology in functional segments. *Cell* 1980; 22:197–207.
11. Chuchana P, Blancher A, Brockly F, et al: Definition of the human immunoglobulin variable lambda (IGLV) gene subgroups. *Eur J Immunol* 1990; 20:1317–1325.
12. Dariavach P, Lefranc G, Lefranc MP: Human immunoglobulin Cλ6 gene encodes the $Kern^{+}Oz^{-}$ lambda chain and Cλ4 and Cλ5 are pseudogenes. *Proc Natl Acad Sci USA* 1987; 84:9074–9078.
13. Ghanem N, Dariavach P, Chibani J, et al: Polymorphism of immunoglobulin lambda constant region genes in populations from France, Lebanon and Tunisia. *Exp Clin Immunogenet* 1988; 5:186–195.
14. Hieter PA, Hollis GF, Korsmeyer SJ, et al: Clustered arrangement of immunoglobulin λ constant region genes in man. *Nature* 1981; 294:536–540.
15. Taub RA, Hollis GF, Hieter PA, et al: Variable amplification of immunoglobulin λ light-chain genes in human populations. *Nature* 1983; 304:172–174.
16. Vasicek TJ, Leder P: Structure and expression of the human immunoglobulin λ genes. *J Exp Med* 1990; 172:609–620.
17. Berman JE, Mellis SJ, Pollock R, et al: Content and organization of the human Ig V_H locus: Definition of three new V_H families and linkage to the Ig C_H locus. *EMBO J* 1988; 3:727–738.
18. Kodaira M, Kinashi T, Umemura I, et al: Organization and evolution of variable region genes of the human immunoglobulin heavy chain. *J Mol Biol* 1986; 190:529–541.
19. Lee KH, Matsuda F, Kinashi T, et al: A novel family of variable region genes of the human immunoglobulin heavy chain. *J Mol Biol* 1987; 195:761–768.
20. Buluwela L, Albertson DG, Sherrington P, et al: The use of chromosomal translocations to study human immunoglobulin gene organization: Mapping D_H segments within 35 kb of the Cμ gene and identification of a new D_H locus. *EMBO J* 1988; 7:2003–2010.
21. Ichihara Y, Matsuoka H, Kurosawa Y: Organization of human immunoglobulin heavy chain diversity gene loci. *EMBO J* 1988; 13:4141–4150.
22. Matsuda F, Shin EK, Hirabayashi Y, et al: Organization of variable region segments of the human immunoglobulin heavy chain: Duplication of the D_5 clus-

ter within the locus and interchromosomal translocation of variable region segments. *EMBO J* 1990; 8:2501–2506.
23. Siebenlist U, Ravetch JV, Korsmeyer S, et al: Human immunoglobulin D segments encoded in tandem multigenic families. *Nature* 1981; 294:632–635.
24. Flanagan JG, Rabbitts TH: Arrangement of human immunoglobulin heavy chain constant region genes implies evolutionary duplication of a segment containing γ, ϵ and α genes. *Nature* 1982; 300:709–713.
25. Lefranc MP, Lefranc G, de Lange G, et al: Instability of the human immunoglobulin heavy chain constant region locus indicated by different inherited chromosomal deletions. *Mol Biol Med* 1983; 1:207–217.
26. Lefranc MP, Lefranc G, Rabbitts TH: Inherited deletion of immunoglobulin heavy chain constant region genes in normal human individuals. *Nature* 1982; 300:760–762.
27. Walter MA, Surtt U, Hofker MH, et al: The physical organization of the human immunoglobulin heavy chain gene complex. *EMBO J* 1990; 10:3303–3313.
28. Early P, Huan H, Davis M, et al: An immunoglobulin heavy chain variable region gene is generated from three segments of DNA: CH, D and JH. *Cell* 1980; 19:981–992.
29. Ravetch JV, Siebenlist U, Korsmeyer S, et al: Structure of the human immunoglobulin μ locus: Characterization of embryonic and rearranged J and D genes. *Cell* 1981; 27:583–591.
30. Max EE, Seidman JG, Leder P: Sequences of five potential recombination sites encoded close to an immunoglobulin κ constant region gene. *Proc Natl Acad Sci USA* 1979; 76:3450–3454.
31. Sakano H, Maki R, Kurosawa Y, et al: Two types of somatic recombination are necessary for the generation of complete immunoglobulin heavy chain genes. *Nature* 1980; 286:676–683.
32. Abe M, Shiku J: Isolation of an IgH gene circular DNA clone from human bone marrow. *Nucleic Acids Res* 1989; 17:163–170.
33. Alt FW, Baltimore D: Joining of immunoglobulin heavy chain gene segments: Implications from a chromosome with evidence of three D-JH fusions. *Proc Natl Acad Sci USA* 1982; 79:4118–4122.
34. Toda M, Hirama T, Takeshita S, et al: Excision products of immunoglobulin gene rearrangements. *Immunol Lett* 1989; 21:311–316.
35. Brack C, Hirama M, Lenhard-Schuller R, et al: A complete immunoglobulin gene is created by somatic recombination. *Cell* 1978; 15:1–14.
36. Weigert M, Perry R, Kelley D, et al: The joining of V and J gene segments create antibody diversity. *Nature* 1980; 283:497–499.
37. Hieter PA, Korsmeyer SJ, Waldmann TA, et al: Human immunoglobulin κ light-chain genes are deleted or rearranged in λ-producing B cells. *Nature* 1981; 290:368–372.
38. Korsmeyer SJ, Hieter PA, Ravetch JV, et al: Developmental hierarchy of immunoglobulin gene rearrangements in human leukemic pre-B-cells. *Proc Natl Acad Sci USA* 1981; 78:7096–7100.
39. Davis MM, Kim SK, Hood LE: DNA sequences mediating class switching in a α-immunoglobulins. *Science* 1980; 209:1360–1365.
40. Davis MM, Kim SK, Hood LE: Immunoglobulin class switching: Developmentally regulated DNA rearrangements during differentiation. *Cell* 1980; 22:1–2.
41. Dunnick W, Rabbitts TH, Milstein C: An immunoglobulin deletion mutant with implications for the heavy chain switch and RNA splicing. *Nature* 1980; 286:669–675.

42. Cory S, Adams JM: Deletions are associated with somatic rearrangement of immunoglobulin heavy chain genes. *Cell* 1980; 19:37–51.
43. Honjo T, Kataoka T: Organization of immunoglobulin heavy chain genes and allelic deletion model. *Proc Natl Acad Sci USA* 1978; 75:2140–2144.
44. Rabbitts TH, Forster A, Dunnick W, et al: The role of gene deletion in the immunoglobulin heavy chain switch. *Nature* 1980; 283:351–356.
45. Iwasato T, Shimizy A, Honjo T, et al: Circular DNA is excised by immunoglobulin class switch recombination. *Cell* 1990; 62:143–149.
46. Matsuoka M, Yoshida K, Maeda T, et al: Switch circular DNA formed in cyto kine-treated mouse splenocytes: Evidence for intramolecular DNA deletion in immunoglobulin class switching. *Cell* 1990; 62:135–142.
47. Krawinkel U, Rabbitts TH: Comparison of the hinge-coding segments in human immunoglobulin gamma heavy chain genes and the linkage of the gamma 2 and gamma 4 subclass genes. *EMBO J* 1982; 1:403–407.
48. Flanagan JG, Rabbitts TH: The sequence of human immunoglobulin epsilon heavy chain constant region gene, and evidence for three non-allelic genes. *EMBO J* 1982; 1:655–660.
49. Max EE, Battey J, Ney R, et al: Duplication and deletion in the human immunoglobulin ϵ genes. *Cell* 1982; 29:691–699.
50. Battey J, Max EE, McBride WO, et al: A processed human immunoglobulin ϵ gene has moved to chromosome 9. *Proc Natl Acad Sci USA* 1982; 79:5956–5960.
51. Rabbitts TH, Forster A, Milstein CP: Human immunoglobulin heavy chain genes: Evolutionary comparisons of $C\mu$, $C\delta$ and $C\gamma$ genes and associated switch sequences. *Nucleic Acids Res* 1981; 9:4509–4524.
52. Milstein C, Deverson EV, Rabbitts TH: The sequence of the human immunoglobulin μ-δ intron reveals possible vestigial switch segments. *Nucleic Acids Res* 1984; 12:6523–6535.
53. Ellison J, Hood L: Linkage and sequence homology of two human immunoglobulin γ heavy chain constant region genes. *Proc Natl Acad Sci USA* 1982; 79:1984–1988.
54. Rabbitts TH, Flanagan JG, Lefranc MP: Flexibility and change within the human immunoglobulin gene locus, in Helm C (ed): *Genetic Rearrangement.* Fifth John Innes Symposium, 1983, pp 143–154.
55. Lefranc G, Chaabani H, Van Loghem E, et al: Simultaneous absence of the human IgG1, IgG2, IgG4 and IgA1 subclasses: Immunological and immunogenetical considerations. *Eur J Immunol* 1983; 13:240–244.
56. White MB, Shen AL, Word CJ, et al: Human immunoglobulin D: Genomic sequences of the delta heavy chain. *Science* 1985; 228:733–737.
57. Huck S, Fort P, Crawford D, et al: Sequences of a human immunoglobulin gamma 3 heavy chain constant region gene: Comparison with the other C gamma human genes. *Nucleic Acids Res* 1986; 14:1779–1789.
58. Huck S, Lefranc G, Lefranc MP: A human immunoglobulin IGHG3 allele (Gmb0, b1, c3, c5, u) with an IGHG4 converted region and three hinge exons. *Immunogenetics* 1989; 30:250–257.
59. Ellison J, Berson BJ, Hood LE: The nucleotide sequence of a human immunoglobulin $C\gamma1$ gene. *Nucleic Acids Res* 1982; 10:4071–4079.
60. Flanagan JG, Lefranc MP, Rabbitts TH: Mechanisms of divergence and convergence of the human immunoglobulin $\alpha1$ and $\alpha2$ constant region gene sequence. *Cell* 1984; 36:681–688.
61. Bensmana M, Huck S, Lefranc G, et al: The human immunoglobulin pseudo-gamma IGHGP gene shows no major structural defect. *Nucleic Acids Res* 1988; 16:3108.

62. Ellison J, Buxbaum J, Hood L: Nucleotide sequence of a human immunoglobulin Cγ4 gene. *DNA* 1981; 1:11–18.
63. Bensmana M, Chuchana P, Lefranc G, et al: Sequence of the CH1 and hinge-CH2 exons of the human immunoglobulin IGHA2 A2m(2) allele: Comparison with the nonallelic and allelic IGHA genes. *Cytogenet Cell Genet* 1991; 56:128.
64. Bensmana M, Lefranc MP: Gene segments encoding membrane domains of the human immunoglobulin gamma 3 and alpha chains. *Immunogenetics* 1990; 32:321–330.
65. Kehry M, Ewald S, Douglas R, et al: The immunoglobulin μ chains of membrane-bound and secreted IgM molecules differ in their C-terminal segments. *Cell* 1980; 21:393–406.
66. Kemp DJ, Morahan G, Cowman AF, et al: Production of RNA for secreted immunoglobulin μ chains does not require transcriptional termination 5′ to the μ_m exons. *Nature* 1983; 301:84–86.
67. Sakano H, Rogers JH, Huppi K, et al: Domains and the hinge region of an immunoglobulin heavy chain are encoded in separate DNA segments. *Nature* 1979; 277:627–633.
68. Lefranc MP, Lefranc G: Délétion de gènes de la région constante des chaines lourdes des immunoglobulines humaines. *Med Sci* 1966; 2:508–513.
69. Lefranc MP, Lefranc G: Human immunoglobulin heavy chain multigene deletions in healthy individuals. *FEBS Lett* 1987; 213:231–237.
70. Ghanem N, Bensmana M, Dugoujon JM, et al: BamHI and SacI RFLPs of the human immunoglobulin IGHG genes with reference to the Gm polymorphism in Africa people: Evidence for a major polymorphism. *Hum Genet* 1989; 83:37–44.
71. Ghanem N, Dugoujon JM, Bensmana M, et al: Restriction fragment haplotypes in the human immunoglobulin IGHG locus and their correlation with the Gm polymorphism. *Eur J Immunol* 1988; 18:1067–1072.
72. Ghanem N, Lefranc MP, Lefranc G: Definition of the RFLP alleles in the human immunoglobulin IGHG gene locus. *Eur J Immunol* 1988; 18:1059–1065.
73. Hammarström L, Ghanem N, Smith CIE, et al: RFLP of human immunoglobulin genes. *Exp Clin Immunogenet* 1990; 7:7–19.
74. Huck S, Keyeux G, Ghanem N, et al: A gamma 3 hinge region probe: First specific human immunoglobulin subclass probe. *FEBS Lett* 1986; 208:221–230.
75. Lefranc MP, Lefranc G: Molecular genetics of immunoglobulin allotype expression, in Shakib F (ed): *Molecular Aspects of Immunoglobulin Subclasses.* Oxford, Pergamon Press, 1990, pp 43–78.
76. Lefranc MP, Rabbitts TH: Human immunoglobulin heavy chain A2 gene allotype determination by restriction fragment length polymorphism. *Nucleic Acids Res* 1984; 12:1303–1311.
77. Soua Z, Ghanem N, Ben Salem M, et al: Frequencies of the IGHA2*M1 and IGHA2*M2 alleles corresponding to the A2m(1) and A2m(2) allotypes in the French, Lebanese, Tunisian and Black African populations. *Nucleic Acids Res* 1989; 17:3625.
78. Keyeux G, Lefranc G, Lefranc MP: A multigene deletion in the human IGH constant region locus involve homologous hot spots of recombination. *Genomics* 1989; 5:431–441.
79. Keyeux G, Ghanem N, Lefranc G, et al: Identification of the PvuII RFLPs from the switch alpha (IGSA) regions. *Nucleic Acids Res* 1989; 17:3623.

80. Keyeux G, Lefranc G, Lefranc MP: A specific switch alpha probe of the human immunoglobulin IGHA locus. *Nucleic Acids Res* 1989; 17:3624.
81. Keyeux G, Nusbaum P, Alexandre D, et al: New RFLPs of immunoglobulin switch alpha region in mesangial IgA glomerulonephritis. *Hum Genet* 1991; 86:624.
82. Lefranc MP, Hammarström L, Smith CIE, et al: Gene deletions in the human immunoglobulin heavy chain constant region locus: Molecular and immunological analysis. *Immuno defic Rev* 1991; 2:265–281.

Molecular Approaches to the Relationships Between HLA and Susceptibility to Diseases

Laurent Degos, M.D., Ph.D.
INSERM U93, Hôpital Saint-Louis, Paris, France
Iman Khalil
Groupe d'Etudes des Oligonucléotides de Diagnostic, Hôpital Saint-Louis, Paris, France
Odile Blanchet, M.D.
INSERM U93, Hôpital Saint-Louis, Paris, France
Virginia Lepage, M.D.
Laboratoire Universitaire, Groupe d'Etudes des Oligonucléotides de Diagnostic, Hôpital Saint-Louis, Paris, France
Pascale Paul, Ph.D.
INSERM U93, Hôpital Saint-Louis, Paris, France
Jacques Hors, M.D.
INSERM U93, Groupe d'Études des Oligonucléotides de Diagnostic, Hôpital Saint-Louis, Paris, France

The histocompatibility leukocyte antigen (HLA) was defined with functional and structural tools. The first includes elements involved in the allogeneic reaction: antibodies and educated cells, either proliferative or cytotoxic lymphocytes. These reagents bind to specific epitopes on the HLA molecule. Polyclonal reagents bind to several epitopes, while monoclonal reagents bind to a specific site on the molecule. The first description of HLA used polyclonal tools, and HLA specificities were defined by one group of sera or by a population of cells recognizing several epitopes simultaneously.

Thus, an HLA type generally includes the expression of several concomitant epitopes and could not be recognized by one monoclonal antibody. Only specificities restricted to one variable epitope are defined with monoclonal antibodies or clonal cells. Conversely, monoclonal antibodies often appear to be polyspecific, recognizing a similar epitope shared by several HLA specificities.

What is an HLA specificity? Is it a precise epitope on the molecule or a combination of several epitopes often found together in a population? The latter concept is more useful for grouping individuals to undergo transplantation, and this HLA definition is based on the results obtained with polyclonal tools. This synthetic (and not analytic) definition will be considered.

Structural methods brought more details on the analytical definition of all variable regions and their sequences. Biochemical tools helped distinguish the various chains and the variability at the amino acid level by demonstrating the molecular weight and the electric charge. Molecular biology specifies the base pair variation, either in the coding or in the noncoding regions, leading to great polymorphism. These techniques are useful for better stratification of the population, generally applied in genetic studies, in population genetic models, or for HLA and disease relationships. The repertoire of the small variations is now known and, for instance, three subregions of the first domain of the HLA-DR β chain include almost all the polymorphism. Some sequences in one of these hypervariable regions could be common to several specificities, but the combinations including all the three variabilities lead to the HLA-DR definition. These analytical results could be converted to the classic HLA definition. With the use of a dictionary of combinations, such a conversion is useful for oligonucleotide typing.

The shape of the HLA molecule is marked by a cavity with two lips. For the HLA class I molecule, the cavity is encoded by one gene,[1] while for the HLA class II molecule, the cavity is made of two chains encoded by two genes.[2] The class II receptacle is made by an association of two kinds of chains, α and β. The role of these class I and class II molecules is to present peptides at the cell surface for the T cells via the T-cell antigen receptor.

According to its polymorphism, each type of cavity presents some peptides and not others. Thus each cavity possesses a repertoire of presented peptides. In addition, each type of cavities could present the same peptide in different ways, exposing separate parts of the peptide. Following the HLA type, that is to say following the collection of cavities, an individual perceives the world as a personal and unique manner, which is the signature of his biologic identity.

In this chapter, we shall restrict our discussion to two examples taken as models for the other relationships between HLA and diseases: first, the precise definition of a cavity in the susceptibility to insulin-dependent diabetes mellitus; and second, the acquired regulation defect in the expression of the HLA molecule in cancer.

Structure of HLA Class II Molecule in Insulin-Dependent Diabetes Mellitus

HLA-DR

Susceptibility to almost all types of autoimmune disease is related to HLA class II polymorphism. Studies in the past decade have shown that HLA-DR3 and/or HLA-DR4 are present in approximately 90% of patients with insulin-dependent diabetic mellitus (IDDM).

Relative risk is dramatically increased for individuals who are heterozygous (HLA-DR3/DR4) in comparison to other types of heterozygosity or even to homozygosity (HLA-DR3/DR3 or HLA-DR4/DR4). The combination HLA-DR3/DR4 is found in 30% of patients with IDDM and only in 1% of the healthy population.[3] This observation suggests the role of two genetic factors.

HLA-DQ

It has been shown that HLA-DQ genes, which are in linkage disequilibrium with HLA-DR, are more strongly associated with IDDM. Recently Tood et al.[4] reported that susceptibility to the disease correlates with the absence of an aspartic acid residue at position 57 of the DQ β chain. However, Asp 57-negative haplotypes do not always confer susceptibility. HLA-DR3 haplotypes, like HLA-DR7 haplotypes, often have a DQw2 specificity, which lacks the Asp 57 amino acid. DR3-DQw2 haplotypes are positively associated with IDDM, while DR7-DQw2 haplotypes are not. Moreover, analysis of DNA sequences from black patients with IDDM (DR7–DQ9) indicates that they have the same DQ α chain encoded by the DQ A1 gene as white patients with IDDM. These observations suggest that another gene, probably DQA1, may play a role in IDDM susceptibility. To evaluate this role, we studied unrelated white patients with IDDM and healthy control subjects with extensive oligotyping for DQA1 and DQB1 genes.[5] We identified eight alleles for the DQA1 series and 12 alleles for the DQB1 series. Comparing frequencies of alleles in 50 patients and 73 control subjects and comparing the sequences of the alleles, we determined a new feature for the susceptibility on the DQ α chain, by the presence of Arg 52.[5]

From the Molecule to the Genotype

The molecular structure[2] now proposed for class II molecules is made by analogy with HLA-A2 class I crystallographic results. The three-dimensional conformation of the DQ molecule shows a cavity in the external part, for the presentation of the antigen to T cells. In this model, residues on the α helices and β sheets, encoded by the second exon sequences of the A and B genes, form the walls and floor of a cavity.

The arginine residue (position 52) on the α chain and the aspartic resi-

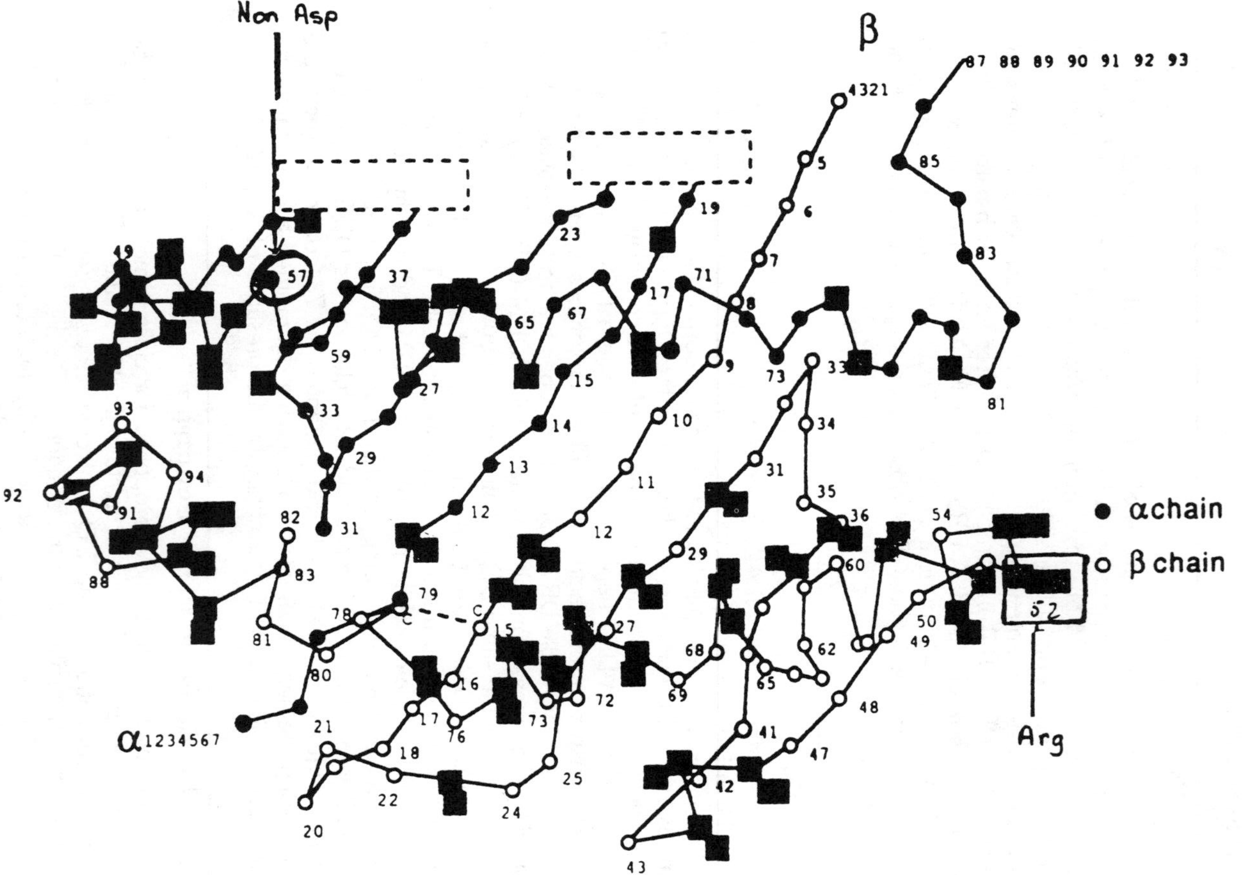

FIG 1.
Molecular description of HLA-DQ groove localization of DQα52 and DQβ57.

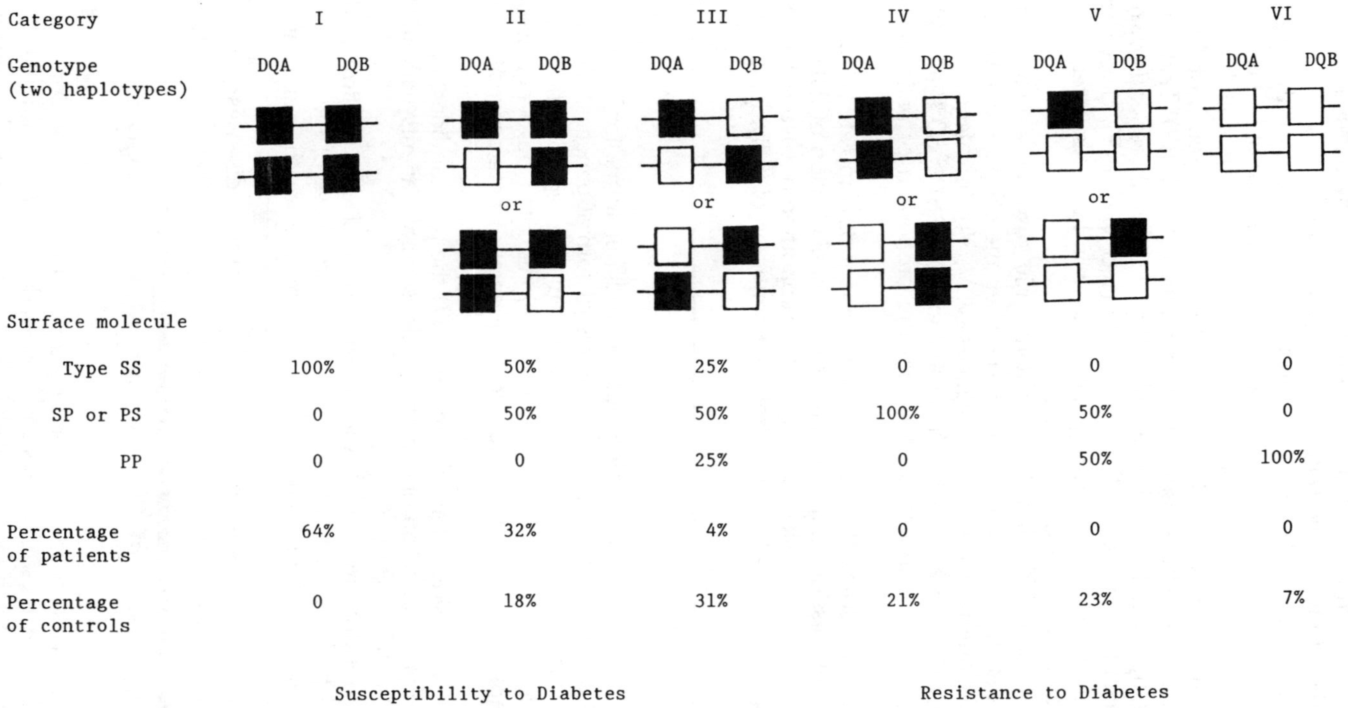

Category	I	II	III	IV	V	VI
Genotype (two haplotypes)	DQA DQB	DQA DQB or	DQA DQB or	DQA DQB or	DQA DQB or	DQA DQB
Surface molecule						
Type SS	100%	50%	25%	0	0	0
SP or PS	0	50%	50%	100%	50%	0
PP	0	0	25%	0	50%	100%
Percentage of patients	64%	32%	4%	0	0	0
Percentage of controls	0	18%	31%	21%	23%	7%

Susceptibility to Diabetes — Resistance to Diabetes

FIG 2.
Risk of IDDM according to DQ molecules deduced from genotypes. DQA (solid box) = 52 Arg+ (susceptible-S), DQB (solid box) = 57 Asp− (susceptible = S); DQA (open box) = 52 Arg− (protective = P); DQB (open box) = 57 Asp+ (protective = P).

due (position 57) on the β chain are located at opposite extremities of the α helical sides of the groove (Fig 1).

Given our results, we propose a molecular model based on the expression at the cell surface of a DQ α-β heterodimer consisting of DQ α Arg 52 positive and DQ β Asp 57 negative (αS and βS, S for susceptible). Conversely, the absence of Arg 52 on the α chain or the presence of Asp 57 on the β chain would be considered as protective (αP and βP). Taking into account all the possible assembled DQ α-β molecules, three kinds of heterodimers can be detected at the cell surface (S-S, S-P, P-P). Since these molecules are coded by A and B genes in *cis* or in *trans,* six categories of genotypes could be considered (Fig 2).

Our results show that individuals having only susceptible heterodimer (αS-βS) are all affected (category I), while when the αS-βS are absent, no affected individuals were found (categories IV, V, VI). In categories II and III, the proportion of susceptible heterodimers (αS-βS) is 50% and 25% respectively, which is in accordance with the proportion of patients with IDDM.

These results indicate the absolute requirement of complete susceptible heterodimer expression at the cell surface for manifestation of IDDM, and the gradient of relative risk according to the proportion of susceptible molecules at the cell surface deduced from the genotype of individuals.

Questions

Are all α and β chains equivalent for heterodimer formation? Do some preferential associations exist? On the basis of formal genetics, all the *cis* and *trans* combinations could equally occur, but with regard to the specific goal of antigen presentation, some combinations could be better associated, perhaps explaining the increased frequency of heterozygosity DR3/DR4.

Are these two residues (Arg 52 and Asp 57) the real candidates for susceptibility? For instance among mongoloids, several patients with IDDM are DQ B Asp 57 positive.

Are other residues involved? A large series is needed to confirm or disprove these findings. In the future, complete sequences of the genes will be needed, since different sequences could encode for the same amino acid.

Could this model be extended to other autoimmune diseases?

Altered Expression of Class I Molecules and Tumoral Progression

Hereditary diseases are known to induce a defect in the expression of class I (or class II) molecules. Cell lines with such a defect are also known. Class II expression has been explored well in these two situations. The defect of class I in the DAUDI cell line was explained by the absence of β2 microglobulin.

Class I molecules play a key role in the recognition of target cells by cytolytic T lymphocytes.

In cancer, the malignant cell and not other cells of the body can have an acquired defect of class I expression.[6] The downregulation of class I molecules facilitates escape from immunosurveillance. Complete loss of class I antigen expression has been reported in a variety of human tumors including neuroblastoma, small cell lung carcinoma, choriocarcinoma, lymphoma, breast cancer, colorectal carcinoma, and melanoma.

Differential expression of class I molecules in primary tumor and metastasis is correlated with the tumorigenic potency in case of melanoma. In mice, the lack of class I in cells derived from lung cancer is related to a strong metastatic effect, while reexpression of class I of the same cells by gene transfection, or by modulation, suppresses the metastatic potency.

Viral oncogenes or cellular oncogenes are able to downregulate the class I expression. The first example is the adenovirus 12 (tumorigenic virus), which induces a lack of class I, while the adenovirus 5 (nontumorigenic) does not. The tumorigenic activity is due to the E1A oncogene of Ad 12. The reduction of HLA class I is caused by the EA1 oncogene in this case. N-*myc* oncogene is involved in the metastatic formation in neuroblastoma. Again, N-*myc* is also involved in the downregulation of class I. Amplification of N-*myc* induces a dramatic decrease in class I expression.

The expression of class I major histocompatibility complex (MHC) genes is tightly regulated, and these elements (viral or cellular oncogenes) could affect this expression. An enhancer element, well known in mice,[7] is conserved in the promotors of human genes that are thought to be a major determinant of MHC class I expression (Fig 3).

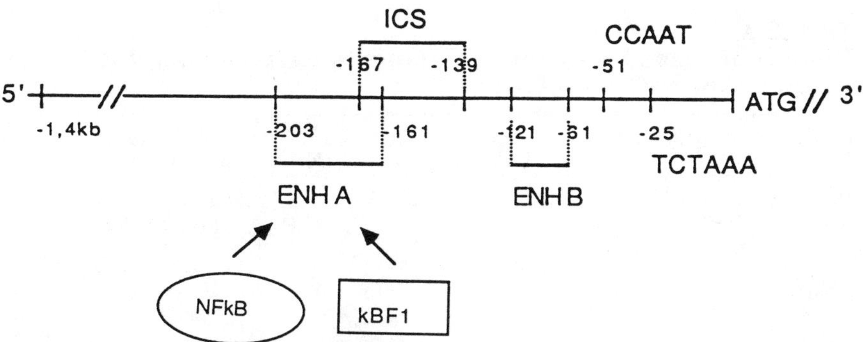

FIG 3.
Description of 5′ region of class I genes. *ENH A* = enhancer A; *ENH B* = enhancer B; *ICS* = consensus sequences for interferon; *ATG* = initiation site of transcription; *CCAAT* = CAAT box; *TCTAAA* = TATA box; *NFkB* and KBF1 are two factors of transactivation on enhancer A.

Lack of Expression of Class I Molecules at the Cell Surface in Human Lymphoma

A previous report on 66 B lymphoma showed a relationship between grades of severity deduced by the pathologic features and expression of class I antigens.[8]

We have studied class I expression at the cell surface of 108 patients with non-Hodgkin lymphomas. Lack of class I is not rare (16 among 108 patients), and this result is probably underestimated since locus-specific defects are not included. We do not find a correlation with the pathologic grade, and it is too early to evaluate the relationship with survival.

Absence of Expression on Human Cancer Cell Lines

Among 26 cell lines from various types of cancer, 13 lack class I at the cell surface. Five others have a locus-specific defect or decreased expression. Among the 13 cell lines without class I, seven have no detectable mRNA, probably resulting from a transcription defect.

Altered Binding of Regulatory Factors to HLA Class I Enhancer Sequence

In five of seven cases without expression of HLA class I mRNA, two related factors (KBFI and NFkB) are missing. These two factors bind to the major regulatory element, so-called enhancer A (see Fig 3). The defect is not due to a mutation of the sequence of the regulatory element but to the lack of DNA binding protein.

TABLE 1.
Profiles of Class I Regulatory Factors in Relationship With Class I Expression on Tumor Cell

Profile of Regulatory Factors	No. of Cell Lines	RNA	Cell Surface Expression
Absence NFkB Absence KBFI	5 tumoral cell lines	−	Deficiency in HLA class I expression
Presence NFkB Absence KBFI	5 tumoral cell lines	+	Normal expression or locus-specific deficiency
Presence NFkB Presence KBFI	16 tumoral cell lines	+: 14 lines	Normal expression or overexpression
		−: 2 lines	No expression of class I

KBFI is a ubiquitous factor that binds strongly on enhancer A, inducing an increase in transcription. It was suggested that a defect of KBFI was the cause of the absence of HLA class I transcription.[9]

In this study, KBFI is absent when HLA class I genes are not transcribed, but in some cases, HLA class I are expressed while KBFI is absent (Table 1).

Another factor, NFkB, also binds to enhancer A. In the present panel of cell lines, combined deficiency of NFkB and KBFI correlated with the absence of class I mRNA.

These results suggest that in the absence of KBFI, NFkB is able to promote MHC class I gene transcription and that a defect of both factors can cause a pleiotropic lack of class I gene expression.

The regulation of class I expression must be sought at the level of the gene of these two factors. Both of the factors are encoded by the same gene.[10]

Better understanding may help in modulating the expression of class I molecules to restore sensitivity of these malignant cells to immune surveillance.

Conclusion

Two directions are being explored in the molecular approach to relationships between HLA and diseases: the molecular structure of the groove presenting the antigen, and the regulation of the genes. This step in our understanding of HLA could open a new orientation for the treatment of diseases acting either on the cavities by ligands or by synthetic peptides, and on the modulation of the transcription of the genes.

References

1. Bjorkman PJ, Saper MA, Samraoui B, et al: The foreign antigen binding site and T cell recognition regions of class I histocompatibility antigens. *Nature* 1987; 329:512–518.
2. Brown JH, Jardetsky T, Saper MA, et al: A hypothetical model of the foreign antigen binding site of class II histocompatibility molecules. *Nature* 1988; 332:845–850.
3. Deschamps I, Lestradet H, Marcelli-Barge A, et al: Facteurs de risque du diabète insulino-dependant. *Pathol Biol* 1986; 34:767–772.
4. Todd JA, Bell JI, McDevitt HO: HLA-DQβ gene contributes to susceptibility and resistance to insulin-dependent diabetes mellitus. *Nature* 1987; 329:599–604.
5. Khalil I, d'Auriol L, Gobet M, et al: A combination of HLA-DQβ Asp 57 negative and HLA DQα Arg 52 confers susceptibility to insulin-dependent diabetes mellitus. *J Clin Invest* 1990; 85:1315–1319.
6. Paul P: Modification de l'expression des molécules de classe I du CMH et progression tumorale. *Med Sci* 1990; 6:449–455.
7. Israel A, Kimura A, Kieran M, et al: A common positive trans-acting factor

binds to enhancer sequences in the promoters of mouse H-2 and beta 2-microglobulin genes. *Proc Natl Acad Sci USA* 1987; 84:2653–2657.
8. Moller P, Herrmann B, Moldenhauer G, et al: Defective expression of MHC class I antigens is frequent in B-cell lymphoma of high-grade malignancy. *Int J Cancer* 1987; 40:32–39.
9. Israel A, Yano O, Logeat F, et al: Two purified factors bind to the same sequence in the enhancer of mouse MHC class I genes: One of them is a positive regulator induced upon differentiation of teratocarcinoma cells. *Nucleic Acid Res* 1989; 17:5245–5247.
10. Kieran M, Blank V, Logeat F, et al: The DNA binding subunit of NF-κB is identical to factor KBF1 and homologous to the rel oncogene product. *Cell* 1990; 62:1007–1018.

Genetic Factors in IgA Nephropathy (Berger's Disease)

Micheline Lévy, M.D.

INSERM U155, Château de Longchamp, Bois de Boulogne Paris, France

Philippe Lesavre, M.D., Ph.D.

Department of Nephrology, INSERM U90, Necker Hospital, Paris, France

At the meeting of the French Society of Nephrology on February 3, 1968, Jean Berger and Nicole Hinglais[1] reported for the first time the presence of IgA containing mesangial deposits by immunofluorescence study of kidney biopsy specimens of 25 patients. A novel nephropathy, now recognized as the most frequent glomerular nephropathy in a large number of countries, was thus defined clinically and histologically and was called Berger's disease or IgA nephropathy (IgAN). According to Drs. Berger and Hinglais,

> Half of the cases were histologically defined by focal glomerulonephritis (GN). In other cases, unclassified GN, chronic nephritis, isolated arteriolar lesions or normal kidney were observed. Moderate proteinuria and microscopic hematuria were present in all patients. Half of them expressed one or more episodes of macroscopic hematuria usually closely associated with an episode of pharyngitis. The renal function was normal in a large majority of patients. Arterial hypertension was present in three cases. The interval between the apparent onset and the kidney biopsy varied from a few months to 12 years.

Only two major clinical observations have since been added to this original report: progression to renal death in 25% of cases[2] and recurrence of the mesangial IgA deposits in the transplanted kidney.[3] Mesangial deposition of IgA is also observed in Henoch-Schönlein purpura (HSP) nephritis, which thus shares similarities with Berger's disease.[3a] In addition, mesangial IgA deposits are present in some patients with alcoholic liver cirrhosis and in an increasing number of patients with immune diseases, including ankylosing spondylitis, coeliac disease, ulcerative colitis, and myasthenia gravis.

Numerous studies on the immune abnormalities present in patients have made real progress in our understanding of the disease but the exact origin and mechanism of deposition of mesangial IgA remains largely unknown. This is unfortunate because the disease is frequent and sometimes severe.

It is most common in young adults and affects men twice more often than women. In a majority of countries, IgA nephropathy is the single most frequent type of primary GN with a prevalence of about 25%. The annual incidence per 1,000,000 inhabitants varies from 19 in the province of Limburg in Holland[4] to 27 or 30 in France in the Rhône Alpes region[5] and in Brittany,[6] respectively. IgA nephropathy is the single most frequent cause of end-stage renal failure (ESRF), as shown in a prospective study conducted in Brittany on a total population of 400,000 inhabitants. End-stage renal failure is due to IgA nephropathy in 0.85 patients per 100,000 inhabitants and is a more frequent cause of ESRF than diabetes mellitus and polycystic kidney disease.[7]

A role of environmental factors such as dietary habits and viral and bacterial infections has been proposed without conclusive findings. As for many immune disorders, Berger's disease can be considered to be a complex etiology disease. This term is applied to diseases that are the result of a complex network of causes, some of them genetic, others environmental. Because of the rareness of multiplex families or rather the failure to recognize them, the possibility of genetic susceptibility had long been ignored. Accumulating data, however, concerning geographical variations in the frequency of the disease, multiplex families and large pedigrees, immune abnormalities in healthy relatives, and the association of the disease with histocompatibility leukocyte antigen (HLA), all favor a hypothesis of genetic susceptibility. It is time to investigate whether some genes coding for products functionally related to the disease, or candidate genes, represent risk factors for the disease.

Immune Mechanisms in Berger's Disease

Extensive reviews of the immune abnormalities observed in IgA nephropathy have been recently published[8–15]; we will focus here on the results that relate to immunogenetics.

Serum and Mesangial Immunoglobulins Class Distribution

The composition of mesangial IgA deposits has been analyzed with subclass specific monoclonal antibodies; the deposits contain predominantly if not exclusively IgA1.[16] IgG, present in the mesangium in about one third of the biopsy specimens, are almost exclusively of IgG1 and IgG3 subclasses.[17] This IgG subclass restriction of mesangial deposits was not accompanied by a major imbalance in IgG1 and their serum levels[17] but was very different from what is observed in other cases of immune glomerulonephritis (membranous nephropathy and anti-GBM nephritis), in which the deposited IgG are essentially IgG1 and IgG4.[18] Conversely, the IgG1-IgG3 restriction observed in IgA nephropathy may favor the hypothesis that the deposited IgG could represent antibodies to viral proteins known to be of IgG1 and IgG3 isotypes.

The serum levels of IgA are elevated in about half of the patients (IgG and IgM serum levels are normal). This elevation is mainly due to monomeric IgA1.[19] The IgA2 serum level and the percentage of polymeric IgA are comparable to that in control subjects.[20, 21] The increase in serum level may reflect the hyperactivity of the IgA immune response observed after systemic immunization.

Furthermore, a predominance of λ light chain IgA in the mesangial deposits as well as in serum has been shown. Chen, in our group, has recently confirmed and extended this observation by studying specifically the κ/λ light chain distribution of IgA1. Her study revealed that the IgA1 increased serum level is almost exclusively due to an increase in IgA1λ, since the IgA1κ serum level was normal. We found a normal synthesis of IgA1λ by peripheral blood mononuclear cells. This may indicate an increase in the bone marrow production of IgA1λ or alternatively an abnormal catabolism possibly related to physicochemical abnormalities of IgA.

Physicochemical Abnormalities of IgA

By direct analysis of the mesangial IgA after elution from kidney biopsy specimens, Monteiro et al. have shown that mesangial IgA was predominantly dimeric (60%) but also monomeric (40%).[22] By contrast with their heterogeneous molecular weight, the eluted mesangial IgA was remarkably homogeneous in charge and anionic.[22] This negative charge restriction of IgA may be related to its affinity for the mesangium, as has been shown in experimental models.

Many investigators have found evidence of high-molecular-weight circulating IgA in IgA nephropathy.[21, 23] This may be due to immune complex formation, although the putative antigen(s) remain unknown, to increased interaction of IgA with fibronectin,[24] to the presence of IgA-rheumatoid factor (IgA-RF) activity or to idiotype-antiidiotype interactions. We have shown the presence of both anionic IgA and IgA rheumatoid factor in the serum of the majority of the patients.[25] The crucial point of this study was the statistically significant detection of either negatively charged serum IgA or IgA-RF in patients with transplants only in the case of recurrence of mesangial IgA deposits without any correlation between these two variables.[25] These results suggest that, although independent, both negatively charged IgA and IgA-RF may play a role in the formation of the mesangial IgA deposits.

Polyclonal Activation and Autoantibody Activity of IgA

In vitro IgA production by lymphocytes has been studied by many investigators and has led to controversial results.[26] Spontaneous IgA production has been reported as normal[27] or raised.[28] Apart from a few studies, pokeweed mitogen (PWM)-stimulated cultures have not produced more IgA than control cultures. A decrease of total and IgA-specific T-suppressor function[29] and an increase of helper T cells with specific receptors for IgA have been reported. Thus, these studies have not consistently established an abnormal production of IgA by peripheral blood mononuclear cells. On the other hand, the production of IgA by bone marrow lymphocytes has been studied by Van den Wall Bake et al.[27] They showed an increase in IgA-producing plasma cells in the bone marrow of patients with IgA nephropathy with a bias toward IgA1 plasma cells and increased IgA1 production in spontaneous culture. Finally, the percentage of IgA-producing plasma cells was increased in tonsils[30] but not in small bowel mucosa.[31]

More recently the role of autoimmunity has been suggested by several factors[32, 33]: IgM antinuclear cold antibodies,[34] IgA class autoantibodies directed against IgG,[25, 35] laminin,[36] and type I collagen.[37] However, the binding of IgA to collagen type I observed in IgAN may be in fact due to the affinity of patient's IgA for fibronectin which in turn binds to collagen.[37] Finally, IgG class autoantibodies to mesangial cells have been observed.

Origin of the Mesangial IgA Deposits

The central question of the origin of the IgA deposited in the mesangium is not yet clearly answered. In healthy adults, the daily production of serum and secretory IgA exceeds that of other immunoglobulin classes. Secretory and serum IgA are produced by two systems that are functionally largely independent (Fig 1).[38] The secretory IgA-producing plasma cells are localized in the lamina propria of mucosal tissues. The precursor B cells of the IgA plasma cells are stimulated in Peyer's patches or in their equivalents of the respiratory system by environmental antigens. They differentiate in IgA plasma cells, leave the peripheral blood, localize in the lamina propria of mucosal tissue, and produce IgA of the IgA1 subclass (60%) and IgA2 (40%), mainly in polymeric form (90%).[39] The active transport of secretory IgA through the mucosal epithelia is driven by the secretory component for which secretory IgA have affinity. Thus, local immunization (for example in the gut) induces a secretory IgA immune response in remote tissue that has not been directly stimulated by the antigen.

Conversely, serum IgA is mainly monomeric (>85%) and mainly of the IgA1 subclass (90%). Serum IgA is almost exclusively produced by bone marrow plasma cells[40] with a synthesis rate analogous to that of IgG. Only humans and the primates have elevated levels of monomeric IgA, the evolutionary benefit of which is not clear. Serum IgA of bone marrow origin may act as a second barrier by eliminating the environmental antigens entering the body in particular through the gut and by inhibiting the inflammatory response to them.

In humans the functional independence of the two systems is supported by the fact that serum IgA (monomeric or polymeric) are not excreted, and that polymeric IgA produced by the mucosal-associated lymphoid tissues (MALT) only contribute marginally to the serum IgA pool. The absence of parallelism between the IgA antibody responses of the two systems confirms this functional independence. It is not absolute, however, since, in individuals primed with the same antigen by the mucosal route, systemic im-

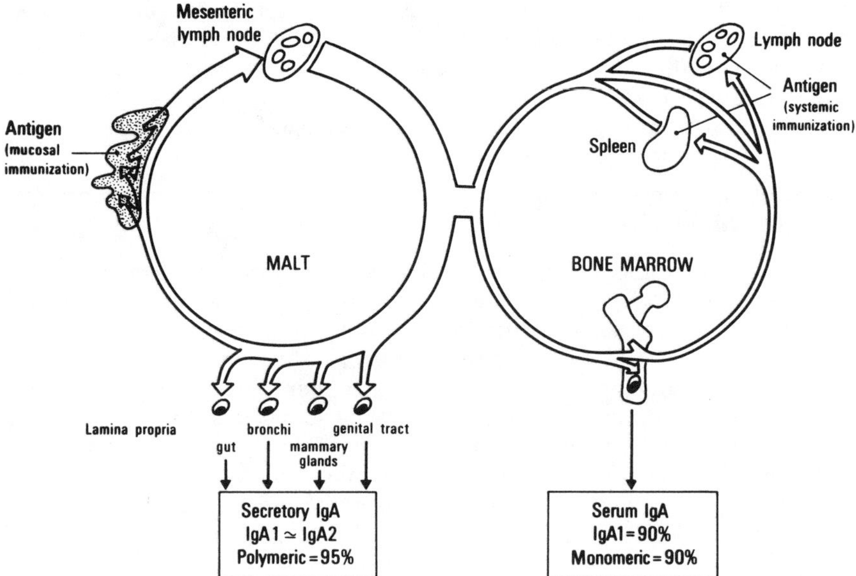

FIG 1.
Circulation of the IgA plasma cell precursor B cells in the human. The mucosa-associated IgA system (MALT) and the bone marrow IgA system are largely distinct functionally and produce secretory IgA and serum IgA, respectively.

munization may induce a secretory IgA response. Finally, although antigenic stimulation by the mucosal route essentially leads to localization of activated B lymphocytes in mucosal tissue, a minority of these cells localize in the bone marrow after repeated stimulation.[38]

In IgA nephropathy, the origin of the mesangial IgA is not clearly known. However, an increased IgA response is observed in both the mucosal and the medullary compartments. Evidence supporting a bone marrow origin includes the IgA1 subclass of the mesangial IgA, increased serum level of IgA, mainly monomeric,[19, 20] and increased IgA1 plasmocytes in bone marrow.[27] Evidence supporting hyperactivity of the mucosal-associated IgA system is increased IgA plasma cells in the tonsils,[30, 41] but not in the gut,[31] and increased serum level of polymeric IgA.

The Role of the Complement System

Besides the mesangial IgA, which defines the disease, complement C3 and properdin are usually present in the deposits. The absence of classical pathway proteins is an indirect argument for a role of the alternative pathway in the disease. Indeed, aggregated IgA activate the alternative pathway. In 75% of the cases studied, Wyatt et al. showed an increase in the plasma level of C3 fragments (iC3b-C3d), with no detectable activation of the classical pathway.[42] However, the presence of C3 fragments in plasma was not associated with a particular clinical situation during the course of the disease. Independently it has been shown that kidney tissue from patients activates the alternative pathway. Finally, it is plausible that assembly of the terminal complex C5b-C9 and insertion in the mesangium may have a lytic role and/or activate the mesangial cells.[43]

Geographical Variations

Although epidemiologic studies stricto sensu concerning glomerular diseases are rare, all authors conclude that Berger's disease is more frequent in Asia than in Australia and Europe and that the disease is not frequent in North America.[44] Pathology departments' files are most often the only sources of information on the number of patients with Berger's disease among those with primary glomerulonephritis. Consequently, the observed percentages do not represent the prevalence of the disease in a given country. The differences among countries may reflect differences in diagnostic strategies. For example, the increased frequency noted in the United Kingdom, which rose from 7% before 1978 to 21% for the period between 1979 and the end of 1986, was interpreted by British authors as largely due to an increase in the number of biopsied patients with microscopic hematuria.[45] The highest percentages of Berger's disease were observed in Singapore (54%) and in Japan (40% to 47%). In both countries, routine screening for urinary abnormalities is carried out in all young men before their military service in Singapore[46] and in all schoolchildren in Japan.[47] It should be mentioned, however, that the frequency of Berger's disease is not identical in all Asian populations. For example, it is less than 10% in Thailand (Boonpucknavig, personal communication) and in India,[48] around 20% in Malaysia,[49] and 30% in China[50] and in Korea.[51]

Similarly, variations are noted in different European countries where percentages vary between 20% and 30% of primary glomerulonephritis; the highest percentages are observed in Spain, Italy, and France.

Variations of the prevalence among well-defined ethnic groups could be arguments in favor of the existence of shared factors, genetic and/or environmental, playing a role in the etiology. For these reasons, data concerning the low frequency of the disease in American and South African black populations and in Polynesians and its high frequency in native Americans are interesting.

Berger's Disease in Blacks

In North America, it is currently accepted that Berger's disease is rare in blacks. Of the 341 patients compiled in various reports, only 12 were black.[52, 53] However, it should be noted that American blacks, descendants of Africans brought from all regions of Africa and sold as slaves (and undoubtedly mixed with both whites and native Americans) do not form an ethnically homogeneous group.[54, 55]

Few data are available from Africa, first because patients with microscopic hematuria do not currently undergo biopsy and second, because immunofluorescent studies are rarely performed. However, two recent studies carried out in South Africa have shown that the number of black patients with Berger's disease is low. In Durban, only 2 of 252 black patients with primary glomerulonephritis had Berger's disease.[56] This low frequency is perhaps due to the fact that black patients only receive medical attention for severe symptoms. According to Seedat et al.,[56] although the incidence of Berger's disease in the white population is not known, it is an important cause of primary glomerulonephritis.

Similarly, in Cape Town, 34 of the 872 biopsy specimens obtained over a period of 7 years showed Berger's disease, but none came from black patients.[57] This biopsy sample was representative of the population and comprised 11.9% of South African black patients. If this low incidence is confirmed, it is reasonable to think that infections, often observed in blacks, may not be involved in the etiology of Berger's disease.[56] It is interesting that anaphylactoid purpura also is rare in South Africa.[58]

Berger's Disease in American Indians

Indian populations are supposed to have been derived from Asian populations, and therefore the high percentage of Berger's disease was compared to the high percentage noted in Japan. On the basis of anthropologic and genetic studies, it is agreed that American Indians are descendants of small human groups, who, coming from the northeast extremity of Asia, entered the New World 25,000 years ago during the last ice age by way of a land bridge in the Behring Sea.[59]

Renal disease due to type II diabetes mellitus is an alarming problem among southwestern American Indians. In Zuni, the incidence of end-stage renal disease is 14.0 times higher than in white Americans and 6.2 times higher than in black Americans.[60] The Zuni are Pueblo Indians, descendants of the earliest inhabitants of the American southwest, living on reservations in New Mexico and Arizona. In nondiabetic patients, renal insufficiency is related to a mesangiopathic glomerulonephritis, marked by the association of mesangial hypercellularity and mesangial electron-dense deposits. In Zunis, this type of glomerulonephritis has some peculiar features. The number of affected men and women is equal, and family clustering is common. The immune composition of the mesangial deposits varies. In a few cases, immunofluorescent microscopy was negative. Staining for IgA (always associated with staining for IgM) was observed in two thirds of the cases whereas IgM was the only immunoglobulin in 10% of cases. Disparate immunofluorescent findings are found among close relatives in a given family. The appearance or the disappearance of IgA in sequentially studied kidneys of several subjects has been noted. Therefore, Hoy et al.[61] have suggested that early mesangiopathic glomerulonephritis may be immunofluorescent negative or show only deposition of IgM with IgA deposits superimposed later.

The proportion of mesangiopathic glomerulonephritis, including those with IgA deposition, is extremely high (64%) in Navajo Indians, the largest Indian tribal group in the United States.[62] A high frequency of Berger's disease was also detected in Indian children from Manitoba.[63]

American Indians, like Australian Aborigines in whom family clustering of Berger's disease has been described, form homogeneous ethnic groups with a high level of consanguinity. They have been subject to rapid westernization, with changes in diet and activity, high rates of unemployment and alcoholism, and high rates of recently acquired obesity, type II diabetes mellitus, and renal disease. According to Hoy et al.[61] and to O'Connell,[64] the high prevalence of glomerulonephritis in both groups probably results from the combined effects of environmental factors such as alcohol and of a genetic predisposition accentuated by consanguinity.

Berger's Disease in Polynesians

Native Australians and Polynesians, indirect though their route may be, came from Southeast Asia. The similarity in DNA haplotype patterns in Polynesians and Southern Chinese is consistent with a common ancestral origin.

During recent years, Polynesians (predominantly Maoris) were found to have a higher overall incidence of glomerulonephritis than New Zealanders of European descent.[65] More specifically, they had a higher incidence of mesangiocapillary glomerulonephritis, postinfectious glomerulonephritis, and focal glomerulosclerosis, but a reduced incidence of Berger's disease. Only 9 of 153 biopsy specimens from Polynesian patients showed Berger's disease vs. 120 of 650 from non-Polynesian patients.

Family Studies

Following the report of de Werra et al.,[66] many large studies of patients have mentioned a history of renal disease in some of the patients' relatives.[15] Subsequently, multiple instances of familial biopsy-confirmed IgA nephropathy have been identified. To our knowledge, more than 30 multiplex families

TABLE 1.
Summary of Published Reports on Multiplex Families

First Author (reference)	Kinship Between Affected Individuals
Okada[67]	Brother and sister (+ relatives)
Tolkoff-Rubin[68]	2 brothers*
Katz[69]	2 brothers (+ relatives)
Montoliu[70]	Brother and sister
Tomizawa[71]	Brother and sister (+ relatives)
Gutierrez Millet[72]	Father and son

Sinniah[73]	Mother and son
	2 sisters
	Mother and son
de Glas-Vos[74]	2 brothers
Kashiwabara[75]	Mother and son
Hene[76]	Father and son
Wyatt[77]	Brother and sister† (+ relatives)
Nomoto[78]	Brother and sister
Feehally[26]	Father and son
Miura[79]	2 sisters (+ relatives)
Ohzono[80]	Mother and son (+ relatives)
Fitzsimmons[81]	Mother and son‡ (+ relatives)
Garcia-Hoyo[82]	2 brothers
	Brother and sister (+ relatives)
	Brother and sister
O'Connell[64]	Father, 3 sons, and cousin (+ relatives)
Scolari[83]	2 brothers and two relatives (+ relatives)
	Aunt, nephew and first cousin (+ relatives)
	Father, son, and daughter
Charlesworth§	Mother and 4 children
Koegel§	Mother and son
Brensilver[84]	2 brothers*
Wyatt[85]	Father, son, and daughter¶ (+ relatives)
Chahin[86]	2 patients (no data) ‖
Rambausek§	Father and son
	Brother and sister (+ relatives)
	Mother and son (+ relatives)
	Mother and son (+ relatives)
	Aunt and nephew (+ relatives)
Schena§	Brother and sister
	2 brothers
Nagata[87]	Mother and son (AP)
Furuse[88]	2 brothers (one with AP)
Meadow[89]	Identical twins (one with AP)
Waldo[90]	No data on this family
Osawa[91]	Mother (AP) and son
Miyagawa[92]	2 daughters (one with AP) and mother
Roodhoft§	Brother and sister (AP)
Montoliu[93]	Father (AP) and son
Rambausek§	Mother and son (AP)

*One of the brothers had end-stage renal failure; the other was asymptomatic but kidney transplanted to his brother had IgA deposits.
†In this family, partial H deficiency was found in affected individuals.
‡In this family, affected individuals show spastic paraplegia, bilateral sensorineural deafness, and intellectual retardation.
§Personal communication.
¶C4B deficiency was found in both sibs.
‖ In this family, the nephropathy is associated with neurosensorial deafness; (AP) = patient presenting with anaphylactoid purpura; (+ relatives) = other relatives show clinical glomerulonephritis.

have been reported. In these families, affected relatives are either parent-offspring or siblings and, in addition, other relatives frequently show clinical glomerulonephritis. Finally, the occurrence of Berger's disease and anaphylactoid purpura in the same family has also been reported (Table 1).[64, 67–94]

Multiplex Families: French Society of Nephrology Collaborative Study

This retrospective study, conducted by French nephrologists, showed that multiplex families are more frequent than previously imagined.[94, 95] Our survey revealed 35 families with two (or more) members having biopsy-confirmed Berger's disease (Fig 2). In addition, in 5 of these 35 families, one or two relatives presented with anaphylactoid purpura with or without renal involvement. An autosomal dominant mechanism of inheritance might explain the families with affected parents and offspring. The main characteristics of these patients are the predominance of affected men (77%), their young age at the apparent onset (47% less than 16 years of age at onset), and the severity of the disease (13 patients developed end-stage renal failure and 9 show moderate renal failure). The long interval, up to 15 to 10 years, frequently observed between the apparent onset of the disease in various family members favors the existence of a genetic predisposition rather than the influence of environmental factors.

In our opinion, the number of multiplex families may be even higher since we collected 90 more families in which one patient with Berger's disease had relatives presenting a renal disease, often severe. Although in many of these patients the diagnosis of Berger's disease was strongly suspected, it could not be proven in the absence of renal biopsy. Several published reports[80, 96] as well as our study clearly show that two different glomerular diseases may be encountered in the same family.

Large Pedigrees From Kentucky and Australia

Julian et al.[97–100] noted that most of their white patients resided in the eastern part of Kentucky. The discovery of a previously unknown first cousin relationship between two patients led the authors to pursue their genealogical investigation in eight generations. They discovered six patients with a common ancestor and eight other patients with potentially related pedigrees.

They also discovered 17 more patients with clinical glomerulonephritis and 6 for whom chronic nephritis was indicated on the death certificate. Further studies showed that their birthplaces and those of their parents, grandparents, and great-grandparents clustered in the far eastern portion of the state. A founder effect would explain the geographical clustering. Ancestors of these patients would be the early settlers who, coming from south Virginia, entered the region after the departure of Indians at the end of the eighteenth century. These data suggest that gene(s) causing susceptibility to Berger's disease would have been carried by one or several of the original settlers.

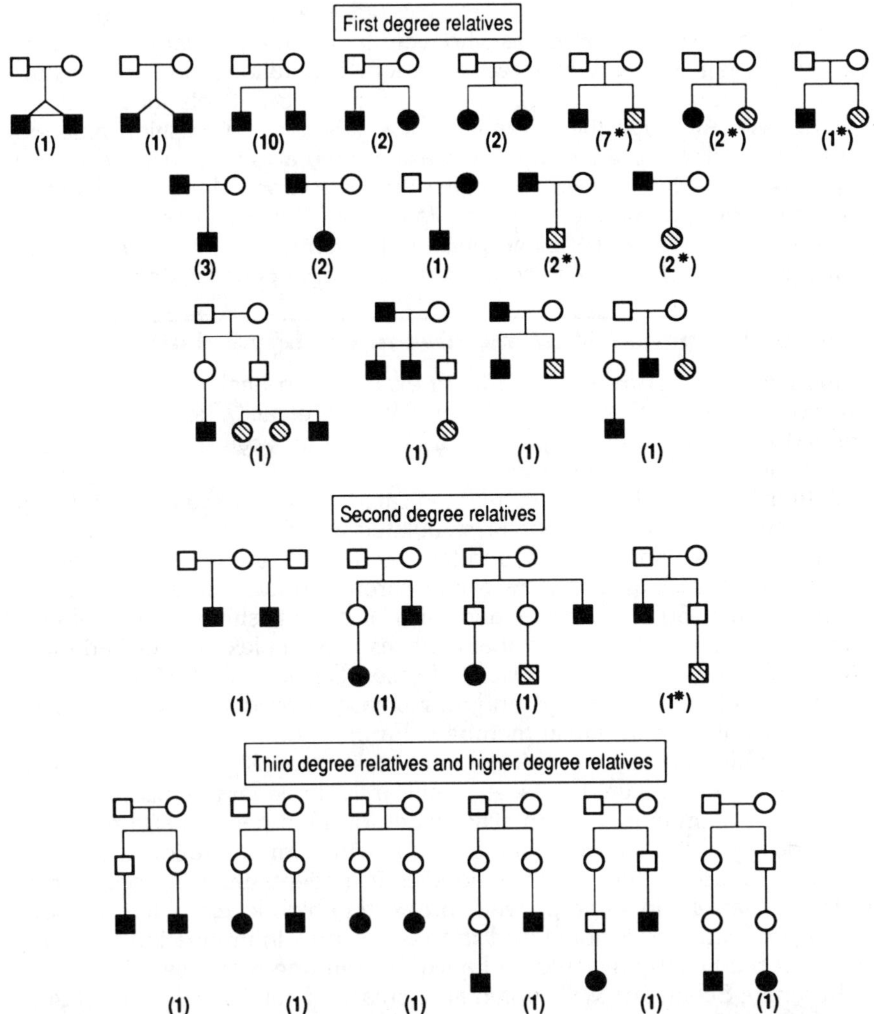

FIG 2.
French Society Nephrology Collaborative study. Familial configurations. Dark symbols indicate patients with biopsy-confirmed Berger's disease; hatched symbols, patients with anaphylactoid purpura. Numbers in brackets indicate the number of families with the given configuration. The *asterisk* indicates the 15 families with only one relative with Berger's disease, the second relative presenting with anaphylactoid purpura. The other 35 families are multiplex families with Berger's disease. Only affected relatives are shown on the configurations. The indicated kinship refers to the two closest relatives.

Similarly, O'Connell et al.[64] investigated the family of 2 Aboriginal brothers from New South Wales who were found to have Berger's disease. Of the 114 family members screened in four generations, 28 had hematuria or proteinuria. Biopsy specimens from 5 of the 8 patients showed Berger's disease. Although the hypothesis of a genetic predisposition may explain the familial clustering of the disease, it may also be explained by the exposure of family members to a common environmental antigen. The fact that some, but not all, members of a family develop Berger's disease suggests a variable response to the presumptive environmental stimulus and that this supposed variability could be under some genetic control.[64]

Immune Response Abnormalities in Healthy Relatives

Immunologic abnormalities have been examined in healthy relatives. Garcia Hoyo et al.,[82] Sakai et al.,[101] and Waldo et al.[90] demonstrated increased synthesis of IgA by peripheral blood lymphocytes, whereas results from Hale et al.[28] were negative.

With the use of different tests that indicate the percentage of IgA-bearing lymphocytes, the spontaneous or stimulated in vitro synthesis of IgA, the percentage of T4 and T8 cells, and the T4/T8 ratio, the group in Madrid[82] noted that all siblings and 77% of the parents showed at least one alteration, and that 50% of siblings and 44% of parents showed three abnormalities. Moreover, they noted that relatives in multiplex families had more abnormalities than relatives of isolated cases. Sakai et al.[101] showed a significant increase in serum IgA and an increase in production of polyclonal IgA in patients and in family members. Furthermore, following immunization with influenza vaccine, IgA class antibodies against influenza virus and rheumatoid factors were increased significantly. In general, similar trends in the pattern of immune abnormalities were found in patients and relatives.

Waldo et al.[102] showed that oral poliovirus immunization induces a greater increase in serum IgA antibodies in patients than in control subjects. Conversely, in some patients, preexisting high levels of IgA antibodies to poliovirus were noted and the response to immunization was low. Some of the healthy relatives had a similar immune response.

Recently, Schena et al.[103] noted an increase of cytokines IL2 and IL4 in patients and first-degree relatives. Serum IgA was similarly increased in patients and relatives.

Is Berger's Disease a Complex Etiology Disease?

Difficulties of Genetic Investigations

To decide whether a given disease has a genetic component, three questions have to be raised successively.[104]

A search for familial aggregation is the initial step. It is generally agreed that a disease clusters in families when the prevalence of the disease is higher among the relatives of affected individuals than in the general population. But it must be emphasized that multiple cases of the same disease in a family may simply occur by chance, or the cases may be due to exposure to the same environmental factors such as infectious agents or dietary habits. In the case of Kuru, initially interpretated as a genetic disease, viral agents have proven to be responsible for familial aggregation.[105]

Once familial aggregation is established, the second step is to try to separate genetic from environmental effects. Some of the methods available for this purpose (twin studies, adoption studies) have been widely used in some disorders, establishing that at least a part of family clustering is due to genetic factors.

When there is good evidence for the role of genetic factors, segregation analysis (examining the distribution of a disease status among members of randomly sampled families) is the common way of testing a mode of inheritance. The majority of familial diseases, however, do not follow a simple mode of transmission. Consequently, further analysis has to determine whether the genetic component is related to a major gene or to a large number of independent genes, each having a small effect, or to both a major gene and polygenes being involved in the etiology of the disease. Unlike monogenic diseases in which a defective gene, such as a rare mutated allele, is responsible for the disease, in complex etiology diseases such a disease gene may not exist. Rather common genetic risk factors are more likely to be implicated. When studying the large family in Kentucky, Asamoah et al.[106] attempted to demonstrate the role of a major gene in the familial aggregation of plasma IgA concentration. With pedigree segregation analysis, they were able to suggest the existence of a recessive allele for high plasma concentration, but it only seems to play a minor role in the etiology of Berger's disease.

Because multiplex families were rare, this strategy has not been applied to Berger's disease. To our knowledge, no study of familial aggregation has been carried out. However, it seems that such families are more frequent than previously thought. In addition to the usual difficulties encountered in this type of analysis, difficulties in interpretation arise from variation in age at onset, variability of the symptoms, possibility of clinical remission, and asymptomatic forms.[107,108] Furthermore, there is no reliable clinical or biologic criterion for the diagnosis of Berger's disease, and the immunohistochemical examination of a kidney biopsy specimen is always required. Finally if one supposes that a genetic susceptibility exists, it will be important to determine whether susceptibility is identical in multiplex families and in isolated cases.

Although Berger's disease was not considered familial, many studies have looked for an association between the disease and a genetic system, usually, the highly polymorphic HLA system. Thanks to molecular technology, DNA polymorphisms may now be used as markers. Since a difference in the distribution of marker alleles may be due to a stratification in the population, one must be cautious in interpreting an association between a marker allele and a disease. The strict homogeneity in geographic origin of both patients and control subjects is an important point. Excluding such errors, a positive association between a disease and a genetic marker may be explained by the role of the marker itself or by the existence of a disease susceptibility locus very close to the marker. It is possible to imagine that a disease is associated with different marker alleles in different populations and that the discrepancies observed in the different studies reflect genetic heterogeneity.

To ascertain the involvement of a marker in the etiology of the disease, association tests at a population level have to be followed by studies performed at a family level (linkage studies) testing the independent transmission of the disease and the marker in a family sample. For the reasons previously mentioned, formal linkage analysis is difficult in Berger's disease. The study of affected siblings from different families or the sib-pair method, derived from the method proposed by Penrose,[109] may be used to understand the mode of inheritance of the disease.

Environmental Factors

Although the strategy developed here indicates a first step to identify the genetic risk factors and to demonstrate their role, it will also be necessary to study interactions with environmental factors.

Among the environmental factors, the role of infectious agents, both bacterial (pneumococcal polysaccharides, *Escherichia coli*) and viral (herpes simplex virus, cytomegalovirus, Epstein-Barr virus, hepatitis B virus) has been proposed. In addition, dietary antigens (bovine serum albumin, ovalbumin, lactoglobulin, gliadin) have also been incriminated.[110] It has been suggested that the pathogen effect could be greater when the intestinal mucosa is previously modified by alcohol.

Demonstrating such antigens has led to various therapies, including tonsillectomy and gluten-free diet. However, the role of these environmental factors is still a matter of discussion. For example, the role of cytomegalovirus is at present debated.[111, 112]

The Candidate Genes

The HLA System

An association between IgAN and HLA antigens was widely studied with classic serologic methods during the 1980s. Variations in the incidence of the disease, as well as the heterogeneous distribution of HLA alleles in France, constitute two difficulties in this type of study. Heterogeneity of the HLA allele frequency is wide in the various French regions: for example, DR4 frequency in Brittany (22.8%) is twice that in Corsica (9.9%).[113] An association between IgAN and HLA B35 has been observed in France,[114] the United States,[115] and Australia.[116] An association with HLA B12 has been reported in the United States,[117] with HLA B37 in Japan,[118] with HLA DR1 in England,[26] and with HLA DR4 in France,[119, 120] and in Japan.[75, 121, 122] Other reports from the United States, Japan, Singapore,

Hungary, the Netherlands, Germany, France, Italy, Spain, England, and Finland[15] did not reveal associations. The most recent studies in Japan showed an association with HLA B35 (30.0% vs. 15.5%) and with HLA-DR4 (60.0% vs. 41.6%). Recently, an association with DQw7 was found in England (Pusey, personal communication, 1991). Conversely, recent studies in France, in Brittany,[123] in the Rhône-Alpes region,[124] in England (London and Newcastle),[125] and in Taiwan[126] found no difference.

The prognostic value of HLA antigens is controversial. Kashiwabara et al.[75] found that HLA DR4 was associated with a severe form of nephropathy. In a first report, Hiki et al.[127] concluded that DR4 was predictive of favorable outcome; subsequently, study of the same group of patients after a longer follow-up showed no influence of DR4 on prognosis. Berthoux et al.[124] observed that HLA B35 was associated with evolution to end-stage renal failure.

Table 2 shows data on HLA haplotype sharing in affected siblings. Twenty-one sibling pairs, one triplet, and one quartet were available for

TABLE 2.
Sib-Pair Method

First Author (reference)	Number of Shared Haplotypes*								
	2 Affected Sibs			3 Affected Sibs			4 Affected Sibs		
	2	1	0	2	1	0	2	1	0
Okada[67]	—	—	1	—	—	—	—	—	—
Tolkoff Rubin[68]	1	—	—	—	—	—	—	—	—
Katz[69]	1	—	—	—	—	—	—	—	—
Montoliu[70]	—	—	1	—	—	—	—	—	—
Tomizawa[71]	1	—	—	—	—	—	—	—	—
de Glas Vos[74]	—	—	1	—	—	—	—	—	—
Wyatt[77]	—	—	1	—	—	—	—	—	—
Miura[79]	1	—	—	—	—	—	—	—	—
Miyagawa[92]	—	—	1	—	—	—	—	—	—
Wyatt[85]	1	—	—	—	—	—	—	—	—
Nomoto[78]	—	1	—	—	—	—	—	—	—
Scolari[83]	—	1	1	—	—	—	—	—	—
Charlesworth†	—	—	—	—	—	—	3	3	—
Brensilver[84]	1	—	—	—	—	—	—	—	—
Collaborative study[94, 128]	4	2	1	—	2	1	—	—	—

*In five families, only HLA-A and -B were available. Sibship with three of four affected sibs are statistically dependent. All possible pairs were considered and weighted by a correcting factor.[129] The observed distribution of sibs having 2, 1, or 0 common haplotypes differs significantly ($P < .05$) from the expected distribution (1/4, 1/2, 1/4) under independence.[130]
†Personal communication, 1986.

study. The observed distribution differs significantly from the expected distribution ($P < .05$). But these results must be interpreted with caution since undoubtedly there could have been some bias in the publishing of HLA-identical pairs. Further systematic studies on a large number of HLA-typed affected sibling pairs are therefore needed before it can be concluded that there is a definite linkage between HLA and Berger's disease.

Molecular genetic studies will lead to new insights in this field. In a group of British patients, Moore et al.[125] found a strong association with a particular HLA DQB RFLP pattern. These Taq1 fragments, designated T2 and T6 after their respective 2 kb and 6 kb size, could not be attributed to DQB alleles.[125] T2 corresponds to an allotype of the DQB type and the nature of the T6 fragments is not clear but may correspond to an allele of DQB or DXB. The simultaneous presence of T2 and T6 defines a subgroup of patients with DR4 who are predisposed to autoimmune diseases. The T2+/T6+ phenotype is present in IgAN in 49% of patients vs. 15% of control subjects. Seventy-two percent of patients having DR4 are also T2+/T6+ (vs. 29% of control subjects). The association is similar to that previously observed in diabetes mellitus (where 15% of patients are T2+/T6+), in pemphigus, in rheumatoid arthritis, and in myasthenia gravis. This similarity supports the hypothesis that autoimmunity may play a role in IgAN. However, the association T2+/T6+ was not confirmed in Finnish and Italian patients in a more recent study of Moore et al.[131]; in this study, there was nevertheless a weak negative association with DQα in Finnish and British patients, but not in Italians. Last, preliminary results suggest that the polymorphism of DQA and DQB genes may play a functional role since there is, in Italian patients, a relationship between DQA and DQB alleles and some immunologic abnormalities such as elevated IgA levels or IgA rheumatoid factor.[132]

Immunoglobulin Genes

The association with heavy chain allotypes (Gm)[133] and κ light chain allotypes has been observed in a group of patients with membranous nephropathy and IgAN.[134] In addition, macroscopic hematuria was found to be associated with the heavy chain Gm allotype.[134]

IgA2 heavy chains have two alleles, A2m(1) and A2m(2), the frequency of which varies among ethnic groups. The A2m(2) allele, present on the Fc portion of the IgA2 heavy chain, differs from the A2m(1) allele by the existence of a disulphide bridge linking the heavy and light chains. Neelakantapa et al.[135] suggested that individuals having the A2m(2) allotype may have a better IgA immune response than those with the A2m(1) allotype, which is probably less stable. This hypothesis was supported by the low frequency of the A2m(1) allele in black (36%), compared to white Americans (98%), given the fact that IgA nephropathy is rare in black Americans. Crowley-Nowick et al.[136] have further studied this hypothesis by restriction fragments length polymorphism (RFLP) analysis of the Cα2 gene in 19 black patients with IgAN vs. black control subjects. This study disproves the hypothesis of Gallo's group and shows that the frequency of A2m alleles is similar in the two groups and that the homozygosity of A2m(2) did not protect from IgAN.

The genes coding for the heavy chain of the different Ig classes are located on chromosome 14. Each Ig constant domain, with the exception of IgD, is preceded by a gene region called the switch region. These switch regions are homologous and contain repetitive sequences able to coassociate and allow the deletion of the intermediate genes between two switch regions. Thus it allows a single antibody site to associate with different constant regions. The preferential IgA1 expression observed in IgAN prompts investigators to study the RFLP fragments of IgA1 and IgA2 switch regions (Sα1 and Sα2). Two groups observed contradictory results with the same probe[137] and the same restriction enzyme, SstI. The probe was homologous to the IgM switch region (Sμ) and revealed RFLPs from Sμ as well as from the switch IgA1 region (Sα1). Demaine et al.[138] have shown that the heterozygous Sμ genotype 2.6;2.1 kb is significantly diminished in patients (33% vs. 56% in control subjects). For the Sα1 region, they found an increase of the 7.4-kb allele frequency and of the 7.4-kb homozygous genotype in patients (62.5% vs. 32.7%). More recently, the same investigators observed that homozygosity for the 7.4-kb allele was associated with an increased probability of unfavorable evolution (end-stage renal failure, nephrotic syndrome, and/or interstitial fibrosis).

Moore et al.[139] studied patients of other geographical origins (Finland and Italy) as well as British patients. They found no differences with control subjects. This discordance could be explained by the facts that, in both studies, the number of patients is limited; the groups are ethnically heterogeneous, in particular in the study of Demaine a group of patients partly of German origin was compared to a group of control subjects partly of English origin; and the composition of the groups was not clinically homogeneous, which is critical in view of the fact that IgA nephropathy is probably composed of several subentities.[140]

We have studied, in collaboration with G. Keyeux and M.P. Lefranc,[141] the RFLPs of the switch region Sα1 and Sα2. The probe used (pSαSH2.1) was isolated by G.D. Keyeux et al.[142] and is different from that used in the two previous studies, having the advantage of hybridizing strongly with Sα1 and Sα2 regions and weakly with Sμ and Sϵ. After digestion with Sac 1, the Sα1 and Sα2 RFLPs can be determined unambiguously. The alleles observed in the control population are present in patients with IgAN with analogous frequency (Table 3). Surprisingly, a much larger polymorphism was found in patients with IgAN; we described two new alleles for the Sα1 region and six for the Sα2 region in a group of 41 patients of French origin with IgAN. Allele transmission was Mendelian. The size of the rare RFLPs observed in patients was close to that observed in control subjects. In this study, 12 of 41 patients (27%) expressed at least one rare allele for either Sα1 or Sα2. These rare alleles are totally absent in the control group; thus, we found a new polymorphism for patients, particularly in the Sα2 region, which had not been studied by others. The statistical study in our patients

TABLE 3.
Restriction Fragments in Switch α Regions in Berger's Disease

	Allele Frequency	
	Control Subjects[142]	Patients
No. of Alleles	70	64
IGSA1 S1 (7.1 kb)	0.685	0.687
S2 (6.6 kb)	0.314	0.250
S3 (6.5 kb)	—	0.047
S4 (6.3 kb)	—	0.016
IGSA2 S1 (4.5 kb)	0.942	0.812
S2 (5.1 kb)	0.028	0.047
S3 (4.2 kb)	0.028	—
S4 (4.4 kb)	—	0.062
S5 (4.7 kb)	—	0.016
S6 (4.8 kb)	—	0.016
S7 (5.0 kb)	—	0.016
S8 (5.5 kb)	—	0.016
S9 (6.7 kb)	—	0.016

showed that the vascular lesions (glomerular capillaries and small arterioles) were more frequent in the patients with usual alleles (22/27) than in patients with rare alleles (5/12) ($P < .05$). This coincides with the fact that renal failure was less frequent, although not significantly, in the group of patients with rare alleles. Finally, rare alleles are very unusual since they were present in only 2 of 32 children with Henoch-Schönlein purpura, studied with P. Niaudet (Hôpital des Enfants-Malades, Paris).

The apparent discordances among these three studies in different ethnic groups deserve further work. Family case analysis will allow to specification of the exact role of the switch α region in IgAN. We have to date studied four families with two affected first-degree relatives. None of these families had individuals with rare alleles and none was informative with regard to Sα1 and Sα2 regions. However, it is very likely that the switch α region plays a major role in IgAN, given the fact that we found a high frequency of rare alleles, particularly for the Sα2 region, and their total absence in the control group.

Complement Protein Genes

Rare association with complement deficiency has been reported. Wyatt et al.[77] observed the association of IgAN with partial factor H deficiency, a complement control protein of the alternative pathway. A single case of association with properdin was reported.[143] The main observations concern the polymorphism of factor B, C3, C4, and C7 since its distribution is different between IgA nephropathy and control subjects. In this regard, it is worth noting that C4 and factor B are coded in the HLA region and constitute, with C2, the HLA class III genes.

Complement Component C4

C4 is coded by two loci (C4A and C4B) within the major histocompatibility complex. C4A and C4B proteins are highly homologous but differ in biologic properties. C4A interacts more efficiently than C4B with immune complexes and therefore its deficiency may affect the solubilization and/or clearance of immune complexes.[85, 144]

Complete C4 deficiency (four null alleles) is rare and is commonly associated with systemic lupus erythematosus. Lhotta et al.[145] have recently observed a 17-year-old man with complete C4 deficiency and Henoch-Schönlein purpura progressing to end-stage renal failure.

Conversely, partial deficiency is frequent in the normal population because of the high frequency of the null alleles C4AQ0 and C4BQ0. Several authors have reported an increased frequency of null alleles in IgAN.[146] Wyatt's group in Kentucky first underlined an increase in one of the two null genes in patients of European origin, whereas an association with C4BQ0 was demonstrated in patients from Cincinnati, Ohio. Subsequently, Wyatt et al.,[147] reinvestigating their group of patients from Kentucky and the mid-South (parts of Tennessee, Alabama, and Mississippi), as well as another group of patients from the region of Puglia, Italy, and reanalyzing the results published in Ohio and Madrid, Spain, concluded that there is no increased incidence of C4AQ0 or C4BQ0 in any of the populations studied. Ali Ad'Hia et al. in Cardiff, U.K.,[148] found an increased frequency of C4AQ0 and of complotype BfS C2C C4AQ0 C4B1.

Welch et al.[149] studied by RFLP analysis five patients with complete C4B deficiency and showed that it was genetically more heterogeneous than C4A deficiency. The multiple genetic basis for C4 deficiency (C4B and 21-hydroxylase gene deletion, or C4A3 duplication) may constitute an argument against a linkage between the C4B deficiency with a locus coding for a susceptibility gene and reinforced the hypothesis that the functional deficiency itself may favor the occurrence of the disease. Recently Abe et al.,[150] studying a Japanese group of patients, showed a C4 deletion in 9/56 patients (16% vs. 2.9% in control subjects). In this study, no association with a particular HLA haplotype was noted.

Factor B of the Alternative Pathway

Factor B of the alternative pathway is genetically polymorphic, as revealed by agarose gel electrophoresis. Three major phenotypes are observed: homozygous BfFF (fast), BfSS (slow) and heterozygous BfFS. The hemolytic activity varies for each allotype (BfFF>BfFS>BfSS).[151, 152] Rambausek et al.[153] observed an increase in the homozygous BfFF phenotype in IgAN (10.4% vs. 0%). The frequency of the BfF gene was also increased (33% vs. 20%), and the rare allotypes BfF1 and S1 had a frequency comparable to that of control subjects. Because of the association between the BfFF phenotype and the HLB Bw35 antigen, it was suggested by these authors that both alleles may be genetic markers in disequilibrium linkage with a third gene, namely a susceptibility gene for the disease. Finally, they observed that the homozygous BfFF phenotype was more frequent in patients with severe forms of the disease complicated by kidney failure and elevated blood pressure. A more recent Japanese study found no association between factor B polymorphism and IgAN.[154]

Complement C3

C3 plays, together with factor B, a major role in the activation of the alternative pathway. The coding gene for C3 is located on chromosome 19 and is polymorphic with two main alleles: F and S.[155] Rambausek et al. studied German and Dutch patients and observed C3 allele frequency different from that of other forms of glomerulonephritis and control groups.[153] Homozygous C3FF or C3SS phenotype alleles are elevated in patients with IgAN; the frequency of C3F and C3S phenotypes, however, was normal. Nevertheless, the electrophoretic analysis used to determine these alleles is unable to distinguish between homozygous F or S and eventual heterozygous C3 deficient individuals. By contrast, Wyatt et al. in Kentucky[156] found increased frequency of the C3F gene in IgAN. There is no simple interpretation for the difference observed in these two studies. One may conceive that the distribution of the genes is not random in the group of patients from Kentucky, where patients are frequently related. The effect of partial consanguinity is unlikely in the European study since the C3 allele frequency was comparable in the two groups of German and Dutch patients.

It is possible that the heterozygous C3FS may be protective against the occurrence of mesangial deposits. The advantage provided by heterozygosity may be due to better defense against bacterial infection, as has been suggested in cystic fibrosis. However, there is no major functional difference between C3F and C3S with regard to immune adherence[157] or hemolytic activity.[158, 159] Yet, it seems that C3FF could have a higher affinity than C3SS for the monocyte/macrophage receptor.[157] It may be noted that association of the C3F allele with atherosclerosis,[160–162] essential hypertension,[161] rheumatoid arthritis,[163, 164] or renal failure whatever the cause[165] has been reported but remains to be interpreted.

C6 and C7 Complement Fractions

Nishimukai et al.[166] studying C6 and C7 allotypes in Japanese patients observed a striking association between the C7 5 allotype and IgA nephropathy (10.7% vs. 2% of control subjects).

Conclusion

Given the high frequency of isolated cases and the rare observation of multiplex families, the possibility of genetic susceptibility in Berger's disease has long been ignored, but the recent observation of more frequently than previously thought familial cases suggests seeking genetic factors. In our opinion, Berger's disease is not the result of defective gene(s), with a rare mutated allele, as observed in monogenic diseases. More likely, Berger's disease is a complex etiology disease, resulting from the combined effects of environmental causes and genetic factors, each gene being normal if considered alone. It is interesting to consider whether some genes coding for products functionally related to the disease, or candidate genes, represent risk factors for the disease. The observation of associations (at the population level) and of linkage (at the family level) between candidate gene markers and the disease may make evident the role of a given gene.

The demonstration of an association with serologically defined HLA antigens was the first argument in favor of the genetic susceptibility hypothesis. Recent analysis at the genomic level with the study of restriction fragment length polymorphisms suggests that DQB polymorphism may be important in determining susceptibility to Berger's disease as well as to other immune diseases. The preferential expression of IgA1 in mesangium and in serum has led to the study of the switch α region of immunoglobulin in patients with Berger's disease. Association with rare alleles in the switch α region, particularly in the switch $\alpha2$ region, may also be important in determining susceptibility. Finally, the role of complement proteins has also been suggested.

These complex data suggest that different genes, all implicated in immune response, could contribute to the appearance of the disease. Interestingly, genes not implicated in the immune response could also play a role in the progression of the nephropathy.[167] Further studies in patients and their relatives should attempt to determine the interactive roles of several candidate genes and the risk for a relative to develop the disease according to the available information on gene markers.

Acknowledgments

The authors would like to thank the members of the Cooperative Group of the French Society of Nephrology who participated in the study on multiplex families. Françoise Clerget-Darpoux contributed fruitful discussion on genetic epidemiology. Our deep thanks also go to Marie-Alice Monod for her invaluable contribution in preparing the manuscript. This work was supported by a 1990 INSERM clinical research grant.

References

1. Berger J, Hinglais N: Les dépôts intercapillaires d'IgA-IgG. *J Urol Nephrol* 1968; 74:694–695.
2. Berger J, Yaneva H, Crosnier J: La glomerulonéphrite à dépôts mésangiaux d'IgA: Une cause fréquente d'insuffisance rénale terminale. *Nouv Presse Med* 1990; 9:219–221.

3. Berger J, Yaneva H, Nabarra B, et al: Recurrence of mesangial deposition of IgA after renal transplantation. *Kidney Int* 1975; 7:232–241.
3a. Berger J: IgA glomerular deposits in renal disease. *Transplantation Proc* 1969; 1:939–944.
4. Tiebosch ATMG, Wolters J, Frederik PFM, et al: Epidemiology of idiopathic glomerular disease: A prospective study. *Kidney Int* 1987; 32:112–116.
5. Berthoux F et les néphrologues de la région: Incidence annuelle des glomérulonéphrites en 1987/1988 dans la région Rhône Alpes élargie. *Presse Med* 1990; 19:1417.
6. Simon P, Ramée MP, Ang KS, et al: Evolution de l'incidence annuelle des glomérulonéphrites primitives dans une population de 400,000 habitants au cours d'une période de 10 ans (1976–1985). *Nephrologie* 1986; 5:185–189.
7. Simon P, Ang KS, Cam G, et al: Epidémiologie de l'insuffisance rénale terminale traitée par dialyse et options thérapeutiques dans une population de 400,000 habitants (1975–1986). *Nephrologie* 1987; 8:293–299.
8. Béné MC, Faure G: Revue: Néphropathies à dépôts mésangiaux d'IgA: aspects étiopathogéniques. *Nephrologie* 1988; 9:109–115.
9. Berthoux FC: Immunopathologie de la glomérulonéphrite à dépôts mésangiaux d'IgA. *Nephrologie* 1989; 10:169–174.
10. Egido J, Julian BA, Wyatt RJ: Genetic factors in primary IgA nephropathy. *Nephrol Dial Transplantation* 1987; 2:134–142.
11. Egido J, Sancho J, Blasco R, et al: Immunopathogenetic aspects of IgA nephropathy. *Adv Nephrol* 1983; 12:103–137.
12. Emancipator SN, Lamm ME: IgA nephropathy: Pathogenesis of the most common form of glomerulonephritis. *Lab Invest* 1989; 2:168–183.
13. Feehally J: Immune mechanisms in glomerular IgA deposition. *Nephrol Dial Transplantation* 1988; 3:361–378.
14. Lesavre P, Noël LH, Monteiro R, et al: La maladie de Berger: Une néphro pathie à IgA. *Med Sci* 1989; 5:286–292.
15. Lévy M: Do genetic factors play a role in Berger's disease? *Pediatr Nephrol* 1987; 1:447–454.
16. Russel MW, Mestecky J, Julian BA, et al: IgA-associated renal diseases: Antibodies to environmental antigens in sera and deposition of immunoglobulins and antigens in glomeruli. *J Clin Immunol* 1986; 6:74–86.
17. Aucouturier P, Monteiro RC, Noël LH, et al: Glomerular and serum immunoglobulin G subclasses in IgA nephropathy. *Clin Immunol Immunopathol* 1989; 51:338–347.
18. Noël LH, Aucouturier P, Monteiro RC, et al: Glomerular and serum immunoglobulin G subclasses in membranous and anti-glomerular basement membrane nephritis. *Clin Immunol Immunopathol* 1988; 46:1–9.
19. Van den Wall Bake AWL, Daha MR, Van Der Ark A, et al: Serum levels and in vitro production of IgA subclasses in patients with primary IgA nephropathy. *Clin Exp Immunol* 1988; 74:115–120.
20. Delacroix DL, Elkon KB, Geubel AP, et al: Changes in size subclass and metabolic properties of serum immunoglobulin A in liver diseases and in other diseases with high serum immunoglobulin A. *J Clin Invest* 1983; 71:358–367.
21. Lesavre P, Digeon M, Bach JF: Analysis of circulating IgA and detection of immune complexes in primary IgA nephropathy. *Clin Exp Immunol* 1982; 48:61–69.

22. Monteiro RC, Halbwachs-Mecarelli L, Roque-Barreira MC, et al: Charge and size of mesangial IgA in IgA nephropathy. *Kidney Int* 1985; 28:666–671.
23. Valentijn RM, Radl J, Haajman JJ: Circulating and mesangial secretory component-binding IgA-1 in primary IgA nephropathy. *Kidney Int* 1984; 26:760–766.
24. Cederholm B, Wieslander J, Bygren P, et al: Circulating complexes containing IgA and fibronectin in patients with primary IgA nephropathy. *Proc Natl Acad Sci USA* 1988; 85:4865–4868.
25. Monteiro RC, Chevailler A, Noël LH, et al: Serum IgA preferentially binds to cationic polypeptides in IgA nephropathy. *Clin Exp Immunol* 1988; 73:300–306.
26. Feehally J, Dyer PA, Davidson JA, et al: Immunogenetics of IgA nephropathy: Experience in a UK centre. *Dis Markers* 1984; 2:493–500.
27. Van den Wall Bake AW, Daha MR, Evers-Schouten J, et al: Serum IgA and the production of IgA by peripheral blood and bone marrow lymphocytes in patients with primary IgA nephropathy: Evidence for the bone marrow as the source of mesangial IgA. *Am J Kidney Dis* 1988; 12:410–414.
28. Hale GM, McIntosh SL, Hiki Y, et al: Evidence for IgA-specific B cell hyperactivity in patients with IgA nephropathy. *Kidney Int* 1986; 29:718–724.
29. Chevailler A, Monteiro RC, Daëron M, et al: Induction of Fc receptors for IgA on murine T cell hybridoma by human monoclonal IgA and by high molecular weight IgA in IgA nephropathy. *Clin Exp Immunol* 1987; 67:114–123.
30. Béné MC, Faure G, Hurault de Ligny B, et al: Immunoglobulin A nephropathy. Quantitative immunohistomorphometry of the tonsillar plasma cells evidences an inversion of the immunoglobulin A versus immunoglobulin G secreting cell balance. *J Clin Invest* 1983; 71:1342–1347.
31. Westberg NG, Baklien K, Schmekel B, et al: Quantification of immunoglobulin-producing cells in small intestinal mucosa of patients with IgA nephropathy. *Clin Immunol Immunopathol* 1983; 26:442–445.
32. Frampton G, Harada T, Cameron JS: IgA autoantibodies in Berger's disease. *Nephrol Dial Transplantation* 1988; 3:510.
33. Oliveira DBG, Peters DK: Autoimmunity and the kidney. *Kidney Int* 1989; 35:923–928.
34. Nomoto Y, Miura M, Suga T, et al: Cold reacting anti-nuclear factor in families of patients with IgA nephropathy. *Clin Exp Immunol* 1984; 58:63–67.
35. Sinico RA, Fornasieri A, Oreni N, et al: Polymeric IgA rheumatoid factor in idiopathic mesangial IgA nephropathy (Berger's disease). *J Immunol* 1986; 137:536–541.
36. Matsiota P, Dosquet P, Louzir H, et al: IgA polyspecific autoantibodies in IgA nephropathy. *Clin Exp Immunol* 1990; 79:361–366.
37. Cederholm B, Wieslander J, Bygren P, et al: Patients with IgA nephropathy have circulating anti-basement membrane antibodies reacting with structures common to collagen I, II and IV. *Proc Natl Acad Sci USA* 1986; 83:6151–6155.
38. Mestecky J, Russel MW, Jackson S, et al: The human IgA system: A reassessment. *Clin Immunol Immunopathol* 1986; 40:105–114.
39. Kett K, Brandtzaeg P, Radl J, et al: Different subclass distribution of IgA-producing cells in human lymphoid organs and various secretory tissues. *J Immunol* 1986; 136:3631–3635.
40. Conley ME, Delacroix DL: Intravascular and mucosal immunoglobulin A:

Two separate but related systems of immune defense? *Ann Intern Med* 1987; 106:892–899.

41. Nagy J, Brandtzaeg P: Tonsillar distribution of IgA, IgG immunocytes and IgA subclasses in IgA nephropathy. *Contrib Nephrol* 1988; 67:107–110.
42. Wyatt RJ, Kanayama Y, Julian BA, et al: Complement activation in IgA nephropathy. *Kidney Int* 1987; 31:1019–1023.
43. Rauterberg FW, Lieberknecht HM, Wingen AM, et al: Complement membrane attack (MAC) in idiopathic IgA glomerulonephritis. *Kidney Int* 1987; 31:820–829.
44. Lévy M, Berger J: Worldwide perspective of IgA nephropathy. *Am J Kidney Dis* 1988; 12:340–347.
45. Ballardie FW, O'Donoghue DJ, Feehally J: Increasing frequency of adult IgA nephropathy in the UK? *Lancet* 1987; ii:1205.
46. Woo KT, Chiang GSC, Edmonson RPS, et al: Glomerulonephritis in Singapore: An overview. *Ann Acad Med Singapore* 1986; 15:20–31.
47. Kitagawa T: Lessons learned from the Japanese nephritis screening study. *Pediatr Nephrol* 1988; 2:256–263.
48. Date A, Raghavan R, Jacob JT, et al: Renal disease in adult Indians: A clinicopathological study of 2827 patients. *Q J Med* 1987; 248:729–737.
49. Cheong IKS, Chong SM, Suleiman AB, et al: Pattern of adult primary glomerular disease in Malaysia (abstract). Xth International Congress of Nephrology, London, 1987, p 84.
50. Li L, Li LS, Chen HP, et al: Primary glomerulonephritis in China. Analysis of 1001 cases. *Chin Med J* 1989; 102:159–164.
51. Lee HS, Koh HI, Lee HB, et al: IgA nephropathy in Korea: A morphological and clinical study. *Clin Nephrol* 1987; 27:131–140.
52. Galla JH, Kohaut EC, Alexander R, et al: Racial differences in the prevalence of IgA-associated nephropathies. *Lancet* 1984; 2:522.
53. Jennette JC, Wall SD, Wilkman AS: Low incidence of IgA nephropathy in blacks. *Kidney Int* 1985; 28:944–950.
54. Jackson FLC: HLA diversity within the context of general human heterogeneity: Anthropological perspectives. *Transplantation Proc* 1989; 21:3869–3871.
55. Johnson AH: The black population in the United States. *Transplantation Proc* 1989; 21:3880.
56. Seedat YK, Nathoo BC, Parag KB, et al: IgA nephropathy in blacks and Indians of Natal. *Nephron* 1988; 50:137–141.
57. Swanepoel CR, Madaus S, Cassidy MJD, et al: IgA nephropathy—Groote Schuur hospital experience. *Nephron* 1989; 53:61–64.
58. Coovadia HM: Henoch-Schönlein purpura in black and Indian children in Natal. *S Afr Med J* 1982; 62:433–434.
59. Langaney A: *Les Hommes.* Armand Colin, Paris, 1988.
60. Hughson MD, Megill DM, Smith SM, et al: Mesangiopathic glomerulonephritis in Zuni (New Mexico) Indians. *Arch Pathol Lab Med* 1989; 113:148–157.
61. Hoy W, Smith SM, Hughson MD, et al: Mesangialproliferative glomerulonephritis in Southwestern American Indians. *Transplantation Proc* 1989; 21:3909–3912.
62. Meleg Smith S, Hoy WE, Pathak D, et al: Pathologic findings in mesangiopathic glomerulonephritis in Navajo Indians. *Arch Pathol Lab Med* 1989; 113:158–163.
63. Casiro OG, Stanwick RS, Walker RD: The prevalence of IgA nephropathy in IgA Manitoba native Indian children. *Can J Public Health* 1988; 79:308–310.

64. O'Connell PJ, Ibels LS, Thomas MA, et al: Familial IgA nephropathy: A study in an Australian Aboriginal family. *Aust NZ J Med* 1987; 17:27–33.
65. New Zealand Glomerulonephritis Study Group: The New Zealand Glomerulonephritis Study: Introductory report. *Clin Nephrol* 1989; 31:239–246.
66. Werra de P, Morel-Maroger L, Leroux-Robert C, et al: Glomérulites à dépôts d'IgA diffus dans le mesangium. Etude de 96 cas chez l'adulte. *Schweiz Med Wochenschr* 1973; 103:761–768.
67. Okada M, Tsuchida H, Yamamoto S: Familial mesangial IgA nephropathy, in Yoshitoshi Y, Ueda Y (eds): *Glomerulonephritis.* Tokyo, University of Tokyo Press, 1979, pp 201–223.
68. Tolkoff-Rubin NE, Cosimi AB, Fuller T, et al: IgA nephropathy in HLA-identical siblings. *Transplantation* 1978; 26:430–433.
69. Katz A, Karanicolas S, Falk JA: Family study in IgA nephritis: The possible role of HLA antigens. *Transplantation* 1980; 29:505–506.
70. Montoliu J, Darnell A, Torras A, et al: Familial IgA nephropathy. Report of two cases and brief review of the literature. *Arch Intern Med* 1980; 140:1374–1375.
71. Tomizawa S, Tsabouchi H, Matsui A, et al: Mesangial IgA nephropathy in HLA-identical siblings with similar blood types (abstract). *Pediatr Res* 1980; 14:995.
72. Gutierrez Millet V, Navas Palacios JJ, Ortega Ruano R, et al: Glomerulonefritis mesangial con depositos de IgA, familiar y hereditaria. *Med Clin (Barcelona)* 1981; 76:1–7.
73. Sinniah R, Javier AR, Ku G: The pathology of mesangial IgA nephritis with clinical correlation. *Histopathology* 1981; 5:469–490.
74. Glas-Vos de JW, Krediet RT, Balk AG, et al: IgA nephropathy in one family. (abstract). *Kidney Int* 1981; 20:538.
75. Kashiwabara H, Shishido H, Tomura S, et al: Strong association between IgA nephropathy and HLA-DR4 antigen. *Kidney Int* 1982; 22:377–382.
76. Hene RJ, de Glas-Vos JW, Valentin R, et al: Aspects sérologiques et génétiques dans deux familles atteintes de néphropathie primitive à IgA (abstract). *Nephrologie* 1982; 3:94.
77. Wyatt RJ, Julian BA, Weinstein A, et al: Partial H (βIH) deficiency and glomerulonephritis in two families. *J Clin Immunol* 1982; 2:110–117.
78. Nomoto Y, Endoh M, Miura M, et al: IgA nephropathy associated with HLA-DR4 antigen. *Am J Nephrol* 1984; 4:184–187.
79. Miura M, Tomino Y, Suga T, et al: Siblings with IgA nephropathy and diffuse proliferative glomerulonephritis, without mesangial IgA deposits associated with identical HLA antigens. *Clin Nephrol* 1984; 22:269–270.
80. Ohzono Y, Hiratani K, Matsuo S, et al: A case of familial IgA nephropathy. *Nippon Jinzo Gakkai Shi* 1985; 27:533–540.
81. Fitzsimmons JS, Watson AR, Mellor D, et al: Familial spastic paraplegia, bilateral sensorineural deafness, and intellectual retardation with a progressive nephropathy. *J Med Genet* 1988; 25:168–172.
82. Garcia-Hoyo R, Lozano L, Egido J: Immune abnormalities in six families with IgA nephropathy, in McGhee J, Mestecky J, Ogra PL, Bienenstock J (eds): *Recent Advances in Mucosal Immunology,* part B. New York, Plenum Press, 1987, pp 1499–1505.
83. Scolari F, Amoroso A, Savoldi S, et al: Familial IgA nephropathy: Immunological and immunogenetical studies (abstract). XXVIth Congress EDTA-ERA, Göteborg, 1989, p 38.
84. Brensilver JM, Mallat S, Scholes J, et al: Recurrent IgA nephropathy in living-

related donor transplantation: Recurrence or transmission of familial disease? *Am J Kidney Dis* 1988; 12:147–151.
85. Wyatt RJ, Schneider PD, Alpers CE, et al: C4B deficiency in two siblings with IgA nephropathy. *Am J Kidney Dis* 1990; 15:66–71.
86. Chahin J, Mendez L, Gallego E, et al: Nefropathia IgA familiar asociada a sordera neurosensorial (abstract). *Nefrologia* 1990; 10:41.
87. Nagata K, Yamabe H, Waga S, et al: A family of IgA nephropathy in mother and Henoch-Schönlein purpura nephritis in son (abstract). 9th International Congress of Nephrology, Los Angeles, 1984.
88. Furuse A, Hiramatsu M, Adachi N, et al: Dramatic response to corticosteroid therapy of nephrotic syndrome associated with IgA nephropathy. *Int J Pediatr Nephrol* 1985; 6:205–208.
89. Meadow SR, Scott DG: Berger disease: Henoch-Schönlein syndrome without the rash. *J Pediatr* 1985; 106:27–32.
90. Waldo FB, Beischel L, West CD: IgA synthesis by lymphocytes from patients with IgA nephropathy and their relatives. *Kidney Int* 1986; 29:1229–1233.
91. Osawa H, Yamabe H, Ozawa K, et al: A family case of IgA nephropathy and Henoch Schönlein purpura nephritis. *Jpn J Nephrol* 1989; 31:1–3.
92. Miyagawa S, Dohi K, Hanatani M, et al: Anaphylactoid purpura and familial IgA nephropathy. *Am J Med* 1989; 86:340–342.
93. Montoliu J, Lens XM, Torras A, et al: Henoch-Schönlein purpura and IgA nephropathy in father and son. *Nephron* 1990; 54:77–79.
94. Lévy M, French cooperative group of the Society of Nephrology: Familial cases of Berger's disease and anaphylactoid purpura: More frequent than previously thought. *Am J Med* 1989; 87:246–248.
95. Lévy M, Cas familiaux de maladie de Berger ou de maladie de Berger et de purpura rhumatoide: Etude coopérative de la Société Française de Néphrologie. *Nephrologie* 1989; 10:175–182.
96. DeSanto NG, Sessa A, Capodicasa G, et al: IgA glomerulonephritis in Wiskott-Aldrich syndrome. *Child Nephrol Urol* 1989; 9:118–120.
97. Julian BA, Quiggins PA, Thompson JS, et al: Familial IgA nephropathy. Evidence of an inherited mechanism of disease. *N Engl J Med* 1985; 312–202–208.
98. Julian BA, Woodford SY, Baehler RW, et al: Familial clustering and immunogenetic aspects of IgA nephropathy. *Am J Kidney Dis* 1988; 12:366–370.
99. Julian BA, Wyatt RJ, Waldo FB, et al: Immunological studies of IgA nephropathy: Familial and racial aspects, in McGhee J, Mestecky J, Ogra PL, et al (eds): *Recent Advances in Mucosal Immunology*, part B. New York, Plenum Press, 1987, pp 1489–1498.
100. Wyatt RJ, Rivas ML, Julian BA, et al: Regionalization in hereditary IgA nephropathy. *Am J Hum Genet* 1987; 41:36–50.
101. Sakai H, Nomoto Y, Tomino Y, et al: Increase of in vivo and in vitro production of polyclonal IgA in patients and in their family members with IgA nephropathy, in McGhee J, Mestecky J, Ogra PL, Bienenstock J (eds): *Recent Advances in Mucosal Immunology*, part B. New York, Plenum Press, 1987, pp 1507–1514.
102. Waldo FB, Cochran AM: Systemic immune response to oral polio immunization in patients with IgA nephropathy. *J Clin Lab Immunol* 1989; 28:109–114.
103. Schena FP, Gesualdo L, Scivittaro V, et al: Role of interleukin (IL)-2 and -4 in primary IgA nephropathy (IGAN) (abstract). *J Am Soc Nephrol* 1990; 1:567.

104. King MC: Genetic epidemiology. *Ann Rev Public Health* 1984; 5:1–52.
105. Harper PS. Mendelian inheritance or transmissible agent? The lesson of Kuru and the Australia antigen. *J Med Genet* 1977; 14:389–398.
106. Asamoah A, Wyatt RJ, Julian BA, et al: A major gene model for the familial aggregation of plasma IgA concentration. *Am J Med Genet* 1987; 27:857–866.
107. Waldherr R, Rambausek M, Duncker WD, et al: Frequency of mesangial IgA deposits in a non-selected autopsy series. *Pathology* 1989; 4:943–946.
108. Julian BA, Cannon VR, Waldo FB, et al: Macroscopic hematuria and proteinuria preceding renal IgA deposition in patients with IgA nephropathy (abstract). *J Am Soc Nephrol* 1990; 1:309.
109. Penrose LS: The detection of autosomal linkage in data which consists of pairs of brothers and sisters of unspecified parentage. *Ann Eugenics* 1935; 6:133–138.
110. Coppo R: The pathogenetic potential of environmental antigens in IgA nephropathy. *Am J Kidney Dis* 1988; 12:420–424.
111. Lai FM, Tam JS, Lo ST, et al: Cytomegalovirus antigens in IgA nephropathy: Fact or artifacts? *Nephron* 1990; 55:87–88.
112. Waldo FB, Britt WJ, Toman M, et al: Non-specific mesangial staining with antibodies against cytomegalovirus in immunoglobulin A nephropathy. *Lancet* 1989; 1:129–131.
113. Betuel H, Gebuhrer L, Lambert J: Marqueurs HLA de classe II dans les Provinces françaises, in Ohayon E, Cambon-Thomsen A (eds): Génétique des populations humaines. *Colloque INSERM* 1986; 142:265–278.
114. Berthoux FC, Gagne A, Sabatier JC, et al: HLA-Bw35 and mesangial IgA glomerulonephritis. *N Engl J Med* 1978; 298:1034–1035.
115. Pardo V, Pardo T, Clerch A, et al: HLA-Bw35 antigen as a marker for segmental sclerosis and progressive disease in IgA mesangial glomerulonephritis (abstract). *Kidney Int* 1981; 19:134.
116. McDonald IM, Dumble LJ, Kincaid-Smith P: The association of HLA-Bw35 and circulating immune complexes in patients with IgA nephropathy (abstract 8.5.36). Fourth International Congress of Immunology, Paris, 1980.
117. Richman AV, Mahoney JJ, Fuller TJ: Higher prevalence of HLA-B12 in patients with IgA nephropathy. *Ann Intern Med* 1979; 90:201.
118. Komori K, Nose Y, Inouye H, et al: Immunogenetical study in patients with chronic glomerulonephritis. *Tokai J Exp Clin Med* 1983; 8:135–148.
119. Fauchet R, Le Pogamp P, Genetet B, et al: HLA-DR4 antigen and IgA nephropathy. *Tissue Antigens* 1980; 16:405–410.
120. Hors J, Grünfeld JP, Noel LH, et al: Strong association between HLA-DRw4 and mesangial IgA nephropathy (Berger's disease) (abstract 8.5 26). Fourth International Congress of Immunology, Paris, 1980.
121. Hiki Y, Kobayashi Y, Tateno S, et al: Strong association of HLA-DR4 with benign IgA nephropathy. *Nephron* 1982; 32:222–226.
122. Kasahara M, Hamada K, Okuyama T, et al: Role of HLA in IgA nephropathy. *Clin Immunol Immunopathol* 1982; 25:189–195.
123. Autuly V, Simon P, Ramée MP, et al: HLA DR4 antigen is not associated with IgA nephropathy (abstract). First Breton Workshop on Autoimmunity, Brest, 1990.
124. Berthoux FC, Alamartine E, Pommier G, et al: HLA and IgA nephritis revisited 10 years later: HLA-B35 antigen as a prognostic factor. *N Engl J Med* 1989; 319:709–710 and 320:748 [Corrections].
125. Moore RH, Hitman GA, Lucas EY, et al: HLA DQ region gene polymor-

phism associated with primary IgA nephropathy. *Kidney Int* 1990; 37:991–995.
126. Huang CC, Hu SA, Lin JL, et al: HLA and chinese IgA nephropathy in Taiwan. *Tissue Antigens* 1989; 33:45–47.
127. Hiki Y, Kobayashi Y, Ookubo M, et al: The role of HLA-DR4 in the long-term prognosis of IgA nephropathy. *Nephron* 1990; 54:264–265.
128. Sabatier JC, Génin C, Assenat H, et al: Mesangial IgA glomerulonephritis in HLA-identical brothers. *Clin Nephrol* 1979; 11:35–38.
129. Hodge SE: The information contained in multiple sibling pairs. *Genet Epidemiol* 1984; 1:109–122.
130. Thomson G: A review of theoretical aspects of HLA and disease associations. *Theor Popul Biol* 1981; 20:168–208.
131. Moore R, Medcraft J, Sinico R, et al: HLA-DQ region gene polymorphism in European IgA nephropathy (IgAN) (abstract). *J Am Soc Nephrol* 1990; 1:564.
132. Moore R, Sinico R, Medcraft J, et al: Functional significance of HLA-DQ gene polymorphism in IgA nephropathy (IgAN) (abstract). XXVIIth Congress of the European Dialysis and Transplant Association, Vienna, 1990, p 64.
133. Demaine AG, Cameron JS, Taube DT, et al: Immunoglobulin (Gm) allotype frequencies in idiopathic membranous nephropathy and minimal change nephropathy. *Transplantation* 1984; 37:507–508.
134. Le Petit JC, Van Loghem EV, de Lange GD, et al: Gm, Am, P1, Km markers in mesangial IgA nephropathy. *J Immunogenet* 1981; 8:415–418.
135. Neelakantappa K, Gallo GR, Baldwin DS: Immunoglobulin A nephropathy in blacks and homozygosity for the genetic marker A2m. *Ann Intern Med* 1986; 104:287–288.
136. Crowley-Nowick PA, Julian BA, Wyatt RJ, et al: IgA2 allotyping in blacks with IgA nephropathy (IgAN) (abstract). *J Am Soc Nephrol* 1990; 1:306.
137. Migone N, Feder J, Cann H, et al: Multiple DNA fragment polymorphisms associated with immunoglobulin μ-chain-switch-like regions in man. *Proc Natl Acad Sci USA* 1983; 80:467–471.
138. Demaine AG, Rambausek M, Knight JF, et al: Relation of mesangial IgA glomerulonephritis to polymorphism of immunoglobulin in heavy chain switch region. *J Clin Invest* 1988; 81:611–614.
139. Moore RH, Hitman GA, Sinico RA, et al: Immunoglobulin heavy chain switch region gene polymorphisms in glomerulonephritis. *Kidney Int* 1990; 38:332–336.
140. Beukhof JR, Kardaun O, Schaafsma W, et al: Toward individual prognosis of IgA nephropathy. *Kidney Int* 1986; 29:549–556.
141. Keyeux G, Nusbaum P, Alexandre D, et al: New RFLPs of the immunoglobulin switch alpha region in mesangial IgA glomerulonephritis. *Hum Genet* 1991; 86:624.
142. Keyeux G, Lefranc G, Lefranc MP: A specific switch alpha probe of the human immunoglobulin IGHA locus. *Nucleic Acids Res* 1989; 17:3624.
143. Wyatt RJ, Julian BA, Galla JH: Properdin deficiency with IgA nephropathy. *N Engl J Med* 1981; 305:1097.
144. Matsuda S, Czerkinsky C, Moldoveanu Z, et al: IgA on the surface of erythrocytes from IgA nephropathy patients. *Adv Exp Med Biol* 1987; 216:1577–1581.
145. Lhotta K, König P, Hintner H, et al: Renal disease in a patient with hereditary complete deficiency of the fourth component of complement. *Nephron* 1990; 56:206–211.

146. McLean RH, Wyatt RJ, Julian BA: Complement phenotypes in glomerulonephritis: Increased frequency of homozygous null C4 phenotypes in IgA nephropathy and Henoch-Schönlein purpura. *Kidney Int* 1984; 26:855–860.
147. Wyatt RJ, Rivas ML, Schena FP, et al: Regional variation in C4 phenotype in patients with IgA nephropathy. *J Pediatr* 1990; 116:72–77.
148. Ad'hiah A, Moore RH, Venning M, Papiha SS: Genetic susceptibility to IgA nephropathy (abstract). XIth International Congress of Nephrology, Tokyo, 1990, p 365.
149. Welch TR, Beischel LS, Choi EM: Molecular genetics of C4B deficiency in IgA nephropathy. *Hum Immunol* 1989; 26:353–363.
150. Abe J, Kohsaka T, Kobayashi N: Increased frequency of C4 gene deletions in IgA nephropathy and Henoch-Schönlein purpura nephritis (abstract). XIth International Congress of Nephrology, Tokyo, 1990, p 111.
151. Mauff G, Adam R, Wachauf B, et al: Serum concentration and functional efficiency of factor B alleles. *Immunobiology* 1980; 158:86–90.
152. Mortensen JP, Lamm LK: Quantitative difference between complement factor-B phenotypes. *Immunology* 1981; 24:505–511.
153. Rambausek M, Van den Wall Bake AW, Schumacher-Ach R, et al: Genetic polymorphism of C3 and Bf in IgA nephropathy. *Nephrol Dial Transplant* 1987; 2:208–211.
154. Nishimukai H, Nakanishi I, Kitamura H, et al: Factor B subtypes in Japanese patients with IgA nephropathy and with idiopathic membranous nephropathy. *Exp Clin Immunogenet* 1988; 5:196–202.
155. Bronnestam R, Cedergren B: Studies of the C3 polymorphism. *Hum Heredity* 1973; 23:214–219.
156. Wyatt RJ, Julian BA, Galla JH, et al: Increased frequency of C3 fast alleles in IgA nephropathy. *Dis Markers* 1984; 2:419–428.
157. Arvilommi H: Capacity of complement C3 phenotypes to bind onto mononuclear cells in man. *Nature* 1974; 251:740–741.
158. Colten HR, Alper CA: Hemolytic efficiencies of genetic variants of human C3. *J Immunol* 1972; 108:1184–1187.
159. Kay PH, Natsuume-Sakai S, Hayakawa J, et al: Different allotypes of C3 degrade at different rates. *Immunogenetics* 1985; 22:563–569.
160. Farhud DD, Ananthakrishnan R, Walter H: Association between C3 phenotypes and various diseases. *Hum Genet* 1972; 17:57–60.
161. Kristenson BO, Peterson GB: Association between coronary heart disease and the C3 F-gene in essential hypertension. *Circulation* 1978; 58:622–625.
162. Sorensen H, Dissing J: Association between the C3 F-gene and atherosclerotic vascular disease. *Hum Heredity* 1975; 25:279–283.
163. Lanchbury JSS, Pal B, Papiha SS: Bf and C3 polymorphisms in rheumatoid arthritis. *Hum Heredity* 1987; 37:144–149.
164. Thomson W, Dyer PA, Sanders PH, et al: Genetic variants of complement component 3 (C3) in DR4 positive and DR4 negative rheumatoid arthritis. *Ann Rheum Dis* 1986; 45:269–271.
165. Welch TR, Berry A: C3 alleles in diseases associated with C3 activation. *Dis Markers* 1987; 5:81–87.
166. Nishimukai H, Nakanishi I, Takeuchi Y, et al: Complement C6 and C7 polymorphisms in Japanese patients with chronic glomerulonephritis. *Hum Heredity* 1989; 39:150–155.
167. Simon P, Ramée MP, Ang KS, et al: Family history of hypertension and the progression of IgA nephropathy (IgAN) (abstract). *J Am Soc Nephrol* 1990; 1:287.

Genetic Susceptibility to Autoimmune Diseases

Henri-Jean Garchon, M.D.

Department of Clinical Immunology, INSERM U25, Hôpital Necker, Paris, France

Christian Boitard, M.D.

Department of Clinical Immunology, INSERM U25, Hôpital Necker, Paris, France

Autoimmune diseases, as a group, affect 5% to 7% of the general population. They often constitute chronic diseases showing a pronounced tendency to spontaneous succession of exacerbation and remission. The genetic background of genetic susceptibility on which various autoimmune diseases occur often include different alleles, although the same genetic regions can be involved. The most important region so far characterized is the major histocompatibility complex (MHC) in which different susceptibility alleles can predispose to different autoimmune diseases. Autoimmune diseases have other common genetic features. Susceptibility to autoimmune diseases is polyfactorial. The study of monozygous twins indicates concordance rates that range from 7% in multiple sclerosis to 36% in insulin-dependent diabetes mellitus. Thus, nongenetic (environmental) factors are likely to play a role in disease dvelopment.

Genetic susceptibility is also polygenic. The MHC is the only region for which available markers have allowed identification of its role in the autoimmune process. Comparison between the concordance rate for a given disease in monozygous twins or histocompatibility leukocyte antigen (HLA)-identical dizygous twins, as well as the analysis of families with several affected siblings, indicate that the MHC is not the only genetic region involved in susceptibility. In animal models of autoimmune diseases, the number of genetic regions that may be involved is considered to be three to six or more[1] on the basis of breeding studies and formal genetic analysis. Besides immunoglobulin genes or genes coding for the T-cell receptor for antigen, no other genetic region has been identified so far. The multifactorial characteristics of autoimmune diseases may explain why they cannot involve simple genetic transmission.

The main genetic factors that may be involved in the susceptibility to development of autoimmune diseases will be discussed in this chapter. The illustrative case of insulin-dependent diabetes mellitus will be analyzed, and MHC genes will be schematically compared to non-MHC genes suspected to be involved.

Advances in Nephrology, vol 21

The Major Histocompatibility Complex

The role of the MHC in susceptibility to various autoimmune diseases was initially indicated by the study of populations affected by such diseases, which provided the first demonstration of HLA-disease associations. It has been further evidenced by the demonstration of a genetic linkage between various autoimmune diseases and the HLA system in families with several affected siblings. The study of association and linkage between the HLA system and autoimmune diseases has indeed been largely dependent on the techniques allowing the characterization of HLA antigen polymorphism and, more recently, MHC gene polymorphism itself.

Serologic Typing

In the early 1970s, the only possible characterization of MHC antigen polymorphism was at the level of class I antigens, which are expressed on all nucleated cells. This allowed describing the association between several diseases with definite class I alleles. An association was thus described between insulin-dependent diabetes mellitus and HLA-A1 and A2, which are encoded by the A locus of the HLA system, and to a greater extent, with HLA-B8 (in linkage disequilibrium with A1), HLA-B15 (in linkage disequilibrium with A2) and, particularly in France, with HLA-B18, which are encoded by the B locus. Actually, the relative risk conferred by each of these alleles is weak, below 2 for the alleles encoded by the A locus, and below 2.7 for alleles encoded by the B locus.

More recently, serologic typing of class II antigens encoded by the DR locus of the D region of the HLA system has become available. The typing of DR antigens has thus allowed to demonstrate the relative risk, which is higher than that defined by serologic typing of class I antigens in most diseases presenting with classical autoimmunity criteria. The association of diabetes mellitus with HLA-DR3 and/or 4 is higher than that associated with HLA-B8, B15, or B18. In the French population, the relative risk is 3.4 in DR3 subjects and 6.4 in DR7 subjects.[2] Ninety percent to 95% of patients with insulin-dependent diabetes mellitus are HLA-DR3 and/or DR4, as opposed to only 40% to 45% in the general population. The relative risks defined in other white populations are similar.[3] A weak association has been observed with HLA-DR1 and DR8. Interestingly, different susceptibility antigens have been defined in nonwhite populations; for instance in Japan, DR4 and DR9, but not DR3, alleles are associated with insulin-dependent diabetes mellitus.

A higher association with class II antigens as compared to class I antigens is a general feature of most autoimmune diseases. Rheumatoid arthritis (DR4), celiac disease (DR3 and DR7), many thyroid diseases (DR3 or DR5), pemphigus vulgaris (DR4 and DRw6), multiple sclerosis (DR2), pernicious anemia (DR3), and myasthenia gravis (DR3) are the most illustrative examples.[4]

The study of diabetes mellitus is also interesting in that two aspects differ from the characteristics found in most other autoimmune diseases. Some class II alleles confer a decreased susceptibility to diabetes mellitus (HLA-DR2, relative risk below 0.2), indicating the existence of protective as well as of susceptibility genes. Moreover, the relative risk conferred by the presence of both HLA DR3 and DR4 in heterozygotes is very high (close to 40 in the French diabetic population),[2, 4] much higher than the relative risk conferred by the presence of either DR3 or DR4 in homozygotes (relative risk below 10). A very high relative risk is known for only one other autoimmune disease, celiac disease, in which DR3 and DR7, or DR7 and DR5 in a small geographic area in Italy, confer a high susceptibility.[5]

Family studies fully confirmed population studies in demonstrating a genetic linkage between autoimmune diseases and the HLA system. In the absence of linkage between a given disease and a genetic marker, when a kindred contains at least two affected subjects, the expected probability that the two affected siblings share two HLA alleles is 25%, one HLA allele is 50%, and no alleles, 25%. Several studies demonstrated that in patients with diabetes mellitus (as well as in other autoimmune diseases), two affected siblings share two or one HLA alleles much more often than would be randomly expected.

All previously described data have been completed due to the recent availability of serologic markers for DP and DQ alleles, The role of the DP locus has been suggested, for instance, in celiac disease. A close association between insulin-dependent diabetes mellitus and HLA-DQ alleles has also been suggested with the use of monoclonal antibodies (TA10 and 2B3), which recognize different HLA-DQ antigens, and more precisely different molecular forms of the DQβ chain (DQw3.1 or DQw7 and DQw3.2 or DQw8). Whatever the HLA-DR typing in a subject with diabetes mellitus, the presence of a DQβ chain recognized by the TA10 antibody is associated with a relative risk that is below 0.10, although no positive association has been reported in a subject expressing the DQβ chain recognized by the antibody 2B3.[6]

As opposed to the various diseases demonstrating a very strong association with antigens of HLA class II, a strong association with those of HLA class I has been observed in other diseases. Two groups of affections have been described, one showing a strong association with HLA-B27 (spondylarthropathy, including ankylosing spondylarthritis, Reiter's syndrome, and reactive arthropathy) and another associated with HLA-B13, B16, and B17 (psoriasis).[4]

Both class I and class II associated diseases are polyfactorial and polygenic. However, these two groups of diseases can be distinguished by the presence of several clinical features. Diseases associated with class II antigens are those which present with the most typical criteria for autoimmune diseases. They are observed with the highest frequency in females. They are characterized by the serologic detection of autoantibodies with often a very high positive predictive value. Their course is favorably affected by immunosuppressive treatments. They often show T lymphocyte abnormalities. Their study is often facilitated by the existence of good animal models in which transfer experiments and induction or disease prevention by immunomanipulation provide very direct criteria for autoimmunity. By contrast, diseases associated with class I MHC antigens are frequently observed in males. Although there is good evidence that an immunologic reaction is involved in class I associated diseases, there is little evidence that this immune reaction is directed toward autoantigens. It has often been suggested that class I-associated autoimmune diseases develop along with infection, in particular bacterial infections. Common epitopes have been defined between HLA class I susceptibility alleles and various infectious agents (*Klebsiella, Yersinia* in case of HLA-B27).[1]

HLA Disease Associations: Genetic Significance

The significance of the association between HLA and disease may not be unique. Examples of an association with HLA antigens (21-hydroxylase deficit, hemochromatosis, etc.), in the absence of any reasonable indication that immune phenomena may be involved in disease mechanisms, underline the fact that observed associations may just point to the role of non-MHC genes localized within the MHC in linkage disequilibrium with HLA antigen encoding genes. Similarly, the stronger association of the many autoimmune diseases with class II than with class I antigens may just reflect the possibility that susceptibility genes are closer to the D region, which encodes the class II antigens, than to the A-B-C region, which encodes for class I antigens.

The presence of many class II alleles within extended haplotypes that may define a genetic susceptibility region larger than that limited to one locus and extend beyond the MHC region has been suggested, for example in case of insulin-dependent diabetes mellitus.[7, 8] To these observations should be added the association between diabetes mellitus and genes encoding for class III MHC alleles (complement proteins),[9, 10] and more recently, in several autoimmune diseases including diabetes mellitus, alleles encoding for tumor necrosis factor β (TNFβ). All these genes are localized in the human on the short arm of chromosome 6 between the MHC region encoding for class I and that encoding for class II antigens. Theoretically, this association with non-class I or class II encoding genes may simply reflect a linkage disequilibrium with HLA-D region genes. Alternatively, these genes may encode for proteins directly involved in the pathophysiologic make-up of autoimmune diseases.

If the association between insulin-dependent diabetes mellitus and complement alleles is related to linkage disequilibrium with HLA-D region genes, the various alleles associated with DR3 and DR4 should be seen with the same frequency in patients with diabetes mellitus and the nondiabetic population. This is not the case so far. Indeed, the relative risk for diabetes mellitus in HLA-DR3 subjects is associated with HLA-B8 BfS C4AQ0 C4B1 DR3 (relative risk 1.9) and B18 Bf-F1 C4A3 C4BQ0 DR3 (relative risk 7.6), but the risk is not increased in subjects carrying the B8

BfS C4Q0 C4A1 DR3 haplotype. Similarly, the association between diabetes mellitus and HLA-DR4 applies to subjects carrying the HLA-B15 BfS C4A3 C4B2 DR4 haplotype (relative risk 17.7), although not to subjects carrying the B15 BfS C4A3 C4βQ0 DR4 haplotype (relative risk 0.6). According to these data, the relative risk for diabetes mellitus in homozygous subjects carrying the B17 BfF1 C4A3 C4BQ0 DR3 is decreased (0.5).[9] These observations indicate that haplotypes including DR3 or DR4 genes imply a higher risk for diabetes mellitus than the HLA-DR3 or DR4 gene alone. This may indicate an interaction between several susceptibility genes located within the MHC region.

The importance of MHC antigens in cellular interactions that allow the development of immune reactions suggests, however, a direct role of class II genes in susceptibility to autoimmune diseases. Although no direct experimental evidence demonstrates that susceptibility genes to diabetes mellitus located within the MHC are indeed the genes encoding for class II antigens, there is convincing evidence favoring such a hypothesis. Dramatic progress in the biochemical characterization of class II antigens[11] allow postulating a direct role of class II antigens in the presentation of autoantigens to specific autoreactive T lymphocytes involved in the development of autoimmune diseases. Moreover, the very high relative risk observed in DR3/DR4 heterozygous patients, in the case of diabetes mellitus, or of DR3/DR7 heterozygous patients in the case of celiac disease, is very likely to point to a direct role of dimeric class II molecules resulting from transcomplementation between genes located on the two paired chromosomes.[12] Such an effect of transcomplementation is difficult to explain by simple linkage disequilibrium with a non-MHC susceptibility gene located close to the MHC-D region.

Molecular Biology Studies of MHC Genes

Class II MHC alleles characterized by serologic typing have been subdivided by various methods that detect polymorphism, undetected by serology. Different specificities can thus be evidenced with mixed lymphocyte culture (MLC) in the absence of serologically detectable differences. MLC defines Dw specificities that correlate with allelic differences at the DRβ1 chain. MLC cellular typing has been very contributive in rheumatoid arthritis, which associates with alleles encoded at the DRβ1 locus.[13] Polymorphism of class II alleles can also be shown by their isoelectrophoretic characteristics of the α and β chain, as evidenced with two-dimensional SDS polyacrilamide gel electrophoresis (SDS-PAGE).[6] Finally, the direct characterization of class II alleles at the level of class II genes has been very fruitful, particularly in diseases associated with DQ or DP alleles, in which differences are hardly evidenced with serologic typing, SDS-PAGE characterization of ab class II dimers, or primary MLC. Molecular biology typing has been especially contributive in insulin-dependent diabetes mellitus. The techniques first described characterized the polymorphism of restriction fragments (RFLP) of DNA recognized by DNA probes specific for DQ,

DR, and more recently, DP genes. Three major DQ antigens were initially defined with serologic typing as DQw1, DQw2, and DQw3, leaving a fourth specificity defined as DQ blank. The specificity DQw1 is indicative of DQα chain polymorphism. The specificities DQw2 and DQw3 are indicative of polymorphism within the DQβ chain. RFLP studies further subdivided DQw1 into at least seven different specificities and DQw3 into three allelic specificities: DQw3.1 (=DQw7), DQw3.2 (=DQw8) and DQw3.3 (=DQw9). Subjects with DR4 are either DQw7, DQw8, or DQ blank. The allele DQw3.1 is recognized with the aforementioned TA10 monoclonal antibody and is thus opposed to DQw3.2. The latter is present in 90% to 95% of DR4 patients with insulin-dependent diabetes mellitus, as compared to 60% to 65% in the general population. Similarly, among HLA-DR2 (=DRw15) subjects, the DQw1.2 (=DQw6) allele confers protection against insulin-dependent diabetes mellitus while the DQw1.AZH (=DQw5) allele observed in DRw16 subjects is associated with increased susceptibility to diabetes mellitus. Sequencing of the most polymorphic external domain of various alleles finally allowed precise definition of the biochemical characteristics associated with susceptibility to autoimmune diseases such as insulin-dependent diabetes mellitus. The comparison of nucleotide sequences indicates the presence of polymorphic residues on the DQβ chain in positions 13, 26, 45, and 57. Alleles that associate with susceptibility to diabetes mellitus DR1-DQw5 (=DQw1.1), DR4-DQw8 (=DQw3.2), DR3-DQw2, DR2-DQw5 (=DQw1.AZH), DRw6-DQw1.19 are characterized by an alanine, serine, or valine residue in position 57. By contrast, alleles that are neutral or confer resistance to diabetes mellitus have an aspartic acid in position 57.[14, 15] With oligonucleotide probes covering positions 54 to 59, DQw8 and DQw7 alleles can be distinguished, taking advantage of the presence or absence of an aspartic acid in position 57. This characterization can be performed on DNA obtained through amplification by the polymerase chain reaction within the studied coding region. A first study showed that among DR4 subjects, 93% of patients with diabetes mellitus were DQw8 (=DQw3.2) (Asp negative) as opposed to only 76% in the nondiabetic population.[14] The study of patients with insulin-dependent diabetes mellitus within multiplex families confirmed these data by indicating a relative risk close to 100 in Asp negative subjects.[16]

Interestingly, HLA-DR4, but also HLA-DR2 and DRw6 haplotypes, possibly associate with different DQ genes on chromosome 6, only some of these containing an aspartic acid in position 57 of the DQβ chain. The analysis of diabetic and control populations carrying the HLA DR4, DR2, or DRw6 haplotypes confirmed the role of the DQβ chain carrying an alanine, serine, or valine in position 57 with respect to diabetes susceptibility.[14] The functional significance of a change in the residues represented in a defined position within the external domain of class II α or β chains, particularly in position 57 of the DQβ chain, is underlined by the study of T cell clones specific for allogeneic epitopes or various antigens. The recent characterization of class I antigens with X diffraction allowed the conceptual visualization of the external domain of class II α and β chains as designing a cleft in which peptides are inserted, stressing the functional importance of polymorphic sites in antigen presentation and very likely in the presentation of autoantigenic peptides.[11]

Exceptions to the role of the DQw8 (=DQw3.2) allele indicate, however, the possible role of other class II MHC antigen chains. The absence of susceptibility to diabetes mellitus in DR7 whites in whom the DQβ chain (DQw2) is identical to that associating with DR3, associating susceptibility to diabetes mellitus, may indicate the role of some DQα chains. The DR7 haplotype is present in the black population, but in contrast with the DR7 haplotype observed in whites, associates with an increased risk for insulin-dependent diabetes mellitus. The external domain of DRβ1, DRα1, and DQβ1 is identical in blacks and whites. The only difference is in the DQα1 external domain, which is indeed identical to that of DR4 subjects.[15, 17]

The frequency of the presence of an arginine in position 52 on the DQα chain has been reported as the biochemical characteristic of white patients with insulin-dependent diabetes mellitus, the significance of which may be identical to that of the absence of aspartic acid in position 57 on the DQβ chain. However, the arginine in position 52 on the DQα chain is directly dependent on the DR3/DR4 heterozygous genotype or the DR3/DR4 homozygous genotypes.[18]

The same DQα and DQβ chains associate on DR9 haplotypes and some DR5 haplotypes in the black population, in whom they associate with an increased susceptibility to diabetes mellitus. In whites, the DR9 haplotype does not show any association with diabetes mellitus but carries a DQa chain that is different from that of the black population and is characterized by the presence of an aspartic acid in position 57. The combination of DQα and DQβ chains identical to those expressed by DR5 and DR9 subjects in the black population is observed in DR3/DR4 heterozygous subjects in the white population in whom the DQα chain characteristic of the DR4 haplotype may associate with the DQβ chain characteristic of the DR3 haplotype. A transcomplementation effect between DQ alleles on paired chromosomes is a possible explanation for the DR3/DR4 heterozygous effect. The same type of association may occur in DR3/DR9 Chinese subjects.[19] In the Japanese population, the strongest association with diabetes mellitus occurs with the DQα1 allele, which has previously been described in the black population and is observed in DR4 subjects. It is also remarkable that in the Japanese population no positive association is observed between diabetes mellitus and the DQβ chain, which associates with the DR4 haplotype, and that positive associations can be observed with antigens that carry a DQβ chain, including an aspartic acid in position 57.[15]

Data obtained by MLC studies also suggest the role of the DR locus by showing the absence of susceptibility in Dw14 subjects, in contrast with a positive association with Dw4 and Dw10, which can all associate with DR4.[20]

The sequencing of class II alleles has been obtained in other autoimmune diseases. The role of critical epitopes in susceptibility to rheumatoid arthritis on the DRP1 chain,[21] celiac disease on the DQβ and DPβ chains,[22, 23] or pemphigus on the DQβ chain[1] has thus been defined. Interestingly, the contribution of either a DQβ chain or a DPβ chain showing an arginine residue in the same position (in 69 and 71 on the external domains of both chains) has been suggested. In pemphigus vulgaris, a different epitope of the DQβ chain (negatively charged amino acids in the third hypervariable region in DR4 subjects, aspartate residue in 57 in DRw6 subjects) may contribute to disease susceptibility.

Animal Models

Animal models of insulin-dependent diabetes mellitus have proved to be very important to our present understanding of the role of the MHC in the development of autoimmunity. Although data obtained from models of experimentally induced diabetes mellitus are still not comprehensive and apply only to diabetes mellitus induced by low-dose streptozotocine, the MHC (the H-2 system in the mouse, the RT1 system in the rat) is one of the genetic susceptibility regions which, as in the human, appears to be determinant in the development of spontaneous diabetes mellitus in the NOD mouse and the BB rat. This is clearly indicated by breeding experiments crossing the NOD mouse with various conventional genetic backgrounds (C3H, NON, C57BL/10 followed by back-crossing of F1 animals with NOD mice). The MHC of the NOD mouse has characteristic features: (1) NOD mice express only I-A antigens (DQ equivalent) and do not express I-E antigens (DR equivalent); and (2) the Ab chain (DQβ equivalent) of I-A of NOD differs from that sequence in conventional laboratory strains by the presence of a serine in position 57, as opposed to an aspartic acid in common laboratory strains.[24] The incidence of diabetes is weak in heterozygous animals that are I-A Asp-57/I-A non-Asp-57. The Aα chain is identical to that of H-2^d mice (for instance DBA/2). Diabetes mellitus appears mostly in homozygous animals for I-A^{NOD}. Breeding studies on the C57BL/10 background, which like the NOD mouse expresses I-A antigens but not I-E antigens, indicate the presence on this background of a resistance gene to diabetes mellitus that is localized within the MHC and is independent of I-E.[25, 26] This observation is very important with regard to the demonstration of protection toward insulitis in animals expressing I-E, as obtained by crossing NOD mice with C57BL/6 mice transgenic for $E\alpha^d$ and expressing I-E^d, followed by back cross on the parental NOD partner.[27] It is clear that the expression of I-A antigens, which include a β chain with an aspartic in position 57, is not in itself protective. (NOD × C57BL/10) F1 chimeras grafted with T-cell-depleted NOD bone marrow cells have a high incidence of diabetes mellitus despite the expression in the recipient thymus of I-A^b (Aβ Asp57) antigens. In the BB rat a gene appears, as in the mouse, to be linked to the MHC, but the sequencing of the B locus encoded β chain of the RT1 system (equivalent to the DQβ in the human or I-Aβ in the mouse) showed the presence of a serine in position 57 in diabetes-prone rat strains (diabetes-prone BB rats) as well as in non-diabetes-prone conventional rat strains. This may distinguish the BB rat model from the previously reported NOD mouse model. The BB rat is also particular since rats heterozygous for a susceptibility haplotype and a protective haplotype with respect to diabetes mellitus have a high incidence of diabetes mellitus. The analysis of class II genes in the rat did not allow identification of the biochemical constraints that may be associated with diabetes mellitus susceptibility so far.

Susceptibility Genes Unlinked to the MHC

While there is no doubt about a role for MHC-linked genes in autoimmune susceptibility, the involvement and the nature of similar genes mapping outside the MHC are still hypothetical.[28–30] The role of non-MHC genes, however, is strongly suggested by epidemiologic analysis of patients' families and by the rate of concordance, which was found to be higher in monozygous twins than in HLA-identical only siblings.[31] It is the study of experimental models that most convincingly demonstrates their existence. With inbreeding of homozygous lines, mostly in the murine species, showing either spontaneous or induced disease following cross-immunization against a self-antigen, it has become possible to follow up the segregation of pathologic traits within crosses between diseased and normal mice. These studies have unraveled a complex genetic control involving many genes with probable interactions between them.

Recent progress in molecular biology has led to the construction of accurate genetic maps in man and soon in the mouse. It now permits an extensive screening of the genome and identification of chromosomal regions that confer an increased susceptibility to autoimmune diseases. This type of approach may be valid in fact mostly in the mouse because parental homozygous genetic constitution greatly simplifies segregation analysis. By contrast, in man, this method has demonstrated its power in the investigation of monogenic diseases but it remains difficult to handle when it comes to polygenic diseases since it requires elaborate statistical tools. Among other approaches of potential interest, examination of the role of candidate genes provides a higly valuable option inasmuch as it can also be guided with immunologic data and by the results of genomic mapping in animal models.

We will first review data available on two logical candidate-genes, the antigen T-cell receptor (TCR) and immunoglobulin (Ig) genes. We will then discuss the lessons that can be drawn from the genetic study of animal models of autoimmune diseases.

The Genes Encoding Lymphoid Cell Antigen Receptors

Among candidate genes, those coding for T-cell antigen receptors and for immunoglobulins, the B-cell counterpart of TCR, hold a special place similar to that of MHC class I and class II genes since their products bind antigen molecules, although in different manners. In this view, autoimmunity results from an abnormal or obviated recognition of self-antigen(s). However, to become functional, antigen-receptor genes undergo somatic rearrangements of their genomic organization in the course of lymphocyte ontogeny. This is not the case for MHC genes, and it bears major consequences for genetic analysis.

The variable domain in all antigen receptor peptidic chains is dedicated to antigen recognition; it is encoded by DNA variable regions resulting from the recombination of two or three DNA segments, V+J or V+D+J (V = variable, J = junction, and D = diversity), in each lymphoid cell clone. All these segments originate from separate sets, whose size varies along with the kind of antigen receptor and may reach several hundred members. Moreover, modifications including nucleotide deletions or additions at the V+D and D+J segment junctions are associated with the process of recombination. This junctional diversity has been shown to play a major role in the fine tuning of antigen recognition. The occurrence of these somatic rearrangements makes the genetic analysis more complex; it imposes examination of their eventual influence on gene product expression in addition to their germ line configuration.

Various types of evidence support a role for either the antigen T-cell receptor or immunoglobulins in autoimmune susceptibility.

The Role of Antigen T-cell Receptor in Autoimmune Susceptibility

Surprisingly, more data about genomic organization of TCR genes are presently available than about the biochemistry and the biology of their protein product. TCR proteins are heterodimers of approximately 90 kDa molecular weight, made of two glycosylated peptidic chains, either αβ or γδ, usually linked by an interchain disulfide bond.[32]

Because little is yet known about the γδ receptor, the following discussion will bear mostly on the αβ heterodimer. The most conspicuous functional property of the αβ receptor lies in the dual recognition of antigen presented in association with the MHC class I or class II gene products after its processing into small peptides.[33] This phenomenon is termed syngeneic restriction. Its structural basis is still poorly understood. Given the central role of T cells in the function of the immune system, this knowledge will be crucial for a clear understanding of self-tolerance and its breakage.

The consequences of α- and β-chain gene somatic modifications appear to be less dramatic than they are for Ig loci. The number of V (100 to 150 Vα, 50 to 60 Vβ in humans) and D (2Dβ, none for the α-chain) segments is limited when compared to that of Ig genes. The number of J segments (50 to 70 Jα, 13 Jβ) is somewhat larger in TCR genes than it is in Ig genes, but the overall number of possible V,D,J combinations to assemble a functional V region was estimated to be much lower in TCR genes than in Ig genes. More importantly, somatic hypermutation, a major means of diversification of Ig V regions, has been found not to occur in TCR V regions. In addition, the heterogeneity of V and J segments used in the response to a variety of antigens including external antigens, peptidic self-antigens such as the basic protein of myelin, MHC class II self-antigens, Mls gene products, and assimilated superantigens[34] was found to be limited. This restricted usage is related to the α-chain or the β-chain or both. For all these reasons, examination of the germinal configuration of α- and β-chain loci is likely to provide informative data about their contribution to autoimmune susceptibility, preparing the ground for more detailed studies at the level of functional rearranged genes.

TCR genes can also be envisioned as immune response genes similar to Ig genes or MHC genes. The TCR α-chain locus was shown to influence the cytotoxic response of the BALB/c strain to male (H-Y) antigen to the same extent as the MHC. In addition, a close linkage between β-chain genes and susceptibility to disease was detected in at least three experimental models including systemic lupus in the NZB mouse strain, collagen-induced arthritis, and Theiler's virus demyelinating encephalomyelitis. In all these models, the contribution of the β-chain locus to the disease was most significant in association with the appropriate haplotype of the MHC; these observations reflect the close interactions that occur between the corresponding peptides in the course of antigen recognition by T cells.

Among human diseases, multiple sclerosis (MS) has been most extensively studied; convincing data about a role for TCR in autoimmune susceptibility are presently available. Beall et al.[35] studied 36 patients with a chronic form of MS and 100 control subjects. They showed an association of the disease with a particular Vβ-haplotype; this association was most significant in DR2+ patients. Another study of 34 multiplex familes with the relapsing remitting form of MS by Seboun et al.[36] revealed a close linkage of the disease with the β-chain locus. A significant association of particular alleles of the α-chain gene with MS and with myasthenia gravis was also detected.[37] Finally, in patients with lupus and anti-Ro (SS-A) antibodies but without anti-La (SS-B) antibodies, a strong increase in a Cβ-haplotype was evidenced.[38] Production of anti-Ro antibodies is known to be closely linked to the heterozygous HLA DQ1/DQ2 phenotype in these patients.

In contrast, contradictory data were obtained in other autoimmune diseases such as type I insulin-dependent diabetes mellitus, Graves' disease, membranous nephropathy, and celiac disease. Difficulties in detecting a significant correlation where it exists may pertain to the variable ethnic origin of the patients, to disease heterogeneity, and, currently, to the availability of a still-limited number of TCR polymorphisms. These difficulties emphasize: (1) the importance of family studies whenever possible; (2) the need for stratifications, for example using HLA phenotypes or associated autoimmune traits such as the production of an autoantibody; and (3) the importance of better knowledge of TCR gene polymorphisms.

The Involvement of Immunoglobulin Genes in Autoimmune Susceptibility

At first sight, immunoglobulin genes seem to raise problems similar to those raised by TCR genes. However, the number of V regions available for recombination is greater than that of TCR genes. Somatic hypermutation also blurs the perception of functional rearranged genes obtained through the mere examination of their germ line configuration. With some exceptions, antibody responses toward exogenous antigens do not show a biased use of V regions. Likewise, autoantibodies do not exhibit either restricted use of V regions or use of dedicated V regions.[39] Moreover, pathogenic autoantibodies seem to undergo somatic hypermutation. This latter finding suggests that autoantibody production could be antigen-driven in addition to being a consequence of polyclonal B-cell activation.

Besides their role in antigen recognition, immunoglobulins are also characterized by effector functions such as complement fixation, placental transfer, etc. Conceivably, altered effector functions could also support the development of an autoimmune process. With the recent introduction of nucleic acid probes, it will be soon possible to determine the respective contributions of the constant and the variable domains of antibodies, as well as of regulatory sequences (promoter, enhancer) in autoimmune diseases.

Until recently, most studies were performed with serologic reagents. Conflicting results have been obtained with regard to a possible role for immunoglobulin genes in autoimmune susceptibility even in diseases in which familial cases permit linkage studies. In fact, in parallel with TCR data, the same factors appear to limit the power of this type of analysis: the low level of polymorphism of immunoglobulin allotypes; the clinical heterogeneity of these diseases; and the ethnic diversity of the patients. The use of nucleic acid probes that are more polymorphic and more finely mapped than serologic reagents, stratification along with other genetic markers such as HLA, TCR, and examination of clinical subsets will be essential to detect significant associations or linkages, especially in diseases that are mediated by autoantibodies such as myasthenia gravis or Graves' disease.

In addition to these diversified lymphoid cell receptors that are primarily involved in antigen recognition, many monomorphic proteins also take part either in antigen recognition and in lymphoid cell activation or in the effector arm of the immune response. They provide potential targets for development of autoimmune susceptibility. Proteins that participate in the complement cascade are examples of such molecules. C2 deficiency is strongly associated with lupus syndromes, probably because of slow clearance of immune complexes. Null alleles at C4A or C4B loci are frequent in type I diabetes mellitus. In this latter case, however, it is difficult to evaluate the actual contribution of C4 genes because of linkage disequilibrium occurring in HLA haplotypes associated with C4 null alleles.

Overall, there is presently a paradoxical situation residing in the contrast between the large number of molecules that are known to be associated with the functioning of the immune system—including differentiation antigens, molecules involved in the migration of lymphoid cells and cytokines—and methods available to evaluate their role in autoimmunity solely based on clinical observations.

The Importance of Genetic Analysis of Animal Models of Autoimmunity

Genetic analysis of experimental models of autoimmunity could help achieve a better understanding of human diseases in many respects. First, it would permit assessment of the likelihood of the involvement of a candidate gene. We have mentioned previously the role that is devoted to antigen T-cell receptors in the spontaneous disease of lupus-prone mice and also in antigen-induced models of arthritis and experimental allergic encephalomyelitis. Similarly, immunoglobulin loci have been implicated in various models of autoimmunity, including autoimmune hemolytic anemia following an injection of xenogeneic erythrocytes, spontaneous production of rheumatoid factors, myasthenic syndrome induced by immunization with acetylcholine receptor from Torpedo. Interestingly, in these two latter cases, the contribution of immunoglobulin polymorphism is fully visible only in conjunction with the appropriate H-2 haplotypes. These experimental observations make immunoglobulin genes reasonable candidate genes in human autoimmune diseases where it remains difficult to ascertain their role directly.

Second, segregation studies can help to identify linkage between the numerous pathologic traits often seen in autoimmune lupus mice. They also help to assess their contribution to morbidity and to mortality. In NZB mice, autoimmune hemolytic anemia and renal disease appear to depend on different gene sets. Similarly, in NOD mice, an experimental model of type I insulin-dependent diabetes mellitus, humoral and cellular manifestations follow distinct patterns of inheritance although it is still unclear whether they are completely or only partially independent. In (NZB × NZW) F1 hybrids and in their crosses, the onset of glomerulonephritis and mortality are well correlated with serum levels of anti-double-stranded DNA antibodies of the IgG class but not with anti-single-stranded DNA antibodies of the IgM class. These few observations exemplify the polygenic control of autoimmune manifestations. They also underscore the importance of genetic studies to seek phenotypic markers with a real predictive value and/or a pathogenetic significance.

Third, segregation studies can help piece together the natural history of a disease. For example, histologic examination of pancreata in animals derived from various crosses between NOD and non-diabetes-prone strains reveals the existence of only few patterns of infiltration by mononuclear cells.[25] Because of their increasing severity, these patterns are also suggestive of a chronologic order: perivascular and periductal infiltration of the pancreas is initially seen; it is followed by periinsulitis and then by insulitis leading to destruction of insulin-secreting β cells, and eventually to diabetes mellitus. This putative sequence of events is indeed compatible with the observation of the spontaneous disease and also with results of transfer experiments of the disease into nondiabetic animals with lymphoid cells from diabetic animals. Such findings suggest the existence of a genetic control that could be associated with each of these morphologically defined steps.

Although multiple genes are clearly involved in the determination of these manifestations, single locus mutations that profoundly influence the course of autoimmune diseases have also been identified. On a genetically predisposed background, these loci including the *lpr* and *gld* mutations and the Y-chromosome linked *Yaa* factor accelerate the onset of the autoimmune disease and dramatically increase its severity. Conversely, the X-linked *xid* mutation is known to determine an immune deficiency bearing mostly on B-lymphocyte development and on humoral response. When back-crossed onto autoimmune-prone backgrounds, the *xid* mutation results in marked delay of the onset of autoimmune manifestations and in a decrease in their severity. These findings suggest the existence of a common pathway of development of autoimmunity on which these genetic factors exert their effect.

Finally, recent progress in mouse genetics will soon permit fine mapping of the aforementioned susceptibility loci. Because of the existence of conserved syntenies between mouse and humans,[40] these animal studies will provide invaluable guidance in the search for disease genes in humans.

Concluding Remarks

Autoimmune diseases are very diverse. Clearly, multiple genetic factors are involved in their control. The major histocompatibility complex contributes a dominant part to autoimmune susceptibility, most likely by means of autoantigen presentation. Other genes whose products are involved in antigen recognition might also play an important role, especially in organ-specific diseases. These include antigen receptors of lymphocytes; antigen itself and molecules associated with the target organ; and adhesion and migration molecules. Additional genes involved in nonspecific regulation of the immune response also influence the course of the disease. They are probably most important in systemic autoimmune diseases including lupus and rheumatoid arthritis.

The large number of these genes and their complex interactions probably explain the enormous diversity of clinical conditions encountered. Non-Mendelian genetic factors such as somatic rearrangements of antigen-receptor genes, somatic hypermutation in immunoglobulin V segments, parental imprinting, and environmental modulation of gene activity bring further complexity to their analysis. However, one may reasonably assume that their identification will soon permit new appraisal and classification of often ill-defined clinical syndromes.

References

1. Sinha AA, Lopez MT, McDevitt HO: Autoimmune diseases: The failure of self tolerance. *Science* 1990; 248:1380–1387.
2. Deschamps I, Lestradet H, Bonaïti C, et al: HLA genotype studies in juvenile insulin-dependent diabetes. *Diabetologia* 1980; 19:189–193.
3. Svejgaard A, Platz P, Ryder LP: Histocompatibility testing 1980, in Terasaki PI (ed): *Report of the 8th International Histocompatibility Workshop*. Los Angeles, 1980, pp 638–656.
4. Svejgaard A, Platz P, Ryder LP: HLA and disease 1982—A survey. *Immunol Rev* 1983; 70:194–218.
5. Sollid LM, Markussen G, Gjerde JEH, et al: Evidence for a primary association of celia response to a particular HLA-DQ α/β heterodimer. *J Exp Med* 1989; 169:345–350.
6. Schreuder GMT, Tilanus MGJ, Bontrop RE, et al: HLA-DQ polymorphism associated with resistance to type I diabetes detected with monoclonal antibodies, isoelectric point differences, and restriction fragment length polymorphism. *J Exp Med* 1986; 164:938–943.
7. Awdeh ZL, Raum D, Yunis EJ, et al: Extended HLA/complement allele haplotypes: Evidence for T/t-like complex in man. *Proc Natl Acad Sci USA* 1983; 80:259–263.
8. Raum D, Awdeh Z, Yunis EJ, et al: Extended major histocompatibility complex haplotypes in type I diabetes mellitus. *J Clin Invest* 1984; 74:449–454.
9. McCluskey J, McCann VJ, Kay PH, et al: HLA and complement allotypes in type 1 (insulin-dependent) diabetes. *Diabetologia* 1983; 24:162–165.
10. Wolf E, Cudworth AG, Markwick JR, et al: The Bf system in diabetes-gene interaction or linkage disequilibrium? *Diabetologia* 1982; 22:85–88.
11. Bjorkman PJ, Saper MA, Samraoui B, et al: Structure of the human class I histocompatibility antigen, HLA-A2. *Nature* 1987; 329:506–518.
12. Nepom BS, Schwartz D, Palmer JP, et al: Transcomplementation of HLA genes in IDDM. *Diabetes* 1987; 36:114–117.
13. Nepom GT, Hansen JA, Nepom BS: The molecular basis for HLA class II associations with rheumatoid arthritis. *J Clin Immunol* 1987; 7:1–7.
14. Todd JA, Bell JI, McDevitt HO: HLA-DQβ gene contributes to susceptibility and resistance to insulin-dependent diabetes mellitus. *Nature* 1987; 329:599–604.
15. Todd JA, Fukui Y, Kitagawa T, et al: The A3 allele of the HLA-DQA1 locus is associated with susceptibility to type I diabetes in Japanese. *Proc Natl Acad Sci USA* 1990; 87:1094–1098.
16. Morel PA, Dorman JS, Todd JA, et al: Aspartic acid at position 57 of the HLA-DQβ chain protects against type I diabetes: A family study. *Proc Natl Acad Sci USA* 1988; 85:8111–8115.
17. Todd JA, Mijovic C, Fletcher J, et al: Identification of susceptibility loci for insulin-dependent diabetes mellitus by trans-racial gene mapping. *Nature* 1989; 338:587–589.
18. Khalil I, d'Auriol L, Gobet M, et al: A combination of HLA-DQβ Asp57-negative and HLA DQα Arg 52 confers susceptibility to insulin-dependent diabetes mellitus. *J Clin Invest* 1990; 85:1315–1319.
19. Todd JA: Genetic control of autoimmunity in type 1 diabetes. *Immunol Today* 1990; 11:122–128.
20. Sheehy MJ, Scharf SJ, Rowe JR, et al: A diabetes-susceptible HLA haplotype

is best defined by a combination of HLA-DR and HLA-DQ alleles. *J Clin Invest* 1989; 83:830–835.

21. Hiraiwa A, Yamanaka K, Kwok WW, et al: Structural requirements for recognition of the HLA-Dw14 class II epitope: A key HLA determinant associated with rheumatoid arthritis. *Proc Natl Acad Sci USA* 1990; 87:20.
22. Bugawan TL, Angelini G, Larrick J, et al: A combination of a particular HLA-DPβ allele and an HLA-DQ heterodimer confers susceptibility to coeliac disease. *Nature* 1989; 339:470–473.
23. Kagnoff MF, Harwood JI, Bugawan TL, et al: Structural analysis of the HLA-DR, -DQ, and -DP alleles on the celiac disease-associated HLA-DR3 (DRw17) haplotype. *Proc Natl Acad Sci USA* 1989; 86:6274–6278.
24. Acha-Orbea H, McDevitt HO: The first external domain of the nonobese diabetic mouse class II I-Aβ chain is unique. *Proc Natl Acad Sci USA* 1987; 84:2435–2439.
25. Wicker LS, Miller BJ, Coker LZ, et al: Genetic control of diabetes and insulitis in the nonobese diabetic (NOD) mouse. *J Exp Med* 1987; 165:1639–1654.
26. Wicker LS, Miller BJ, Fischer PA, et al: Genetic control of diabetes and insulitis in the nonobese diabetic mouse. *J Immunol* 1989; 142:781–784.
27. Nishimoto H, Kikutani H, Yamamura K-I, et al: Prevention of autoimmune insulitis by expression of I-E molecules in NOD mice. *Nature* 1987; 328:432–434.
28. Garchon HJ, Bach JF: The contribution of non-MHC genes to susceptibility to autoimmune diseases. *Hum Immunol,* in press.
29. Shoenfeld Y, Schwartz RS: Immunologic and genetic factors in autoimmune diseases. *N Engl J Med* 1984; 311:1019–1029.
30. Theofilopoulos AN, Dixon FJ: Murine models of systemic lupus erythematosus. *Adv Immunol* 1985; 37:269–390.
31. Spielman RS, Baur MP, Clerget-Darpoux F: Genetic analysis of IDDM: Summary of GAW5 IDDM results. *Genet Epidemiol* 1989; 6:43–58.
32. Davis MM, Bjorkman PJ: T cell antigen receptor genes and T-cell recognition. *Nature* 1988; 334:395–402.
33. Schwartz RH: T lymphocyte recognition of antigen in association with gene products of the major histocompatibility complex. *Ann Rev Immunol* 1985; 3:239–263.
34. Marrack P, Kappler J: The staphylococcal enterotoxins and their relatives. *Science* 1990; 248:705–711.
35. Beall SS, Concannon P, Charmley P, et al: The germline repertoire of T cell receptor β-chain genes in patients with chronic progressive multiple sclerosis. *J Neuroimmunol* 1989; 21:59–66.
36. Seboun E, Robinson MA, Doolittle TH, et al: A susceptibility locus for multiple sclerosis is linked to the T cell receptor β chain complex. *Cell* 1989; 57:1095–1100.
37. Oksenberg JR, Sherritt M, Begovich AB, et al: T-cell receptor Vα and Cα alleles associated with multiple sclerosis and myasthenia gravis. *Proc Natl Acad Sci USA* 1989; 86:988–992.
38. Frank MB, McArthur R, Harley JB, et al: Anti-Ro (SSA) autoantibodies are associated with T-cell receptor β genes in systemic lupus erythematosus patients. *J Clin Invest* 1990; 85:33–39.
39. Tron F, Bach JF: Molecular and genetic characteristics of pathogenic autoantibodies. *J Autoimmunity* 1989; 2:311–320.
40. Nadeau JH, Reiner AH: Linkage and synteny homologies in mouse and man, in Lyon MF, Searle AG (eds): *Genetic Variants and Strains of the Laboratory Mouse.* Oxford, University Press, 1990, pp 506–536.

Genetic Susceptibility to Diabetic Nephropathy

Andrzej S. Krolewski M.D., Ph.D.

Chief, Section on Epidemiology and Genetics, Research Division, Joslin Diabetes Center; Assistant Professor, Department of Medicine, Harvard Medical School, Boston, Massachusetts

James H. Warram M.D., Sc.D.

Investigator, Section on Epidemiology & Genetics, Research Division, Joslin Diabetes Center, Boston, Massachusetts

Lori M.B. Laffel M.D., McPott.

Investigator, Section on Epidemiology & Genetics, Research Division, Joslin Diabetes Center; Instructor, Department of Pediatrics, Harvard Medical School, Boston, Massachusetts

Diabetic nephropathy consists of several distinct stages: an early subclinical stage of microalbuminuria; a clinical stage of persistent proteinuria; and a stage of progressive renal failure.[1] While the pathogenetic mechanisms underlying advancement from one stage to another are not completely understood, genetically determined susceptibility has recently been recognized as an important factor for the development of nephropathy in diabetes mellitus.

This report will review the evidence supporting the importance of genetic factors in the development of diabetic nephropathy. We will also consider specific genes that may be considered as candidates for these factors. At the end, we will review research strategies for testing hypotheses about candidate genes, as well as strategies for locating genes that are involved in the development of diabetic nephropathy even though the functions of the genes are unknown. Mainly data for patients with type I (insulin dependent) diabetes mellitus (IDDM) will be presented, since there have not been many studies conducted among patients with type II (non-insulin dependent) diabetes mellitus (NIDDM).

Epidemiologic and Family Studies

The appearance of persistent proteinuria in patients with IDDM indicates the presence of significant structural damage in the glomeruli.[2] Figure 1 shows the relationship between the appearance of persistent proteinuria

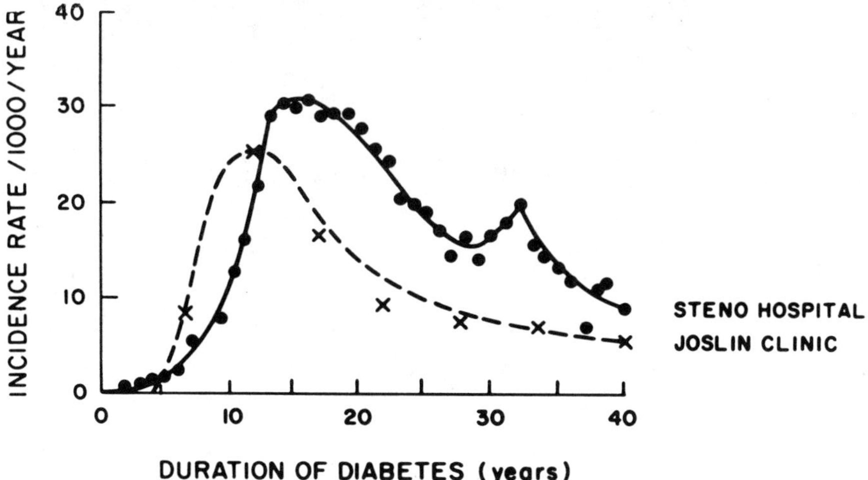

FIG 1.
Incidence rate of persistent proteinuria according to duration of type I diabetes mellitus in two different clinic populations. (Adapted from Andersen AR, Christiansen JS, Andersen JK, et al: *Diabetologia* 1983; 25:496–501, and Krolewski AS, Warram JH, Christlieb AR, et al: *Am J Med* 1985; 78:785–794.)

and the duration of diabetes mellitus among patients with juvenile-onset type I diabetes mellitus in two different populations.[3, 4] Persistent proteinuria did not occur during the first 5 years after diagnosis. Thereafter, its incidence (new cases/1,000 persons per year) rose rapidly, peaked during the second decade of diabetes mellitus, and then declined. Overall, during 40 years of diabetes mellitus, only a third of the patients developed persistent proteinuria.[3, 4]

This pattern of increasing and then decreasing incidence of persistent proteinuria according to the duration of IDDM contradicts the generally held belief that the accumulated exposure to diabetes mellitus (duration) is the major determinant of late diabetic complications. However, this pattern is consistent with the hypothesis that patients comprising a subset of diabetics (fewer than 50%) are susceptible to kidney damage in the presence of diabetes mellitus. Depletion of these susceptible diabetic patients would explain the declining incidence rate after the second decade of diabetes mellitus.

Other evidence for the existence of susceptibility to diabetic nephropathy has recently come from family studies. In two studies, families with a pair of diabetic siblings were classified into two groups according to whether the first diabetic sibling had diabetic nephropathy.[5, 6] After matching on the duration of diabetes mellitus, the second sibling was more likely to have renal complications if the first had nephropathy than if the first sibling had no evidence of renal disease. In another study, conducted among Pima Indians where half of the population has non-insulin dependent diabetes mellitus, having a parent with diabetic nephropathy was significantly more frequent among persons with diabetic nephropathy than it was among persons without nephropathy.[7] Furthermore, having a parent with renal failure, specifically, was more frequent in persons with renal failure. This familial clustering of diabetic nephropathy, found in three different populations, is consistent with the hypothesis that susceptibility to renal complications in diabetes may be determined by genetic factors.

Clinical Studies

Hypertension in patients with IDDM develops mainly in connection with the clinical emergence of nephropathy, and those in whom nephropathy does not develop remain normotensive despite a long duration of diabetes mellitus and advancing age.[8–10] These observations suggested to us that susceptibility to diabetic nephropathy may overlap with a genetic predisposition to hypertension. To test this hypothesis, we studied a group of patients who developed diabetic nephropathy during the first 20 years of diabetes mellitus (case subjects) and a group of patients with the same duration of diabetes mellitus but without nephropathy (control subjects) and compared the frequency of parental history of hypertension and the maximal velocity of Na-Li countertransport (CTT) in red blood cells (presumed markers of predisposition to hypertension). The group of case subjects had a hypertensive parent and elevated Na-Li CTT significantly more frequently than the group of control subjects.[11] Similar observations were reported by others[12, 13] and were obtained by us in a more recent study (Bak et al., unpublished data).

As can be seen in Figure 2, patients with diabetic nephropathy have a higher Vmax of Na-Li CTT in red blood cells than patients with IDDM without renal complications. The most interesting point, however, is the observation that the Vmax of the Na-Li CTT was as elevated in patients with microalbuminuria and no impairment of renal function as it was in patients with overt proteinuria or renal failure. This observation, recently confirmed by others,[14] suggests that the elevated Vmax of Na-Li CTT is a marker of the predisposition for the onset of diabetic nephropathy rather than for its progression. At present, it is not clear whether patients with an elevated Vmax of Na-Li CTT are at risk of diabetic nephropathy because they have elevated systemic blood pressure or because an elevated Vmax of Na-Li CTT indicates an underlying abnormality in the kidneys that predisposes to nephropathy in the presence of diabetes mellitus.

Further confirmation of the role of an elevated Vmax of Na-Li CTT as a marker of genetic susceptibility to diabetic nephropathy has been obtained in a very recent family study. Walker et al.[15] compared the Vmax of Na-Li CTT in a group of patients with diabetic nephropathy and in a group of patients without nephropathy as well as in their respective parents. In findings similar to those of previous reports,[11, 13] they found a higher Vmax of Na-Li CTT in the group of case subjects than in control subjects. Further-

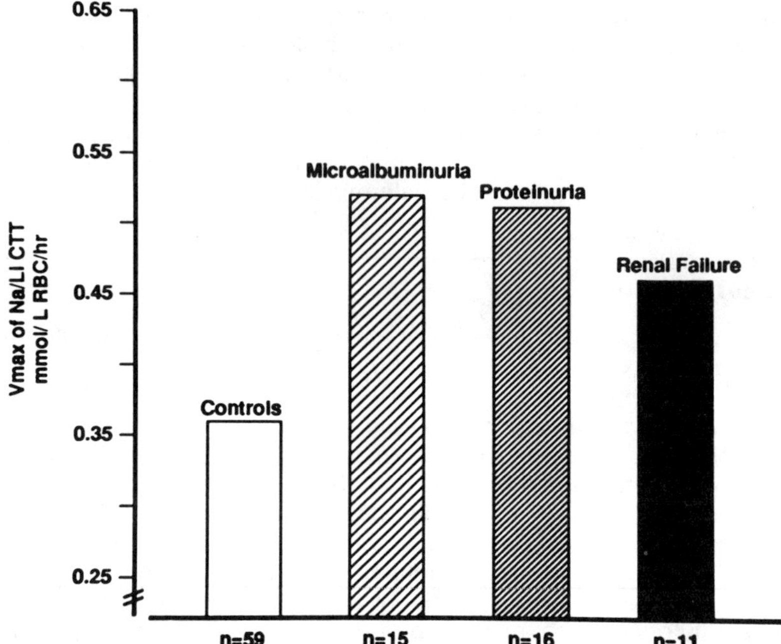

FIG 2.
Mean values of the Vmax of Na/Li CTT in red blood cells in patients with 15 to 20 years duration of juvenile-onset type I diabetes mellitus according to whether diabetic nephropathy was absent (control subjects) or one of the various stages of diabetic nephropathy was present. (Adapted from Krolewski AR, Canessa M, Warram JH, et al: *N Engl J Med* 1988; 318:140–145.)

more, parents of the case subjects also had an elevated Vmax of Na-Li CTT in comparison with the parents of the control subjects.

Although an elevated Vmax of Na-Li CTT in red blood cells (RBC) is a predictor of diabetic nephropathy, it does not cause this complication on its own. As can be seen in Table 1, among patients with a Vmax of Na-Li CTT less than 0.35 (median) mmol/L RBC/hr, not many developed diabetic nephropathy, and those who developed this complication had a similar level of glycemic control as those who remained without it. In the group of patients with an elevated Vmax of Na-Li CTT, however, there were many cases of diabetic nephropathy, but its development was conditional on poor glycemic control. The odds of developing diabetic nephropathy among patients with poor glycemic control were nine times that among patients with good or fair glycemic control. This particular finding provides strong evidence for the existence of an interaction (synergism) between a putative susceptibility factor and poor glycemic control in producing diabetic nephropathy.

At present, the mechanisms involved in the postulated interaction are not clear. However, several indirect pieces of evidence allow us to hypoth-

TABLE 1.
Risk of Diabetic Nephropathy in IDDM According to Vmax of Na-Li CTT in RBCs and the Level of Glycemic Control during the First 10 Years of Diabetes*

	Vmax of Na/Li CTT <.35		Vmax of Na/Li CTT >.35	
Level of Glycemic Control	Control Subjects	Case Subjects	Control Subjects	Case Subjects
Good or Fair	12	4	21	5
Poor†	11	3	10	21
Odds ratio (95% confidence interval)	0.82		8.82	

*Adapted from Krolewski AS, Canessa M, Warram JH, et al: *N Engl J Med* 1988; 318:140–145.
†Includes nonattenders defined as patients with less than five clinic visits.

esize about these mechanisms. First, it has been shown that patients with an elevated Vmax of Na-Li CTT seem to have abnormalities in the regulation of renal blood flow, such as an inability to increase renal blood flow in response to a high salt diet.[16] Further evidence of genetically determined abnormalities in the regulation of renal circulation was obtained in family studies in which renal hemodynamics were compared between normotensive offspring of hypertensive parents and normotensive offspring of normotensive parents. In these studies, offspring of hypertensive parents showed abnormalities in the control of the renal circulation, which manifest as diminished renal blood flow or an exaggerated vasodilation in response to captopril.[17–19] Moreover, similar differences were found in a comparison between patients with IDDM and a family history of hypertension and those without a family history of hypertension.[20]

In a recent study, it was shown that patients with poor glycemic control have significantly lower renal blood flow and a higher filtration fraction than patients with good glycemic control.[21] These abnormalities were normalized with acetylcholinesterase inhibition. Therefore, it is possible that if both factors (abnormalities in regulation of renal blood flow and poor glycemic control) occur together, they produce particularly high intraglomerular pressure, which can be the underlying factor for the onset of diabetic nephropathy.

Elevated Vmax of Na-Li CTT in red blood cells is a marker of predisposition to essential hypertension in the non-diabetic population[22, 23] and of predisposition to nephropathy in patients with IDDM, as previously discussed. However, the biologic meaning of an elevated Vmax of Na-Li CTT in red blood cells is unclear. It has been postulated that this CTT is a mode of operation of Na-H exchanger and that the elevated activity of the former reflects the elevated activity of the latter.[24] A direct test of this hypothesis, however, is complicated.[25] Vmax of Na-Li CTT in red blood cells is determined at intracellular pH 7.4. The Na-H exchanger, on the other hand, is not active at neutral pH.

To study the kinetics of the Na-H exchanger, one must lower intracellular pH to determine the Vmax of Na-H exchanger and its cooperativity with intracellular protons. When we compared these parameters of the Na-H exchanger in red blood cells of patients with and without diabetic nephropathy, we found the same Vmax of the Na-H exchanger in both groups, but patients with diabetic nephropathy had significantly lower cooperativity of the exchanger with intracellular protons.[26] This finding suggests that the defect which is somehow associated with the development of diabetic nephropathy may be in the intracellular part of the Na-H exchanger, which seems to determine cooperativity of this system.[27] Studies of this exchanger in lymphocytes have yielded different findings; patients with diabetic nephropathy had a higher Vmax of the Na-H exchanger in comparison to patients with IDDM without renal complications.[28] At present, it is difficult to reconcile the different findings obtained in red blood cells and lymphocytes. One possibility is that the kinetics of the Na-H exchanger can be influenced by the numbers of these exchangers, per cell, a characteristic that can be modified in nucleated cells (lymphocytes) but not in red blood cells.[27]

Pathologic Studies

Currently available data are insufficient to establish whether the early stage of diabetic nephropathy (i.e., microalbuminuria) is associated with any particular morphologic lesion in the kidney.[2, 29] On the other hand, there is agreement that patients with advanced diabetic nephropathy have significant structural changes in the kidney, notably thickening of the glomerular basement membrane and expansion of the mesangium.[2, 30] Taking these pathologic observations together with the clinical studies that were discussed earlier, one can postulate that the onset of diabetic nephropathy is due to renal hemodynamic abnormalities (elevated intraglomerular pressure) whereas progression to renal failure is determined by the rate of expansion of mesangium and occlusion of glomeruli.

As previously discussed, the level of intraglomerular pressure may vary among patients with IDDM according to the level of glycemic control and according to genetically determined predisposing factors. Similarly, the rate of expansion of the mesangium by accumulating basement membrane-like material may vary among diabetic patients.[2, 30] This variability, perhaps, is responsible for the fact that patients with IDDM who have developed overt proteinuria may need as few as 3 years or as many as 20 years to progress to renal failure.[3, 4] Furthermore, the rate of development of a glomerular pathologic state does not correlate well with several potential risk factors.[30–32]

Thus, it is possible that genetic factors determine the rate of development of these morphologic lesions.

While the mechanisms leading to expansion of the mesangium and widening of the glomerular basement membrane are not clear, it has been shown that a major component of the expanded mesangium and thickened basement membrane is collagen IV.[33] In a mouse model of diabetes mellitus, it has been demonstrated that albuminuric animals had increased expression of mRNA for type IV collagen but not mRNA for other basement membrane components such as laminin and heparan sulfate proteoglycan.[34] It is important to note that increased expression of mRNA for type IV collagen did not occur in diabetic mice in the absence of albuminuria; moreover, it was significantly reduced in the albuminuric animals by treatment with a thromboxane synthase inhibitor, which diminished intraglomerular pressure. These observations suggest that the increased production of collagen IV in kidney cortex occurs in response to damage caused by increased intraglomerular pressure.

At the biochemical level, type IV collagen forms the basic framework to which the other components of basement membrane such as laminin, heparan sulfate, nidogen, and enactin are attached.[35] Type IV collagen is a triple helical molecule with a noncollagenous knob at the C-terminus and the so-called "7 S collagen domain" at the N-terminus. The triple helix consists of two α-1 chains and a single α-2 chain.[36] Recently, other chains such as α-3, α-4, and α-5 have been identified.[37–39] It is postulated that the triple helical molecule of type IV collagen may contain a combination of these chains. In the extracellular space, four such heterotrimers become linked to each other at the N-termini to form tetramers, which are further assembled at the carboxy termini into larger networks.[36] At present, it is unknown whether the expanded mesangium contains an enlarged network of collagen IV or an accumulation of it in a different form. Similarly, it is unclear whether the accumulation of type IV collagen in the mesangium and glomerular basement membrane is due to overproduction or abnormalities in its degradation.

Candidate Genes and Molecular Genetics Studies

From the discussion so far, it appears that genetic factors may contribute to the development of various stages of diabetic nephropathy. Two groups of so-called "candidate genes" can be postulated. The first is related to genetic predisposition to hypertension,[40] and the second is a group of genes that code for components of the glomerular basement membrane (Table 2).[40–44]

From among the candidate genes for predisposition to hypertension, the first that we have studied was the human renin gene. In an animal model, structural abnormalities in this gene have been found to increase the risk of hypertension.[45] In our preliminary study, we compared a group of patients

TABLE 2.
Candidate Genes for Susceptibility to Diabetic Nephropathy

Genes Implicated in the Development of Hypertension	Genes Coding for Components of Basement Membrane
Renin	Type IV collagen α-1
Angiotensinogen	Type IV collagen α-2
Angiotensin converting enzyme	Type IV collagen α-3
Angiotensin II receptor	
Kallikrein	
Na-H exchanger amiloride sensitive	

with diabetic nephropathy and a group of individuals without diabetic nephropathy with regard to the distribution of a Hind III RFLP recognized by a part of the renin gene.[46] The frequency of the Hind III RFLP genotype was similar in both groups. Recently, we applied a new method of denaturing gradient gel electrophoresis blots (Krolewski, unpublished data) to detect additional sequence differences in the renin gene. We found four additional frequent polymorphisms and are now studying their distribution in case subjects and in control subjects. This set of polymorphisms also enables us to study sibling pairs that are affected with diabetic nephropathy to determine whether there is linkage between mutations in the renin locus and the development of diabetic kidney disease.

Recently complementary DNA (cDNA) for the Na-H exchanger was cloned, and the gene has been located on the short arm of human chromosome 1.[44] With the use of several RFLPs that flank the Na-H exchanger locus and studying families with two hypertensive siblings, a role of this locus in the development of essential hypertension was excluded.[47] In more recent studies, it was found that there are at least two genes that code for the Na-H exchanger[48] (J. Pouyssegur, personal communication). The gene that was cloned codes for the so-called "amiloride-sensitive" Na-H exchanger, which is located in the basolateral membrane of the proximal tubules and is present as a housekeeping gene in most nuclear cells (including lymphocytes).[44] The other gene codes for an amiloride-insensitive Na-H exchanger, which is located in the luminal membrane of proximal tubules. The cDNA for this gene has been partially cloned (J. Pouyssegur, unpublished data, 1990). It is possible that abnormalities in regulatory or structural parts of this gene for the second Na-H exchanger contribute to the development of essential hypertension or diabetic nephropathy.

Among the candidate genes that code for the glomerular basement membrane, there are several that have been cloned (see Table 2). Currently, we are investigating whether mutations/sequence differences in coding regions of the gene for the type IV collagen α-1 chain contribute to the development of advanced stages of diabetic nephropathy. We have compared the distribution of a Hind III RFLP recognized by cDNA for type IV α-1 chain in DNA samples from patients with different stages of diabetic nephropathy and in a group of patients without renal complications. Patients with advanced stages of nephropathy were predominantly heterozygotes for the Hind III RFLP, whereas those who remained in the stage of incipient nephropathy, despite a long duration of diabetes mellitus, were mainly homozygotes.[49] This difference was highly significant statistically. The mechanisms responsible for this association are not clear. The Hind III RFLP results from a sequence difference in the intron between exons 42 and 43 and does not have any impact on the splicing of the subsequent exons 43 to 52. We found, however, that this Hind III RFLP is in linkage disequilibrium with a sequence difference in exon 45, which changes glutamine to histidine at position 1318.[50] At present, we do not know whether this mutation is responsible for the increased risk of progression to overt proteinuria and renal failure or if there are other mutations (possibly more important) that are in linkage disequilibrium with the Hind III RFLP as well.

Strategies for Identifying Susceptibilty Gene(s) for Nephropathy

As was discussed previously, mutations in several candidate genes might contribute to the development of different stages of diabetic nephropathy. To identify these mutations, one may use two different study designs: the so-called "case-control" study, and the family study.

A case-control study can be designed to test for an association between the presence of a particular stage of diabetic nephropathy and the presence of a mutation/sequence difference in one of the candidate genes (see Table 2). Mutations or sequence differences in the regulatory or structural parts of a candidate gene are of particular interest. The mutation may be one that is already known, and its frequency is then compared between case and control subjects. Alternatively, the approach may be indirect through a DNA marker that recognizes a polymorphism in noncoding parts of the candidate gene. The distribution of the marker is compared between case subjects and control subjects and if an association is found, the genetic basis for this relationship is investigated (see the example above of the Hind III RFLP in the type IV collagen α-1 gene).

In selecting patients for the case-control study, one needs to control factors that may confound the results, for example ethnicity or level of glycemic control. A mutation/sequence difference may be associated with particular ethnic groups, and if the group of case and control subjects are different in this regard, they will also differ with regard to the distribution of that particular mutation. On the other hand, if a mutation of a particular candidate gene contributes to the severity of diabetes mellitus, it may be present frequently in patients with diabetic nephropathy, not because it increases susceptibility to renal complications, but because that genetic factor underlies the severity of diabetes.

The roles of mutations in candidate genes may be tested in family studies as well. Several types of families can be used for genetic studies. However, in the case of diabetic nephropathy, one can use only families in which at least one parent is studied and there are two or more offspring with diabetes mellitus and one or more of them has diabetic nephropathy. Additional information with regard to this design of family studies can be found in other reviews.[51, 52] In this type of family study, one can test a broad hypothesis such as whether the locus for the candidate gene is involved in any way in the development of diabetic nephropathy (see example in reference 47).

Families such as that described can be used to test an even broader hypothesis. For example, if one cannot find any association (in case-control studies) or linkage (in family studies) between a candidate gene and diabetic nephropathy, one may screen the entire human genome for chromosome segments that contain a susceptibility gene for diabetic nephropathy. At present, the family approach is limited by the availability of families of the type described previously. It will require, perhaps, the pooled effort of several centers to collect a sufficient number of such families.

References

1. Mogensen CE, Christensen CK, Vittinghus E: The stages in diabetic renal disease. With emphasis on the stage of incipient diabetic nephropathy. *Diabetes* 1983; 32:64–78.
2. Mauer SM, Steffes MW, Sutherland DER, et al: Structural-functional relationship in diabetic nephropathy. *J Clin Invest* 1984; 74:1143–1155.
3. Andersen AR, Christiansen JS, Andersen JK, et al: Diabetic nephropathy in type I (insulin-dependent) diabetes: An epidemiologic study. *Diabetologia* 1983; 25:496–501.
4. Krolewski AS, Warram JH, Christlieb AR, et al: The changing natural history of nephropathy in type I diabetes. *Am J Med* 1985; 78:785–794.
5. Seaquist ER, Goetz FC, Rich S, et al: Familial clustering of diabetic kidney disease. *N Engl J Med* 1989; 320:1161–1165.
6. Borch-Johnsen K, Norgaard K, Hommel E, et al: Diabetic nephropathy - an inherited complication? (abstract). *Diabetologia* 1990; 33:30.
7. Pettitt DJ, Saad MF. Bennett PH, et al: Familial predisposition to renal disease in two generations of Pima Indians with type 2 (non-insulin-dependent) diabetes mellitus. *Diabetologia* 1990; 33:438–443.
8. Parving HH, Smidt UM, Frisberg B, et al: A prospective study of glomerular filtration rate and arterial blood pressure in insulin-dependent diabetes with diabetic nephropathy. *Diabetologia* 1981; 20:457–461.
9. Oakley WG, Pyke DA, Tattersall RB, et al: Long-term diabetes: A clinical study of 92 patients after 40 years. *Q J Med* 1974; 43:145–156.
10. Borch-Johnsen K, Nissen RN, Nerup J: Blood pressure after 40 years of insulin-dependent diabetes. *Diabetic Nephropathy* 1985; 4:11–12.

11. Krolewski AS, Canessa M, Warram JH, et al: Predisposition to hypertension and susceptibility to renal disease in insulin-dependent diabetes mellitus. *N Engl J Med* 1988; 318:140–145.
12. Viberti G, Keen H, Wiseman MJ: Raised arterial pressure in parents of proteinuric insulin dependent diabetics. *Br Med J* 1987; 295:515–517.
13. Mangili R, Bending JJ, Scott G, et al: Increased sodium-lithium countertransport activity in red cells of patients with insulin dependent diabetes and nephropathy. *N Engl J Med* 1988; 318:146–150.
14. Jones SL, Trevisan R, Tariq T, et al: Sodium-lithium countertransport in microalbuminuric insulin-dependent diabetic patients. *Hypertension* 1990; 15:570–575.
15. Walker JD, Tariq T, Viberti G: Sodium-lithium countertransport activity in red cells of patients with insulin dependent diabetes and nephropathy and their parents. *Br Med J* 1990; 301:635–638.
16. Redgrave JE, Canessa M, Gleason R, et al: Red blood cell Na-Li countertransport in non-modulating essential hypertensives. *Hypertension* 1989; 13:721–726.
17. Uneda S, Fujishima S, Fujiki Y, et al: Renal haemodynamics and the renin-angiotensin system in adolescents genetically predisposed to essential hypertension. *J Hypertens* 1984; 2:437–439.
18. Blackshear JL, Garnic D, Williams GH, et al: Exaggerated renal vasodilator response to calcium entry blockade in first degree relatives of essential hypertensive subjects. *Hypertension* 1987; 9:384–389.
19. Schalekamp M, von Hooft I, Grobbee D, et al: Abnormal renal blood flow in normotensive offspring of hypertensive parents (abstract). *J Am Soc Nephrol* 1990; 1:512.
20. Hannedouche T, Marques LP, Natov S, et al: Influence of familial history of essential hypertension on renal function in normotensive insulin-dependent diabetics. *Am J Hypertens* 1990; 3:67.
21. Jenkings DAS, Cowan P, Collier A, et al: Blood glucose control determines the renal haemodynamic response to angiotensin converting enzyme inhibition in type I diabetes. *Diabetic Med* 1990; 7:252–257.
22. Canessa M, Adragna N, Solomon HS, et al: Increased sodium-lithium countertransport in red cells of patients with essential hypertension. *N Engl J Med* 1980; 302:772–776.
23. Turner ST, Johnson M, Boerwinkle E, et al: Sodium-lithium countertransport and blood pressure in healthy blood donors. *Hypertension* 1985; 7:955–962.
24. Aronson PS: Red cell sodium-lithium countertransport and essential hypertension. *N Engl J Med* 1982; 307:317.
25. Canessa M: Kinetics properties of the human red cells Na/H and Li/Na exchanges. *Methods Enzymol* 1989; 173:176–191.
26. Bak MI, Canessa ML, Warram JH, et al: Differences in the activity of Na/H exchanger in red blood cells of individuals with and without diabetic nephropathy. *Clin Res* 1989; 37:551.
27. Grinstein S, Rotin D, Mason MJ: Na/H exchange and growth factor-induced cytosolic pH changes. Role in cellular proliferation. *Biochem Biophys Act* 1989; 988:73–97.
28. Ng LL, Simmons D, Garrido MC, et al: Leucocyte Na/H antiport activity in type 1 (insulin-dependent) diabetic patients with nephropathy. *Diabetologia* 1990; 33:371–377.
29. Chavers BM, Bilous RW, Ellis EN, et al: Glomerular lesions and urinary albu-

min excretion in type I diabetes without overt proteinuria. *N Engl J Med* 1989; 320:966–970.
30. Osterby R, Parving HH, Hommel E, et al: Glomerular structure and function in diabetic nephropathy. Early to advanced stages. *Diabetes* 1990; 39: 1057–1063.
31. Mauer SM, Goetz FC, McHugh LE, et al: Long-term study of normal kidneys transplanted into patients with type I diabetes. *Diabetes* 1989; 38:516–523.
32. Bilous RW, Mauer SM, Sutherland DER, et al: Mean glomerular volume and rate of development of diabetic nephropathy. *Diabetes* 1989; 38:1142–1147.
33. Gubler MC, Noel LH, Mounier F, et al: Immunohistochemical study of extracellular matrix components in diabetic glomerulosclerosis, in Gubler MC, Sternberg M (eds): *Progress in Basement Membrane Research. Renal and Related Aspects in Health and Disease.* London, John Libbey Eurotext, 1988, pp 201–204.
34. Ledbetter S, Copeland EJ, Noonan D, et al: Altered steady-state m RNA levels of basement membrane proteins in diabetic mouse kidneys and tromboxane synthase inhibition. *Diabetes* 1990; 39:196–203.
35. Leblond CP, Inoue S: Structure, composition, and assembly of basement membrane. *Am J Anat* 1989; 185:367–390.
36. Timple R, Wiedemann H, Delden V, et al: A newtork model for the organization of type IV collagen molecules in basement membranes. *Eur J Biochem* 1981; 120:203–211.
37. Butkowski RJ, Langeveld JPM, Wieslander J, et al: Localization of the Goodpasture epitope to a novel chain of basment membrane collagen. *J Biol Chem* 1987; 262:7874–7877.
38. Gunman S, Saus J, Noelken ME, et al: Glomerular basement membrane. Identification of a fourth chain, alpha 4, of type IV collagen. *J Biol Chem* 1990; 265:5466–5469.
39. Hostikka SL, Eddy RL, Byers MG, et al: Identification of distinct type IV collagen alpha chain with restricted kidney distribution and assignment of its gene to the locus of X chromosome-linked Alport syndrome. *Proc Natl Acad Sci USA* 1990; 87:1606–1610.
40. Corvol P, Jeunemaitre X, Plouin PF, et al: The application of molecular genetics to the study of familial arterial hypertension. *Adv Nephrol* 1990; 19:31–52.
41. Soininen R, Huotari M, Ganguly A, et al: Structural organization of the gene for the alpha 1 chain of human type IV collagen. *J Biol Chem* 1989; 264:13565–13571.
42. Hostikka SL, Tryggvason K: The complete primary structure of the alpha 2 chain of human type IV collagen and comparison with the alpha 1 (IV) chain. *J Biol Chem* 1988; 263:19488–19493.
43. Morrison KE, Germino GG, Reeders ST: The cloning and sequence of a cDNA encoding the alpha 3 chain of type IV collagen (abstract). *J Am Soc Nephrol* 1990; 1:301.
44. Sardet C, Franchi A, Pouyssegur J: Molecular cloning, primary structure, and expression of the human growth factor-activatable Na/H antiporter. *Cell* 1989; 56:271–280.
45. Rapp RJ, Wang SM, Dene SH: A genetic polymorphism in the renin gene of Dahl rats cosegregate with blood pressure. *Science* 1989; 243:542–544.
46. Frossard PM, Gonzalez PA, Frits LC, et al: Two RFLPs at the human renin gene locus. *Nucleic Acids Res* 2986; 24:4380.
47. Lifton RP, Hunt SC, Williams RR, et al: Exclusion of the Na/H antiporter as a candidate gene in essential hypertension. *Clin Res* 1990; 38:469.

48. Biemesderfer D, Hildebrandt F, Exner M, et al: Cloning and immunolocalization of a Na/H exchanger in LLC-PK1 cells (abstract). *J Am Soc Nephrol* 1990; 1:743.
49. Krolewski AS, Tryggvason K, Warram JH, et al: Diabetic nephropathy and polymorphism in the gene coding for the alpha 1 chain of collagen IV (abstract). *Kidney Int* 1990; 37:510.
50. Krolewski AS, Tryggvason K, Stanton V, et al: Diabetic nephropathy and polymorphism in cDNA of the alpha 1 chain of type IV collagen (abstract). *J Am Soc Nephrol* 1990; 1:634.
51. Elston RC: Genetic Analysis Workshop II. Sib pair screening test for linkage. *Genet Epidemiol* 1984; 1:175–178.
52. Weeks DE, Lange K: The affected-pedigree-member method of linkage analysis. *Am J Hum Genet* 1988; 42:315–326.

Molecular Genetics of Renal Tumors

Claudine Junien, Pharm. D., Ph.D.

Professor of Genetics, INSERM U73, University of Paris V, Paris, France

There is an increasingly large body of evidence that supports the involvement of genetic lesions in the etiology of human cancer. Cancer results from mutations that disrupt the harmonious checks and balances that regulate normal cellular growth and development. The genetic damage found in cancer cells is of two sorts: dominant, with targets known colloquially as protooncogenes; and recessive, with targets known variously as tumor suppressor genes, growth suppressor genes, recessive oncogenes, or antioncogenes. The dominant damage typically results in a gain of function, whereas the recessive lesions cause loss of function.

Genetic mechanisms of tumor suppression operate within the cell and in systemic interactions between the cells of different types. Clearly, within the cell, several properties increase the risk of neoplastic transformation. Among them are chromosome instability, the capacity to undergo terminal differentiation, and the control of proliferation. Systemic interactions include: (1) communication between cells through junctional connections, steroid hormones, or secreted signal peptides; (2) immune surveillance; (3) regulation of angiogenesis; and (4) regulation of tumor invasion, including changes in expression of matrix components, proteases, and antiproteases.

In addition to these, impairment of other systems may be responsible for individual susceptibility to cancer. Among these are a small group of disorders characterized by chromosome breakage and DNA repair abnormalities, which include xeroderma pigmentosum, Fanconi anemia, Bloom's syndrome, and ataxia telangiectasia. These disorders are transmitted as autosomal recessive traits. However, heterozygous individuals may be at increased risk to develop cancer. Due to genetic polymorphism in drug or carcinogen metabolism, certain individuals are more prone to transform chemicals or various types of rays into potent carcinogens. Recognition of environmental factors that reveal this susceptibility would be an important step in cancer prevention.

Many human cancers are known to occur in two different forms: as sporadic tumors in the general population, and as hereditary tumors within families. Thus hereditary tumor syndromes offer unique model systems for isolating the gene mutations that lead to cancer. There is accumulating evidence that hereditary and sporadic tumors are caused by a similar pathogenesis affecting the same gene loci. The cloning and characterization of

Advances in Nephrology,® vol 21

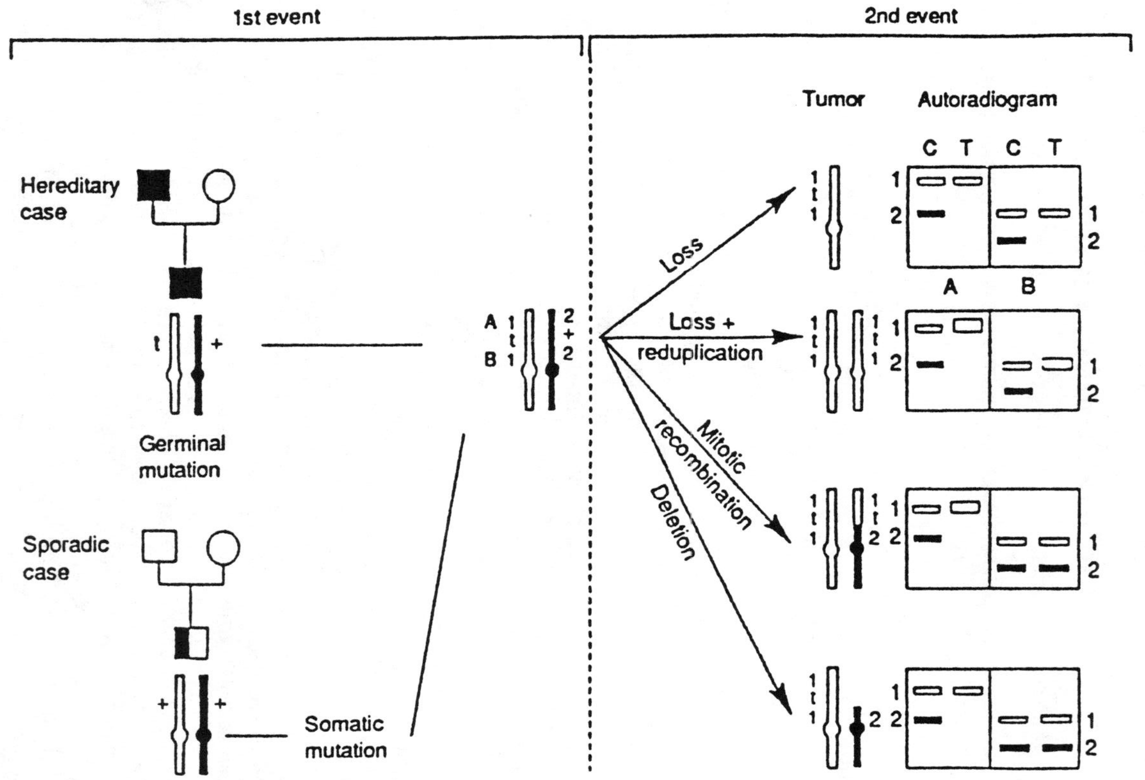

FIG 1.
The two hit theory of Knudson, accounting for hereditary (and sporadic) forms of most types of cancer.

these genes may therefore have important implications for diagnosis and treatment, not only for the relatively rare hereditary tumors but also for their much more common sporadic counterparts.

As yet, none of the known dominant oncogenes have been implicated in the inheritance of cancer. Moreover, the reality of dominant inheritance for cancer has been challenged on several grounds. Perhaps dominant oncogenes do not occur as congenital lesions because their presence precludes survival of the embryo (although mice bearing a variety of transgenic oncogenes do reach maturity without fault). More likely, as proposed by Knudson, the theory of the two hits affecting both alleles of a tumor suppressor gene accounts for hereditary (and sporadic) forms of most types of cancer. To date, predispositions transmitted by heterozygous defects in tumor suppressor genes are the sole form in which inherited mutations that have a direct effect on the growth of cells have been identified. These predispositions have been attributed to the fact that only one allele of a tumor suppressor gene remains to be inactivated before a full deficiency for the gene is achieved. Inheritance of the predisposition follows a dominant pattern, even though the tumors arise due to recessive lesions at the cellular level. The second hit is achieved by somatic mutations or chromosome aberrations revealed as losses of alleles (or loss of heterozygosity) with restriction fragment length polymorphism (RFLP) markers (Fig 1).

The strategy for identification of the genes involved in these inherited disorders is based on reverse genetics. The first goal is not to find the defective protein that is unknown, but rather to isolate the defective gene based on the determination of its chromosome location in the human genome. This can be achieved by tracing both germ line and somatic mutations. First, specific constitutional chromosome aberrations, namely translocations, deletions, or duplications in patients with a cancer predisposing syndrome and linkage analysis with RFLP markers in families with disease can provide a precise chromosome location for a cancer-predisposing gene. Second, karyotyping and investigating somatic losses of alleles with appropriate DNA markers can provide the chromosome location of genes involved in either cancer predisposition or progression.

Renal Cell Carcinoma

Renal cell carcinoma (RCC), which accounts for 3% of adult malignancies, is the most common type of kidney cancer. There are 20,000 new cases in the United States each year and 10,000 deaths. Two different forms occur: a sporadic form and a hereditary form; rarer is a bilateral and multifocal form corresponding either to a familial form or to a hereditary form associated with the von Hippel-Lindau disease (VHL). Present treatments include partial or total nephrectomy and, for the more advanced metastatic states, immunotherapy.

The implication of sequences on chromosomes 3 was initially recognized following two observations: first, a reciprocal translocation 3;8 involving a breakpoint in region 3p14.2 in a family with RCC[1]; second, a familial RCC with a 3;11 chromosome translocation limited to tumor cells. The proximal 3p was translocated on the distal end of 11p.[2] More recently, linkage analysis in families with VHL demonstrated that the gene mapped to 3p25-26.[3] Loss of heterozygosity for 3p markers in hereditary as well as sporadic forms of RCC suggests that the VHL gene may be involved in both forms and thus may behave as a tumor-suppressor gene. However, loss of heterozygosity may be restricted, in some tumors, not to the VHL region in 3p25-26, but to region 3p14-p21, thus suggesting the existence of another gene or genes (Fig 2).

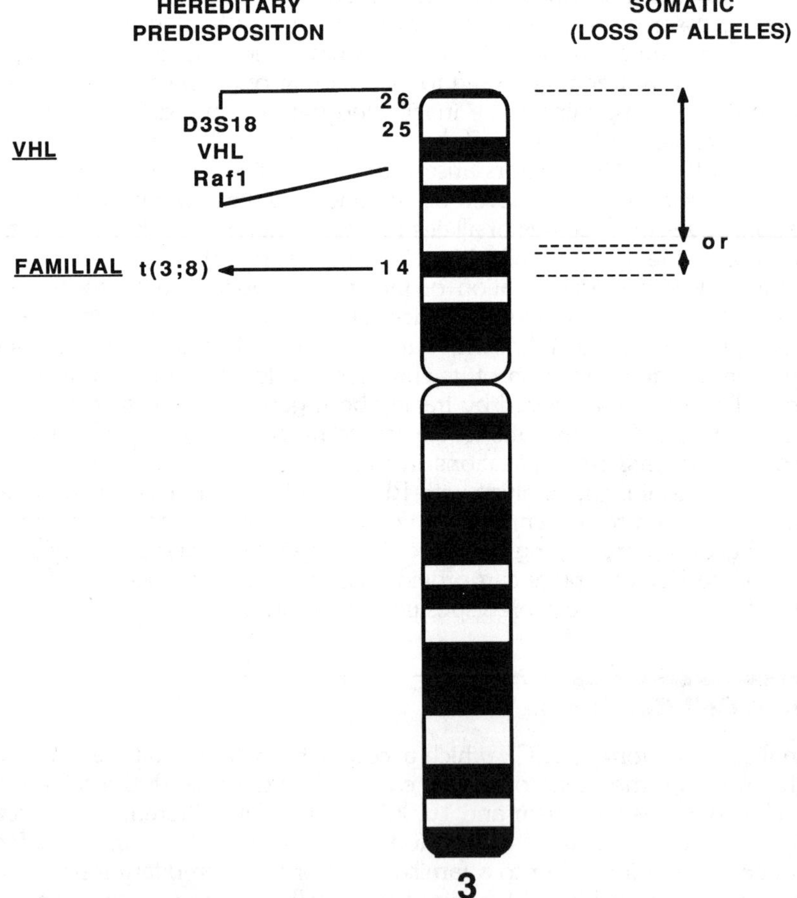

FIG 2.
Chromosome 3. The fact that loss of heterozygosity in some tumors is not restricted to the VHL region in 3p25-26 but to 3p14-21 suggests the existence of a second gene.

Genetic Predisposition

The von Hippel-Lindau disease, a member of the group of phakomatoses, is a devastating disorder associated with various forms of cancer in multiple organ systems. The most common manifestations include tumors of the central nervous system: hemangioblastomas (endothelial-derived tumors) in the cerebellum, retina, and spinal cord; and pheochromocytomas and multiple cysts of the kidney, pancreas, and other organ systems. Thirty-five percent of patients with VHL develop bilateral and multifocal RCC. This tumor thus represents a particularly frequent cause of death in these patients.

Linkage between VHL and a chromosome 3 marker, namely RAF1, was first demonstrated by Seizinger et al. in 1988.[3] New markers[4] and more families have been used to more precisely define the region of the VHL locus.[5] The VHL locus is now flanked by RAF1 on the centromeric side and by D3S18, 64E, and 479H4 on the telomeric side. A new marker 233E2, which, as yet, has failed to detect recombination in VHL families, can be used for genetic counseling.[6]

Analysis of tumors from VHL patients revealed that: (1) in all RCC, as well as in tumors from other tissues, a deletion of chromosome 3 was observed; (2) in a given patient, whatever the type of tumor analyzed, the allele lost is always the same; (3) the allele retained in the tumor comes from the affected parent whereas the lost allele was inherited by the healthy parent; and (4) the VHL gene can thus be considered as a tumor-suppressor gene in agreement with the two-hit theory of Knudson.[7]

Cohen et al.[1] identified a family with a constitutional (3;8) translocation that was associated with the development of RCC. Ninety percent of family members with the translocation developed RCC by age 60. RCC in affected family members was often bilateral and multiple. Brauch et al.[8] used cytogenetic and molecular techniques to test for the presence and source of 3p loss in RCC associated with the t(3;8). They showed that at least three events are responsible for this form of RCC: first, inheritance of the translocated chromosome; second, a somatic mutation of the renal cell carcinoma gene located on the normal chromosome 3; and third, loss of the derivative 8 chromosome bearing the distal portion of 3p (3p14.2 → 3pter).

Chromosome Abnormalities in Tumors

Cytogenetic analyses performed on tumors had already revealed that rearrangements on chromosome 3 were quite frequent.[9] Karyotype analysis of 51 tumors subdivided into four groups comprising: (1) clear cell nonpapillary tumors; (2) papillary carcinomas; (3) nonclear cell, nonpapillary carcinomas; and (4) oncocytomas, revealed a chromosomal abnormality in 57% of the tumors. Deletions of 3p are specific to clear cell nonpapillary carcinomas in which 17p deletions as well as trisomies of 17, 7, and 12 exist. Trisomy 17 is the only characteristic feature of papillary carcinomas.

There was no specific abnormality in the two other types of tumor.[10] The absence of 3p deletion in adenomas shows that this event is crucial in the progression of adenoma to carcinoma.[11] Cytogenetic analysis of tumors from 12 patients with VHL also revealed a specific deletion of the short arm of 3, as well as, in some cases, a monosomy 14, and a partial or total trisomy of 5 or 7.[7]

Specific deletions of the short arm of chromosome 3 were confirmed in 90% of the tumors, with polymorphic markers mapping to this chromosome[12, 13] and more precisely to region 3p14-21[14] or 3p14.2.[10] The latter very precisely corresponds to the region of the breakpoint of the familial translocation t3;8.[1] Should this be confirmed, it implies that apart from the VHL gene, which unambiguously maps to 3p25-26, chromosome 3 harbors a second gene involved in RCC progression and predisposition. This is reminiscent of an analogous situation for Wilms' tumor. Chromosome 11 carries two genes involved in predisposition to Wilms' tumor, WT1 in 11p13 and WT2 in 11p15. Losses of alleles have been observed for each locus.

Among other tumor-suppressor genes already identified, some can be associated with progression to malignancy. This is the case for the retinoblastoma gene (RB, 13q14), the gene coding for the p53 protein (P53, 17p13), and the product of the WT2 gene in 11p15. With appropriate

Chromosome	Tumors	Chromosome	Tumors
Chromosome 1	**56**	Chromosome 13	23
Chromosome 2	26	**Chromosome 14**	**66**
Chromosome 3	**174**	Chromosome 15	19
Chromosome 4	28	Chromosome 16	29
Chromosome 5	**67**	Chromosome 17	36
Chromosome 6	29	Chromosome 18	21
Chromosome 7	**107**	Chromosome 19	9
Chromosome 8	**64**	Chromosome 20	28
Chromosome 9	42	Chromosome 21	17
Chromosome 10	14	Chromosome 22	9
Chromosome 11	10	Chromosome X	23
Chromosome 12	33	**Chromosome Y**	**61**

FIG 3.
Study of 227 tumors in renal cell carcinoma.

DNA markers, loss of heterozygosity was demonstrated for region 11p in 24% of the tumors, for 13q in 34%, and for 17p in 11%. These deletions were only observed in advanced or metastatic stages, suggesting the involvement of RB and WT2 only in tumor progression. In contrast with what has been described for lung cancer, mutations in the p53 gene are rare in RCC.[15]

Losses of alleles for the short arm of chromosome 3 have also been observed in several other types of tumors including small cell lung carcinoma, breast cancer, and testicular tumors. The gene(s) involved in these tumors may be identical to or different from the gene(s) predisposing to RCC (Fig 3).

Chromosome 3 Tumor-Suppressor Gene(s)

The presence of a tumor-suppressor gene in chromosome 3 has also been confirmed by experiments showing that reversion of the neoplastic phenotype and suppression of tumorigenicity of a renal carcinoma cell line could be obtained by introduction of one or two copies, respectively, of a wild type chromosome 3.[16]

Nephroblastoma

Nephroblastoma or Wilms' tumor (WT) of the kidney is an embryonal tumor that affects approximately 1 in 10,000 children. Although sporadic forms are the most frequent (95%), the occurrence of bilateral tumors in 8% of the cases suggests the presence of a predisposing germ line event in an even greater number, probably due to new mutations. The rarity of familial cases (2%) did not facilitate linkage analysis. The first hint for the location of a gene predisposing to WT came from the observation of children (1%) with the complex syndrome WAGR associated with a deletion of band 11p13. Usual treatment is chemotherapy followed by total or partial nephrectomy, especially in hereditary cases.

Genetic Predisposition

Two regions on the short arm of chromosome 11 are involved in malformation syndromes associated with a predisposition to WT. First, the deletion of region 11p13 is associated with a predisposition to WT(W), aniridia (A), genitourinary abnormalities (GU), and mental retardation (R), (the so-called WAGR syndrome).[17] Second, region 11p15 contains a gene involved in the Beckwith-Wiedemann syndrome (BWS), in associated childhood tumors, and in progression of several adult malignancies. BWS is characterized by gigantism, macroglossia, exomphalos, neonatal hypoglycemia, and a tendency (10%) to develop tumors including WT, adrenocortical carcinoma, hepatoblastoma, and rhabdomyosarcoma.[18] The involvement of region 11p15 is based on two observations: (1) more than a dozen reported cases presented with constitutional duplications of region

11p15 resulting either from de novo rearrangements or from malsegregation of balanced paternal translocations; and (2) linkage analysis with 11p15 markers revealed that the locus for the familial form also mapped to this region.[19–21]

When markers for regions 11p13 and 11p15 were used to investigate for the location of the gene involved in familial predisposition, both regions were excluded. This suggests that a third as yet unmapped locus, WT3, is involved in predisposition to WT.[22, 23]

Predisposition to WT is associated with several other malformation syndromes including Drash syndrome,[24] hemihypertrophy,[25] and genitourinary abnormalities[26] (Table 1).

Chromosome Rearrangements in Tumors

Cytogenetics

Cytogenetic analyses of Wilms' tumors have revealed that chromosomes other than 11 play an important role in tumorigenesis. Structural abnormalities of both arms of chromosomes 1, 7, 16, and 17 as well as quantitative abnormalities including trisomy 12, 6, 8, and 18[27] are characteristic features of WT.

Losses of Alleles

By analogy with retinoblastoma,[28] losses of alleles for markers mapping to the same 11p region as the genes for predisposition to WT were described.[29] However, due to the presence of two different loci, and to limited informativeness of the markers, it was not always possible to determine whether the loss of alleles corresponded to the loss of the second allele at the same locus. Some sporadic WT have a loss of alleles limited to region 11p13, while other tumors show a loss of heterozygosity for markers within 11p15 but not 11p13.[25] In four patients with WAGR and a constitutional del11p13, the al-

TABLE 1.
Nephroblastoma (WT) Genes of Susceptibility

Gene	Syndrome	Mode	Location
WT1	WAGR	Deletion	11p13
WT2	BWS	Duplication, families, disomy	11p15
WT3	WT, familial	Families	(unlinked to 11p)
?	Drash	?	?
?	Hemihypertrophy	?	?

lele loss was limited to region 11p15.[30] This may suggest that, as with hereditary and nonhereditary forms of colon carcinoma, a cascade of multiple genetic events is involved in WT. Furthermore in patients with del11p13, the somatic loss of the unique WT1 allele may not be necessary for the tumor to develop. Unlike retinoblastoma, there are only five cases described to date with a homozygously deleted WT1 gene (Fig 4).

The loss of heterozygosity for region 11p15 is a common event to several childhood and adult tumors. This region may thus contain one or several genes involved in rhabdomyosarcomas,[31, 32] testicular tumors,[33] renal cell carcinoma,[14] bladder cancer,[34] and breast cancer.[35]

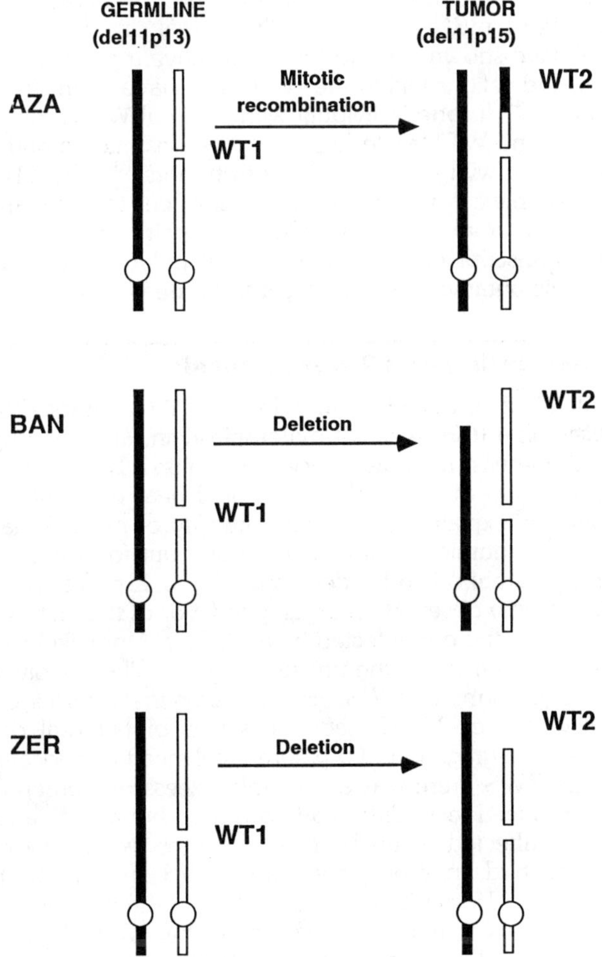

FIG 4.
Sequential involvement in Wilms' tumor.

Isolation and Characterization of the WT1 Gene

Isolation of the WT1 gene mapping to this 11p13 region has revealed a gene encoding a zinc finger protein.[36,37] When intact, this region binds to a DNA sequence that shows a striking homology with the target sequence of EGR1.[38] EGR1 and EGR2 (early growth response genes), which show homology with the zinc finger domain of WT1, are mammalian genes expressed when cells are stimulated by serum or growth factors. The WT1 gene is primarily expressed in blastemal cells of the kidney during a critical period in the development of the glomerulus.[36–39] This relatively restricted pattern of expression is in marked contrast with the ubiquitous expression of the RB gene. In addition, unlike RB the majority of WT express significant levels of WT1 mRNA of apparently normal size. Initial screenings of sporadic WT have shown 1 in 50 tumors to have a gross DNA rearrangement, but small deletions within the WT1 gene have been detected in 1 of 8 Wilms' tumors.[40] In one individual with bilateral Wilms' tumors, a germ line deletion in one WT1 allele has been demonstrated along with a subsequent loss of the wild type allele in both tumors.[40a] The 11p13 locus itself may be complex: a transcript, Wit-1, adjacent to WT1 and encoding an open reading frame of only 276 base pairs, has been isolated.[41] Whether this transcript encodes a functional polypeptide is unclear, and mutations in this putative gene have yet to be demonstrated.

Genomic Imprinting and Tumorigenesis

Whenever identifiable, the 11p alleles lost in Wilms' tumor (26/27) and in rhabdomyosarcoma (6/6) were of maternal origin, and, although not fully demonstrated, the vast majority concerned region 11p15, not 11p13. This preferential retention of paternal alleles could bear different significations: first, this could be explained by hypermutability of paternal gametes; second, differential genomic imprinting could account for these observations. A preferential paternal origin for deletion of band 11p13 appearing as new mutations is the only observation arguing in favor of the first explanation, if the WT1 locus was the one affected by allele loss. More likely, and in favor of the second explanation, is the unusual parental allele involvement in the different etiologic forms of BWS: first, in cytogenetic forms of BWS, the duplicated segment of 11p15 sequences was of paternal origin (11/12 cases), due to malsegregation of a paternal balanced translocation; second, in families with BWS there was a threefold excess of women carriers due not only to a reduced fecundity in affected men but also to a higher probability of being affected when born to a carrier woman (sex-dependent transmission)[42]; third, in sporadic cases of BWS, uniparental paternal disomy limited to 11p15 markers was described in three of eight cases.[43] Altogether, these observations suggest that the BWS locus undergoes genomic imprinting. The isolation of the 11p15 Wilms' tumor locus will be necessary to test this concept and understand the nature of the underlying mechanisms. If a locus involved in tumorigenesis undergoes genomic im-

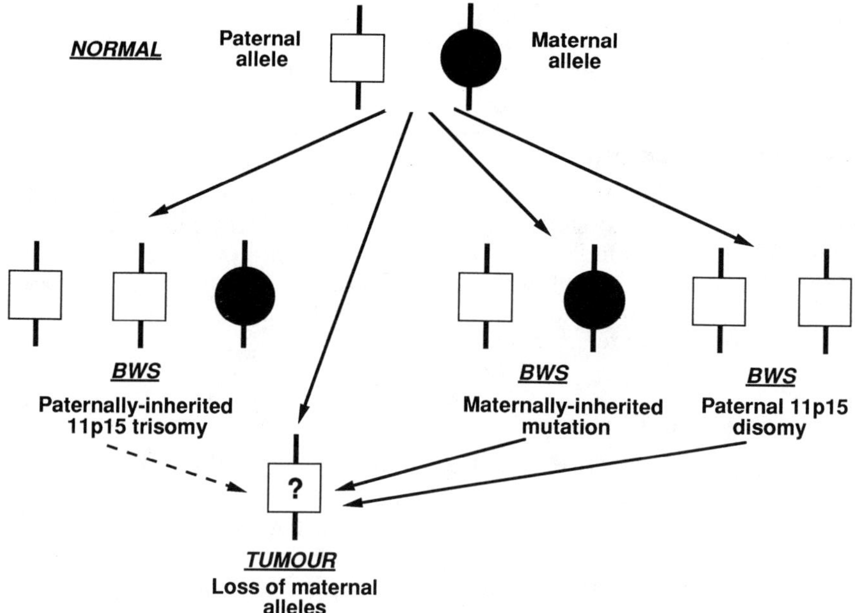

FIG 5.
Beckwith-Wiedemann syndrome.

printing, this would infer that the loss of the second allele is not necessary. Actually this could be argued by the following observations: in Wilms' tumor, Poisson statistical analysis of the frequency of bilateral tumors predicts that 38% of all cases are hereditary[44]; however, familial cases are estimated to represent approximately 2% of observed Wilms' tumors, while 8% of the cases develop bilateral tumors; Knudson's findings thus imply that the vast majority of bilateral cases as well as a portion of unilateral cases represent de novo germ line mutations at either of the three loci for predisposition; alternatively, this may also suggest that imprinting of the 11p15 locus would require only one additional event, the loss of the maternal allele, for the tumor to develop. Imprinting would be the equivalent of the germ line mutation in hereditary cases (Fig 5).

Perspectives

Research of Other Genes

As shown by consistent specific cytogenetic abnormalities in tumors, several loci on the genome are involved in tumor progression. They not only include losses of gene function but also gain of function or gene dosage effects revealed by the occurrence of trisomy for certain regions. The corresponding genes can be further mapped with DNA markers. Alternatively, a more general approach involving construction of subtractive hybridization libraries can lead to isolation of expressed sequences implicated in these pathologic processes.

Genetic Counseling

Linkage analysis in kindreds with the familial form may help discover the location of the gene(s) for hereditary susceptibility. This will allow genetic counseling for at-risk individuals and detection of de novo germ line mutation with predictability of recurrence. Moreover it should be possible through epidemiological surveys to determine the tissue targets of carcinogens and to institute real prevention.

Prognosis and Therapy

One of the main goals of molecular studies on oncogenes and tumor-suppressor genes is to establish correlations between the grade and the stage of the tumor to better define the prognosis and therefore the most appropriate therapy. This requires looking for mutations and testing the level of expression of several genes in the context of a multiparametric analysis of the tumors.

Although in vitro suppression of tumors by means of introduction of tumor-suppressor genes sounds very appealing, its feasibility in vivo has not yet been demonstrated. More likely, a better knowledge of the fundamental chromosome and molecular mechanisms participating in metastasis and angiogenesis is required to devise appropriate tools to fight these processes.

The receptor for protein-tyrosine phosphatase γ has been shown to be a candidate tumor suppressor gene for renal carcinoma and lung carcinoma. This gene maps to 3p21 and is deleted in 3 of 5 renal carcinomas and in 5 of 10 lung cancers.[45]

References

1. Cohen AJ, Li FP, Berg S, et al: Hereditary renal carcinoma associated with a chromosomal translocation. *N Engl J Med* 1979; 301:592–595.
2. Pathak S, Strong LC, Ferrel LE, et al: Familial renal cell carcinoma with a 3;11 chromosome translocation limited to tumor cells. *Science* 1982; 217: 939–941.
3. Seizinger BR, Rouleau GA, Ozelius LJ, et al. Von Hippel-Lindau disease maps to the region of chromosome 3 associated with renal cell carcinoma. *Nature* 1988; 332:268–269.
4. Lerman MI, Latif F, Glenn GM, et al: Isolation and regional localization of a large collection (2000) of single copy DNA fragments on human chromosome 3 for mapping and cloning tumor suppressor genes. *Hum Genet* 1991; 86:567–577.

5. Hosoe S, Brauch H, Latif F, et al: Localization of the von Hippel-Lindau disease gene to a small region of chromosome 3. *Genomics* 1990; 8:634–640.
6. Seizinger BR, Smith D, Klauck JM, et al: Toward the isolation of the gene causing von Hippel-Lindau disease: Identification of tightly linked flanking markers (abstract). *Am J Hum Genet* 1990; 47:A17.
7. Jordan DK, Patil SR, Divelbiss JE, et al: Cytogenetic abnormalities in tumors of patients with von Hippel-Lindau disease. *Cancer Genet Cytogenet* 1989; 42:227–241.
8. Brauch H, Hosoe S, Li F, et al: Loss of the derivative 8 chromosome in hereditary renal cell carcinoma associated with a 3;8 translocation (abstract). *Am J Hum Genet* 1990; 47:A3.
9. Yoshida MA, Ohyashiki K, Ochi H, et al: Cytogenetic studies of tumor tissue from patients with nonfamilial renal cell carcinoma. *Cancer Res* 1989; 46:2139–2147.
10. Presti JC, Rao PH, Chen O, et al: Histopathologic, cytogenetic and molecular characterization of renal tumors (abstract). *Am J Hum Genet* 1990; 47:A15.
11. Wang N, Smith S, Lui W, et al: Molecular analysis of constitutive fragile site mapping at 3p14.2 (abstract). *Am J Hum Genet* 1990; 47:A23.
12. Kovacs G, Erlandsson R, Boldog F, et al: Consistent chromosome 3p deletion and loss of heterozygosity in renal cell carcinoma. *Proc Natl Acad Sci USA* 1988; 85:1571–1575.
13. Kovacs G, Frisch S: Clonal chromosome abnormalities in tumor cells from patients with sporadic renal cell carcinoma. *Cancer Res* 1989; 49:651–959.
14. Zbar B, Brauch H, Talmadge C, et al: Loss of alleles of loci on the short arm of chromosome 3 in renal cell carcinoma. *Nature* 1987; 327:721–724.
15. Whaley JM, Chung RY, Yandell DW, et al: Mutation of the P53 gene is an uncommon event in sporadic human renal cell carcinoma (abstract). *Am J Hum Genet* 1990; 47:A25.
16. Schimizu M, Yokota J, Mori N, et al: Introduction of normal chromosome 3p modulates the tumorigenicity of a human renal cell carcinoma cell line YCR. *Oncogene* 1990; 5:185–194.
17. Francke U, Holmes LB, Atkins L, et al: Aniridia-Wilms' tumor association: Evidence for specific deletion of 11p13. *Cytogenet Cell Genet* 1979; 24:185–192.
18. Wiedemann HR: Tumors and hemyhypertrophy associated with Wiedemann-Beckwith syndrome. *Eur J Pediatr* 1983; 414:129.
19. Turleau C, Grouchy J de: Beckwith-Wiedemann syndrome: Clinical comparison between patients with and without 11p15 trisomy. *Hum Genet* 1985; 28:93–96.
20. Ping AJ, Reeve AE, Law DJ, et al: Genetic linkage of Beckwith-Wiedemann syndrome to 11p15. *Am J Hum Genet* 1989; 44:720–723.
21. Koufos A, Grundy P, Morgan K, et al: Familial Wiedemann-Beckwith syndrome and a second Wilms' tumor locus both map to 11p15.5. *Am J Hum Genet* 1989; 44:711–719.
22. Huff V, Compton DA, Chao LY, et al: Lack of linkage of familial Wilms' tumor to chromosomol band 11p13. *Nature* 1988; 336:377–378.
23. Grundy P, Koufos A, Morgan K, et al: Familial predisposition to Wilms' tumor does not map to the short arm of chromosome 11. *Nature* 1988; 336:374–376.
24. Habib R, Loirat C, Gubler MC, et al: The nephropathy associated with male pseudohermophroditism and Wilms' tumor (Drash syndrome): A distinctive glomerular lesion. Report of 10 cases. *Clinic Nephrol* 1985; 24:269–278.

25. Mannens M, Slater RM, Heyting C, et al: Molecular nature of genetic changes resulting in loss of heterozygosity of chromosome 11 in Wilms' tumor. *Hum Genet* 1988; 81:41–48.
26. Junien C: Les antioncogènes. *Médecine/Science* 1986; 2:238–254.
27. Wang-Wuu S, Soukup S, Bove K, et al: Chromosome analysis of 31 Wilms' tumor. *Cancer Res* 1990; 50:2786–2793.
28. Cavenee WK, Dryja P, Phillips, et al: Expression of recessive alleles by chromosomal mechanisms in retinoblastoma. *Nature* 1983; 305:779–784.
29. Koufos A, Hansen MF, Lampkin BC, et al: Loss of alleles at loci on human chromosome 11 during genesis of Wilms' tumor. *Nature* 1984; 309:170-172.
30. Henry I, Grandjouan S, Couillin P, et al: Tumor-specific loss of 11p15.5 alleles in del11p13 Wilms' tumor and in familial adrenocortical carcinoma. *Proc Natl Acad Sci USA* 1989; 86:3247–3251.
31. Scrable HJ, Witte DP, Lampkin BC, et al: Chromosomal localization of the human rhabdomyosarcoma locus by mitotic recombination mapping. *Nature* 1987; 329:645–647.
32. Scrable HJ, Cavenee W, Ghavimi F, et al: A model for embryonal rhabdomyosarcoma tumorigenesis that involves genome imprinting. *Proc Natl Acad Sci USA* 1989; 86:7480–7484.
33. Lothe RA, Fossa SD, Stenwig AE: Loss of 3p or 11p alleles is associated with testicular cancer tumors. *Genomics* 1989; 5:134–138.
34. Fearon ER, Feinberg AP, Hamilton SH, et al: Loss of genes on the short arm of chromosome 11 in bladder cancer. *Nature* 1985; 318:377–380.
35. Ali IU, Lidereau R, Theillet C, et al: Reduction to the homozygosity of genes on chromosome 11 in human breast neoplasia. *Science* 1987; 238:187.
36. Call K, Jones C, Ito C, et al: Isolation and mapping of cosmid clones and isolation of a candidate gene for Wilms' tumor. Xth International Workshop on Human Gene Mapping. *Cytogenet Cell Genet* 1989; 51:974.
37. Gessler M, Poutska A, Cavenee W, et al: Homozygous deletion in Wilms' tumor of a Zinc-finger gene identified by chromosome jumping. *Nature* 1990; 343:774–778.
38. Rauscher III FJ, Morris JF, Tournay OE, et al: Bonding of the Wilms' tumor locus zinc-finger protein to the EGR-1 consensus sequence. *Science* 1990; 2:1259–1262.
39. Pritchard-Jones K, Fleming S, Davidson D, et al: The candidate Wilms' tumour gene is involved in genitourinary development. *Nature* 1990; 346:194–197.
40. Haber DA, Buckler AJ, Glaser T, et al: An internal deletion within an 11p13 Zinc-finger gene contributes to the development of Wilms' tumor. *Cell* 1990; 61:1257–1269.
40a. Huff V, Miwa H, Haber DA, et al: Evidence for WTI as a Wilms' tumor (WT) gene: Intragenic germinal deletion in bilateral WT. *Genomics* 1991; in press.
41. Huang A, Campbell CE, Bonetta L, et al: Tissue, developmental and tumor specific expression of divergent transcripts implicated in Wilms' tumor. *Science* 1990; 250:991–994.
42. Moutou C, Junien C, Henry I, et al: Segregation analysis in familial Beckwith-Wiedemann syndrome: Explanations of the excess of transmitting females. Submitted for publication.
43. Henry I, Bonaïti-Pellié C, Chehensse V, et al: Uniparental paternal disomy in sporadic Beckwith-Wiedemann syndrome with Wilms' tumor suggests genomic imprinting. Submitted for publication.

44. Knudson AG: Mutation and cancer: Statistical study of retinoblastoma. *Proc Natl Acad Sci USA* 1971; 4:820–823.
45. LaForgia S, Morse B, Levy J, et al: Receptor protein-tyrosine phosphatase γ is a candidate tumor suppressor gene at human chromosome region 3p21. *Proc Natl Acad Sci USA* 1991; 88:5036–5040.

Hypertension and Renal Disease in Blacks: Role of Genetic and/or Environmental Factors?

Stephen G. Rostand, M.D.

Professor of Medicine, Nephrology Research and Training Center, Division of Nephrology, Department of Medicine, University of Alabama School of Medicine, University of Alabama at Birmingham, Birmingham, Alabama

Hypertension is now recognized as one of the leading health problems in the United States, affecting nearly 60 million people and causing or contributing significantly to cardiovascular and renal disease and to premature death. As a result of numerous blood pressure surveillance studies, it has been recognized that blacks have a 30% to 50% greater prevalence of elevated blood pressure than whites, with largest differences noted in women.[1] Moreover, since the United States government established funding for the treatment of end-stage renal disease (ESRD) in 1973, we have learned that primary hypertension is the leading cause of ESRD[2] and that blacks are disproportionally affected by nearly all forms of renal failure, especially hypertensive renal failure (H-ESRD), which occurs six to 17 times more frequently in blacks than in whites.[3–5] The reasons for the apparent increased susceptibility of American blacks to develop hypertension and its renal consequences are not well understood. Understanding this problem is of great scientific and clinical importance and also may have major social and political implications. In this paper I will attempt to place in perspective the problem of hypertension and its renal consequences as they relate to blacks.

Genetic Basis for Racial Differences in Hypertension

Studies analyzing the relationships between race and hypertension are complicated by several factors. First, it must be recognized that race is an arbitrary classification of people that subsumes many overlapping social and cultural traits in addition to genetic characteristics. No clear group of genes distinguishes the races, only relative frequencies of one or another trait.[6] Second, since blood pressure is a continuous variable, there is probably no precise level of blood pressure that defines hypertension. It is quite likely that levels of blood pressure within the currently defined normal range, in certain environmental and physiologic conditions, may be considered elevated. Since studies examining familial associations with hypertension and associations between hypertension and various intermediate phenotypes have defined hypertension differently, they may be flawed as a result. Last, systemic blood pressure is under the complex control of many factors, some still to be recognized, that affect cardiac output and systemic vascular resistance, the major determinants of blood pressure and hypertension. These systemic and cellular functions (intermediate phenotypes) are interrelated, are under variable genetic control, and are strongly influenced by environmental factors (Fig 1). Thus blood pressure variability is not likely to be controlled by a single gene but rather by multiple genes, the expression of which is significantly influenced by the environment.

The development of several strains of hypertensive rats and the long-observed finding that human hypertension aggregates in families has suggested a genetic basis for the disease. Recent genetic linkage studies[7] performed in 31 black and white families show that at least one of the genes responsible for the familial predisposition to essential hypertension may be located at or near the human leukocyte histocompatibility antigen (HLA) complex. To assess the relative contribution of hereditary and environmental influences on blood pressure, statistically derived heritability estimates have been calculated from studies comparing monozygotic (MZ) and dizygotic twins (DZ)[8] and natural and adoptive families[9–11] (Table 1). Depending on the family relationship examined and the setting in which the stud-

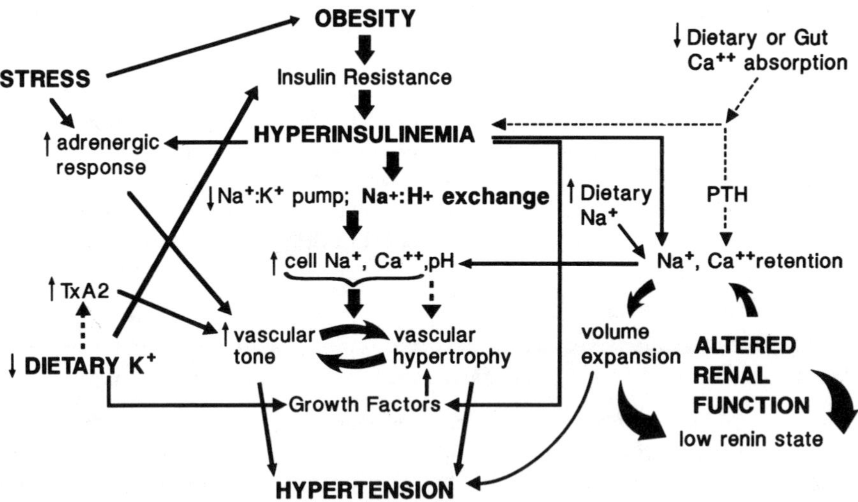

FIG 1.
Scheme of interrelationships of some cellular, systemic, and environmental factors thought to be important in the pathogenesis of hypertension. *Broken line* represents least certain pathogenetic role.

TABLE 1.
Genetic Basis for Hypertension

Family association or aggregation
Concordance in MZ twins >DZ twins
Concordance in parent-natural child >parent-adoptee
Concordance in related sibs living apart >unrelated sibs living together
Heritability estimates: 0.3–0.8 (25%–40%)
Similar heritability estimates for blacks and whites
Concordance between hypertension and intermediate phenotypes
Reduced sodium excretion rates
Salt sensitivity
Nonmodulating essential hypertension
Red blood cell sodium content (membrane cation transport rates)
Body mass index
Darker skin color
Genetic loci (proposed)
Major histocompatibility locus, chromosome 6
Blood type MN locus, chromosome 4
Haptoglobin 1–1 (haptoglobin gene)
Na+: H+ antiporter gene
Renin gene

ies were done, heritability estimates for systolic and diastolic blood pressure vary widely; however, no significant differences between the races have been noted. In fact, careful epidemiologic studies have suggested no statistical association between degree of skin color and level of blood pressure,[12] though this finding is debated.[13] Moreover, the sickle cell gene, strongly associated with blacks, has been correlated in blacks with lower blood pressure and an absence of the expected age-related rise in blood pressure.[14]

The contribution of shared family environment to blood pressure variability has been estimated at between 20% and 40%.[9–11] However, for blacks the influence of shared family environment is less, about 5%. This may be a result of the high frequency of fragmented families among blacks and should not be construed as meaning that blood pressure in blacks is less susceptible to environmental influences. In fact the opposite may be the case, for in the Detroit Project,[10] until statistical adjustments were made for high stress living areas, a genetic basis for blood pressure variability could not be found and it was concluded that unspecified environmental factors alone were responsible. The previously noted studies also demonstrate a strong maternal influence on blood pressure.[9, 11] While this might suggest a strong genetic influence, experimental studies of the spontaneously hypertensive rat (SHR) show that offspring of SHR raised by control mothers do not become hypertensive nor do they show the expected age-associated rise in blood pressure.[15] Thus, these studies show a strong effect of the maternal environment on the genetic expression of hypertension.

Racial Differences in Renal Function and Renal Hemodynamics

Of the many factors controlling blood pressure, alterations in renal function, particularly renal sodium excretion, have been considered essential for the development of hypertension. Guyton et al.[16] have suggested that the primary defect in hypertension is a reduced renal capacity for sodium excretion necessitating a greater systemic pressure to maintain normal sodium and water balance. Such observations have been made in several genetic animal models of hypertension and in human hypertension.[17–19] In keeping with this concept, blacks have been noted to have greater blood pressure responses to saline loading than whites and to excrete sodium more slowly.[20, 21] A similar delay in sodium excretion was noted in first order relatives,[22, 23] and a high concordance for this defect was also observed in MZ twins.[22–24] Thus delayed sodium excretion in essential hypertension is thought to be genetically determined. Moreover, Luft et al.[25] have also shown a strong association between the 1-1 phenotype of haptoglobin and salt sensitivity and have suggested that the haptoglobin gene may play a prominent role in salt-sensitive hypertension.

The blunted sodium excretory response was at first thought to be a consequence of increased activity of the renin-angiotensin system; however, in blacks renin-angiotensin activity is reduced. Since this fundamental racial difference in plasma renin activity (PRA) cannot consistently be explained by differences in blood volume, it may be that an alteration in or near the gene controlling the expression of renin is important in blacks with essential hypertension. Blacks with low PRA, unlike whites, do not show the expected inverse relationship between PRA and plasma volume.[26] Those blacks with hypertension who fail to demonstrate the normal interrelationship between blood pressure, plasma renin activity, and plasma volume may be more volume dependent[26]; thus, they may be similar to patients with nonmodulating essential hypertension. In this form of hypertension in which familial aggregation has been reported,[27] there is a failure to modulate appropriately renal vascular and adrenal responsiveness to angiotensin II in association with changes in volume produced by alterations in sodium intake. Although racial differences have not been examined, the high frequency of this form of disease (nearly 40% of essential hypertension) is similar to the 43% of blacks thought to have abnormal PRA and plasma volume interactions.[26, 27]

The altered sodium excretion pattern seen in blacks with essential hypertension may also be the result of the greater reduction of kallekrein-kinin excretion noted in blacks[28] and may also depend on altered renal hemodynamics, manifested by reduced renal blood flow, increased renal vascular resistance, and attenuation of the renal vasculature compared to whites with hypertension.[29, 30] Since kallikrein catalyzes the formation of bradykinin, a natriuretic and vasodilatory substance, its reduced generation could be responsible for increased renal vascular tone and reduced sodium excretory function noted in blacks.[28] Reduction in kallikrein excretion, however, may not be unique to blacks since it has been observed generally in patients with essential hypertension when compared to normotensives.[31] Moreover, kallikrein excretion has been found to have a strong genetic component in largely white Utah kindreds in whom lower excretory rates are associated with an increased risk of hypertension.[32]

It is unclear if the renal vascular changes noted in blacks are the result of hypertension or precede its onset. Vascular changes have been noted early in the course of hypertension often before structural damage to the vessels is likely to have occurred.[33] Attenuation of the renal vasculature and vascular endothelial and smooth muscle proliferation associated with increased renal vascular resistance may in theory be caused by racial differences in the production or response to endothelium- and platelet-derived growth factors, endothelium-dependent relaxing factors, and/or differences in production and response to vasoconstricting substances, such as endothelin, found to be elevated in the plasma of many patients with essential hypertension.[34] In this regard, the kidneys of the Dahl 'S' strain of rat have recently been noted to have an increased responsiveness to endothelin.[35] Information on the genetic and racial aspects of these substances is presently lacking. However, it is known that the diets of American blacks are low in potassium and protein and as a result may stimulate vascular growth factors and inhibit endothelium-derived relaxing factors.[36, 37]

Insulin is another factor that may contribute to renal sodium retention in hypertension. Hyperinsulinemia has been observed in untreated human hypertension and in genetic animal models of hypertension.[38] Thus, it may serve as a link between essential hypertension, carbohydrate intolerance, obesity, and salt sensitivity[39, 40] (see Fig 1). However, it may also occur independent of obesity.[41] Falkner et al.[42] found higher fasting insulin concentrations in lean black subjects with essential hypertension than in normotensive whites of similar adiposity. Clearly, carbohydrate intolerance occurs more frequently in American blacks than in whites as judged by their increased prevalence of noninsulin dependent diabetes mellitus (NIDDM).[43] However, this increased prevalence of NIDDM is not unique to blacks since Pima Indians also have an increased prevalence of NIDDM when compared to whites and blacks.[44]

Insulin has been shown to enhance renal tubular sodium absorption,[45, 46] presumably by stimulating renal $Na+-K+$ ATPase (sodium pump) activity and $Na+-H+$ exchange.[47] Changes in circulating insulin concentration may be the basis for the natriuresis of fasting and for sodium retention and edema seen with refeeding and suggest that reductions in plasma insulin concentration accompanying weight loss may cause the fall in blood pressure associated with weight reduction. However, the role of insulin in hypertension remains speculative since Hall et al.[48] recently showed no effect of insulin on blood pressure in partially nephrectomized dogs. For all the above reasons, and for others to be elucidated, attenuated renal sodium excretion may be an important factor for the increased prevalence of hypertension in blacks. Moreover, there is a dichotomy between the increased prevalence of NIDDM seen in Mexican-Americans and hypertension in this group. The degree to which this alteration and other differences in renal function noted in blacks are genetically or environmentally influenced have not been determined.

Racial Differences in Systemic Hemodynamics and Sympathetic Nervous System Activity

Messerli et al.[49] have been unable to demonstrate racial differences with regard to cardiac output and total peripheral vascular resistance at rest and in response to blood pressure changes in patients with essential hypertension, and no racial differences have been found in plasma norepinephrine concentrations. Nevertheless, racial differences in sympathetic nervous system responsiveness and systemic vascular reactivity have been noted. Harshfield et al.[50] have noted differences in diurnal blood pressure variation between blacks and whites. Despite blood pressures similar to whites while awake, black adolescents had higher systolic and diastolic blood pressures while asleep. Blacks have a decreased plasma dopamine β-hydroxylase activity, suggesting decreased sympathoadrenal tone.[51] Blacks have been observed to have a greater vascular response to mental stress,[52–54] manifested by reduced skeletal muscle blood flow and increased systolic pressure, but have a reduced cardiac sympathomimetic response, brachycardia. Patients with such responses often have strong family histories of hypertension.[54] Similar observations have been made with respect to exercise.[55] It has been suggested that these effects are the consequence of greater β adrenergic activity with stress-mediated adrenergic activity having a greater effect on peripheral vascular resistance in blacks. Dimsdale et al.[56] found that unlike whites, blacks with hypertension respond to high salt diets with a heightened response to β adrenergic stimulation. They also noted a similar response to infusions of norepinephrine suggesting a heightened α adrenergic sensitivity as well.[57] The cause for increased vascular reactivity seen in blacks in response to sympathetic nervous system stimulation is uncertain. It has been suggested by some that since insulin release can stimulate sympathetic nervous system activity, hyperinsulinemia, which occurs at an early age and at a higher frequency in blacks, may play an important role in altered vascular reactivity.[40, 42, 58] Insulin may also contribute to the enhanced systemic vascular tone through stimulation of cellular cation transport of vascular smooth muscle cells.[39, 47]

Alterations in Cellular Cation Transport

Much attention has been focused on the role of membrane cation transport systems that affect cellular ionic composition and thus, smooth muscle contractility and blood pressure. Although racial differences in cation transport have been described,[59–61] their importance in the pathogenesis of hypertension remains speculative. American and African blacks with essential hypertension have been found to have higher intraerythrocytic sodium concentration than whites.[62, 63] However, studies of African blacks and largely white Utah kindreds show higher red blood cell sodium concentrations in families with hypertension,[62, 64] suggesting that increased red blood cell sodium is not unique to blacks and that the inheritance is polygenetic. In the Utah kindreds, there was also a significant correlation between intraerythrocytic sodium concentration and red blood cell Na+–Li+ countertransport (an analog of Na+–H+ exchange) noted between siblings and between parents and children, again suggesting a genetic linkage.[65] Increased Na+–H+ exchange is thought to work together with reduced rates of sodium pump activity to produce increased cell sodium and calcium concentrations, to alkalinize vascular smooth muscle cells thereby stimulating vascular smooth muscle hypertrophy, proliferation, and vascular tone[66–68] (see Fig 1).

While numerous studies have shown strong associations between red blood cell Na+–Li+ countertransport, hypertension, and level of blood pressure,[60, 61, 63, 65] genetic linkage analysis[69] has revealed that the number of Na+–H+ antiporter alleles shared between hypertensive siblings is no different from random aggregation, suggesting the Na+–H+ antiporter gene may not contribute importantly to the pathogenesis of hypertension. Moreover, in blacks with essential hypertension, red blood cell Na+–Li+ countertransport rates are not different from normotensive control subjects and are similar to normotensive whites.[60, 61] Furthermore, these countertransport rates do not increase with blood pressure as seen in whites.[61] Thus, it appears that the red blood cell Na+–Li+ countertransport rate may not be a suitable marker for hypertension in blacks. There is, however, a strong association in both blacks and whites between diastolic hypertension and increased rates of platelet Na+–H+ exchange.[70] And, recently, Kuriyama et al. have demonstrated greater Na+–H+ antiporter activity in cultured fibroblasts from blacks.[71] Because there is much racial and tissue variability with regard to Na+–H+ antiporter activity, it is uncertain which, if any, of these tissue activities will serve as suitable markers with which to link race and hypertension.

Cellular sodium concentration is largely controlled by rates of sodium pump activity. Because red blood cell sodium concentration is increased in people with hypertension, particularly in blacks, it has been suggested that the activity of the sodium pump is reduced; however, studies of human and experimental hypertension do not show a consistent correlation between Na+–K+ adenosine triphosphatase (ATPase) and blood pressure.[72] One mechanism proposed to explain lower sodium pump activity has been the presence of a circulating inhibitor Na+−K+ATPase, particularly in low renin hypertension seen in blacks.[73] And a recent study[74] has shown an association between black women with family histories of hypertension and a low affinity of sodium pumps for ouabain, suggesting a greater susceptibility in these women to a circulating sodium pump inhibitor. A more consistently observed racial difference in cellular cation transport has been reduced rates of red blood cell Na+−K+ cotransport noted in blacks, which may help explain not only increased red blood cell sodium concentrations but also increased cellular potassium concentrations noted in blacks and not expected from isolated reductions of Na+−K+ ATPase activity.[60] To summarize, all that can be said at present about people with hypertension and their children is that they have a lower capacity to transport sodium against its electrochemical gradient; the specific pumps involved remain to be elucidated.

The variability in sodium pump activity observed in essential hypertension also may be the result of environmental influences known to affect sodium pump activity. Sodium pump activity may be modulated by dietary intake of sodium and potassium.[62, 73] Higher dietary sodium intake has been shown to increase sodium pump activity as has increased dietary potassium. Moreover, reduced dietary potassium intake can reduce sodium pump activity.[73] Obesity may also be associated with reduced red blood cell sodium pump activity,[75] and may link hypertension seen in blacks with reduced cellular cation transport rates and hyperinsulinemia, which accompanies obesity (see Fig 1). While obesity has been shown to have a strong genetic component,[76] there are also associations between obesity and lower socioeconomic status,[77] suggesting an indirect influence of socioeconomic factors on sodium pump activity.

Social and Cultural Influences on Racial Incidence of Hypertension

The foregoing discussion has examined many of the physiologic and cellular factors influencing blood pressure. Although many seem to be controlled genetically, they have uncertain inheritance patterns and as noted (Table 2), their expression is strongly influenced by social and cultural (environmental) factors. Blacks living in western society have a greater prevalence of essential hypertension than American and European whites, and than blacks living in indigenous areas of West Africa and in the West Indies.[78] Within Africa, westernization of communities or migration to large urban centers has often been associated with major social and cultural stresses and with increased blood pressure.[78] Cultural and social disruptions due to migration or westernization of indigenous communities are many and include: changes in work style, dependence on a cash economy, crosscultural interchanges and conflict, variation in physical activity, changes in living and family infrastructure, and alterations in diet. This has been associated with increased body mass and an increased prevalence of

TABLE 2.
Social, Cultural, and Economic (Environmental) Factors Contributing to Hypertension

I. Change in social structure
   A. Westernization
   B. Geographic change
      1. Rural - urban migration
      2. Intercontinental migration
II. Consequences of change in social structure
   A. Increased stress
      1. Altered family structure and support
      2. Cross-cultural interchange and conflict
         a. Suppressed hostility
         b. Changing values
   B. Socioeconomic consequences of changing social structure
      1. Changes in work style
      2. Less secure employment/unemployment
      3. Lower wages
         a. John Henryism
      4. Lower educational level
      5. Reduced access to medical care
   C. Some physical and biologic consequences of geographic and social change
      1. Variations in physical activity
      2. Altered exposure to ultraviolet light
         a. Altered calcium metabolism and rates of vitamin D synthesis
      3. Dietary changes
         a. Reduced potassium intake
         b. ±Reduced calcium intake
         c. Increased sodium and fat intake
            (1) Increased body mass
               a. Increased rate of diabetes mellitus
               b. Increased rate of atherosclerosis
               c. Increased rate of hypertension

NIDDM and hypertension. The impact of cultural disruption on the health and blood pressure of people well adapted to a specific environment is not unique to black populations for it has been observed in the Pima Indians of the southwestern United States desert who have high rates of NIDDM, hypertension, and obesity[43] and in Tokelauan migrants to New Zealand whose blood pressure also increased.[79] In each case, an increased intake of dietary unsaturated fat and calories was at least in part responsible for the increased body mass noted. Moreover, as a consequence of the new living environment, dietary intake of sodium increased and that of potassium decreased compared with former diets.[37, 79, 80] Thus, it seems likely that abrupt changes in diet to which metabolic adaptation had occurred over millenia, may have produced metabolic and physiologic adjustments of varying degree, thus altering body weight, carbohydrate tolerance, and blood pressure. For blacks, increased dietary sodium and fat together with reduced renal sodium excretory rates and many of the possible effects of reduced dietary intake of potassium, such as carbohydrate intolerance, hyperinsulinemia, reduced sodium pump activity, reduced kallikrein production, possible enhancement of platelet- and endothelium-derived growth factors, inhibition of vascular relaxing factors, and increased vascular sympathetic responsiveness may have contributed to the increased prevalence of hypertension.

In blacks, migrations from equatorial regions also may have had a profound effect on calcium metabolism. Since highly pigmented skin protects against the damaging effects of intense and continued exposure to ultraviolet light, migration from equatorial regions in theory should reduce the amount of ultraviolet light penetrating the skin. As a consequence, it has been proposed that there should be less formation of vitamin D in the skin of American and European blacks.[81] In this regard, in comparison to whites, American blacks have been found to have reduced 25-hydroxy vitamin D3 concentrations, increased concentrations of 1,25-dihydroxy vitamin D3 concentrations and parathyroid hormone, and reduced rates of bone formation.[82, 83] These findings in blacks are similar but not identical to changes in vitamin D and parathyroid hormone concentrations observed in the SHR[84] and in low renin human essential hypertension, typical of blacks,[85] suggesting a link between skin color, calcium and vitamin D metabolism, and hypertension.

Although careful epidemiologic studies by Keil et al.[12] have shown only a minimal association between the degree of skin pigmentation and blood pressure when socioeconomic factors and age were controlled for, Harburg et al.[13] have found a very strong association between darker skin and blood pressure in blacks, independent of socioeconomic factors. How altered vitamin D and parathyroid metabolism might relate to hypertension is uncertain. The data suggest the possibility that as a result of blunted intestinal calcium absorption, perhaps a consequence of lactose intolerance found in a majority of blacks, or reduced dietary calcium intake thought to be a feature of the diet of American blacks,[80] secondary hyperparathyroidism develops with subsequent increases in vascular smooth muscle calcium concentration, vascular tone, and hypertension. Increased parathyroid hormone concentrations are also associated with increased insulin concentrations as well as hypertension.[86] Thus, the parathyroid abnormality may link hyperinsulinism, hypertension, and altered calcium metabolism (see Fig 1). The exact role for increased parathyroid hormone is uncertain since parathyroidectomy, while lowering insulin concentrations in humans, does not affect blood pressure.[86, 87]

Socioeconomic status is an important variable that has been examined in relation to hypertension in the United States. There is an inverse relationship between educational level, income, and level of blood pressure for both blacks and whites. Although these associations are similar for both races, blacks still have a nearly twofold greater prevalence of hypertension at all levels of education.[88] The reasons for the increased prevalence of hypertension among lower socioeconomic groups is uncertain but may relate to altered nutrition, insecure employment, limited access to medical care, and to the many social and biologic stresses previously alluded to. Social disorganization resulting from living under continuous stressful circumstances may lead to altered coping mechanisms such as suppressed hostility, frustration, and anger, and John Henryism[89] and may thus contribute to the altered vascular responsiveness to mental stress noted in blacks and to their tendency to hypertension (see Table 2).

Racial Differences in Susceptibility to Developing Renal Disease

Blacks develop renal failure approximately 4 times more frequently than whites[4] and develop H-ESRD 6 to 17 times more frequently.[3–5] Since the prevalence of hypertension is only 50% greater in blacks, the greater prevalence of hypertension has not been thought to explain entirely the differences between blacks and whites in rates of ESRD in the United States.[1, 3] Nevertheless, blacks have higher blood pressures than whites earlier in life and have a blunted diurnal variation in blood pressure, thus placing them at risk for a longer period of time than whites. The sustained high prevalence of H-ESRD in blacks, despite the availability of numerous classes of antihypertensive drugs, suggests that their kidneys may be genetically more susceptible to develop renal disease. In this regard, we studied a group of patients with essential hypertension with serum creatinine concentrations less than 1.5 mg/dL and good blood pressure control and found that blacks had a significant rise in creatinine twice as often as whites.[90] These data suggest that blacks have an early susceptibility to renal damage; however, once renal function reaches a more advanced degree of deterioration, racial differences in the rates of renal deterioration appear to be lost.[91]

Several lines of experimentation suggest that intrinsic (inherited) abnormalities of renal function may contribute to the heightened susceptibility of blacks to H-ESRD. First, Ferguson et al.[92] have found a strong association between hypertension and family histories of renal failure. Second, transplantation with kidneys from normotensive donors corrects hypertension in black patients and normalizes responses to salt restriction and loading, suggesting a defect within the native kidney[93] that may relate to the renin-angiotensin system.[94] These findings also suggest that differences in intrarenal hemodynamics, perhaps causing alterations in tubulo-glomerular feedback and increased single nephron glomerular filtration rates may contribute to the accelerated deterioration of renal function. Observed racial differences in intrarenal hemodynamic responses to hypertension suggest a target organ specificity that may be important for the increased susceptibility of blacks to develop hypertensive renal failure. Evidence for this comes from studies by Levy et al.,[30] who showed that at the same level of glomerular filtration rate and mean arterial pressure, renal blood flow was lower, renal vascular resistance higher, and renal vascularity more attenuated in blacks than in whites. This suggested a greater renal vascular damage in blacks for the same degree of hypertension. Last, increased susceptibility of blacks to develop hypertensive renal failure may relate to their blunted rates of sodium excretion. This tendency toward enhanced sodium absorption may be associated with increased renal metabolic work, which has been proposed by some to cause renal tubular damage,[95] although the mechanisms are not well understood.

We have already emphasized nutritional differences between blacks and whites. In this regard, Tobian and his colleagues[37, 96] found that dietary potassium supplementation confers protection against the renal arteriolar and nephron damage caused by hypertension. These data suggest that inadequate dietary potassium intake may be important in the pathogenesis of hypertensive renal damage. Thus, the lower dietary potassium intake noted in blacks may contribute importantly to their susceptibility to H-ESRD.

The increased prevalence of carbohydrate intolerance and hyperinsulinemia in association with hypertension in blacks may also be important in accelerating the rate of renal failure. Using multivariant analysis, we have found (Qualheim et al., unpublished observations) a strong inverse association between the presence of carbohydrate intolerance and the length of time between patient referral and onset of dialysis therapy in a predominantly black population of patients with primary hypertension. In addition, it is clear that patients with diabetes mellitus and family histories of hypertension develop renal failure more often than those without hypertension.[97] However, it is uncertain if long-term control of plasma glucose or reduction of circulating insulin concentration is achievable or if it has any long-term effect on renal function. Another endocrine abnormality, altered calcium metabolism and increased parathyroid hormone activity seen in blacks, may be important particularly if there is an increased renal accumulation of calcium. In this regard, Harris et al.[98] have shown that calcium channel blockade can decrease renal calcium content and slow the rates of renal failure in animals with experimental renal disease.

In the United States, renal failure appears to be most strongly associated with less well educated and lower income groups. These populations are less likely to receive adequate medical care, are least likely to afford medications, to take time from work for follow-up and are most likely, therefore, to have the hypertension inadequately treated. Although not universally agreed to, several studies show that control of blood pressure and adequate follow-up are associated with a slower rate of decline of renal function in people with hypertension.[99, 100] Since blacks make up a large portion of lower socioeconomic groups in the United States, we may have a partial explanation for their greater rate of H-ESRD. Moreover, cultural and attitudinal differences toward medical care between blacks and whites may also serve as additional barriers to adequate medical care.

In summary, the many factors that affect blood pressure are under the variable control of genetic and environmental forces. Careful assessment of these factors reveals some racial differences in physiology and cell metabolism that may contribute to the increased prevalence of hypertension and increased susceptibility of H-ESRD seen in blacks. However, lack of standardized studies makes it difficult to determine if these differences are intrinsic to the black race or are the result of a different degree of physiologic adaptation to environmental stresses.

References

1. National Center for Health Statistics: Blood pressure levels in persons 18-74 years of age in 1976-80 and trends in blood pressure from 1960 to 1980 in the United States. Vital and Health Statistics. Series 11, No 234. Public Health Service. Washington DC, U.S. Government Printing Office, DHHS publication No. 86-1684, pp 1–68.
2. US Renal Data System: USRDS 1989 Annual Report. Bethesda, Md, The National Institutes of Health, National Institute of Diabetes and Digestive and Kidney Diseases, 1989, pp 1–11.
3. McClellan W, Tuttle E, Issa A: Racial differences in the incidence of hypertensive end-stage renal disease (ESRD) are not entirely explained by differences in the prevalence of hypertension. *Am J Kidney Dis* 1988; 12:285–290.
4. Rostand SG, Kirk KA, Rutsky EA, et al: Racial differences in the incidence of treatment for end-stage renal disease. *N Engl J Med* 1982; 306:1276–1279.
5. Weller JM, Wu S-Ch, Ferguson W, et al: End-stage renal disease in Michigan. Incidence, underlying causes, prevalence and modalities of treatment. *Am J Nephrol* 1985; 5:84–95.
6. Cooper R: A note on the biologic concept of race and its application in epidemiologic research. *Am Heart J* 1984; 103:715–723.
7. Gerbase-DeLima M, DeLima JJG, Persoli LB, et al: Essential hypertension and histocompatibility antigens: A linkage study. *Hypertension* 1989; 14:604–609.
8. Feinleib M, Garrison RJ, Fabsitz R, et al: The NHLBI twin study of cardiovascular disease risk factors: Methodology and summary of results. *Am J Epidemiol* 1977; 106:284–295.
9. Annest JL, Sing CF, Biron P, et al: Familial aggregation of blood pressure and weight in adoptive families. II. Estimation of the relative contributions of genetic and common environmental factors to blood pressure correlations between family members. *Am J Epidemiol* 1979; 110:492–503.
10. Moll PP, Harburg E, Burns TL, et al: Heredity, stress and blood pressure, a family set approach: The Detroit project revisited. *J Chronic Dis* 1983; 36:317–328.
11. Pérusse L, Rice T, Bouchard C, et al: Cardiovascular risk factors in a French-Canadian population: Resolution of genetic and familial environmental effects on blood pressure by using extensive information on environmental correlates. *Am J Hum Genet* 1989; 45:240–251.
12. Keil JE, Tyroler HA, Sandifer SH, et al: Hypertension: Effects of social class and racial admixture: The results of a cohort study in the black population of Charleston, South Carolina. *Am J Public Health* 1977; 67:634–639.

13. Harburg E, Gleibermann L, Roeper P, et al: Skin color, ethnicity and blood pressure: I. Detroit blacks. *Am J Public Health* 1978; 68:1177–1183.
14. Johnson CS, Giorgio AJ: Arterial blood pressure in adults with sickle cell disease. *Arch Intern Med* 1981; 141:891–893.
15. Cierpial MA, McCarty R: Hypertension in SHR rats: Contribution of maternal environment. *Am J Physiol* 1987; 253:980–984.
16. Guyton AC, Coleman TG, Cowley AW Jr, et al: Arterial pressure regulation: Overriding dominance of the kidneys in long-term regulation and in hypertension. *Am J Med* 1972; 52:584–594.
17. Farman N, Bonvalet JP: Abnormal relationship between sodium excretion and hypertension in spontaneously hypertensive rats. *Pfluegers Arch* 1975; 354:39–53.
18. Rostand SG, Lewis D, Watkins JB, et al: Attenuated pressure natriuresis in hypertensive rats. *Kidney Int* 1982; 21:330–338.
19. Tobian L, Lange J, Azar S, et al: Reduction of natriuretic capacity and renin release in isolated, blood-perfused kidneys of Dahl hypertensive-prone rats. *Circ Res* 1978; 43:92–98.
20. Luft FC, Grim CE, Fineberg N, et al: Effects of volume expansion and contraction in normotensive whites, blacks and subjects of different ages. *Circulation* 1979; 59:643–650.
21. Weinberger MH, Miller JZ, Luft FC, et al: Definitions and characteristics of sodium sensitivity and blood pressure resistance. *Hypertension* 1986; 8:127–134.
22. Grim CE, Luft FC, Miller JZ, et al: An approach to the evaluation of genetic influences on factors that regulate arterial blood pressure in man. *Hypertension* 1980; 2:34–42.
23. Luft FC, Weinberger MH, Grim CE: Sodium sensitivity and resistance in normotensive humans. *Am J Med* 1982; 72:728–736.
24. Luft FC, Miller JZ, Cohen SJ, et al: Heritable aspects of salt sensitivity. *Am J Cardiol* 1988; 61:1–6.
25. Weinberger MH, Miller JZ, Finebert NS, et al: Association of haptoglobin with sodium sensitivity and resistance of blood pressure. *Hypertension* 1987; 10:443–446.
26. Frohlich ED: Hemodynamic differences between black patients and white patients with essential hypertension. *Hypertension* 1990; 15:675–680.
27. Lifton RP, Hopkins PN, Williams RR, et al: Evidence for heritability of nonmodulating essential hypertension. *Hypertension* 1989; 13:884–889.
28. Warren SE, O'Connor DT: Does a renal vasodilator system mediate racial differences in essential hypertension? *Am J Med* 1980; 69:425–429.
29. Frohlich ED, Messerli FZ, Dunn FG, et al: Greater renal vascular involvement in the black patient with essential hypertension: A comparison of systemic and renal hemodynamics in black and white patients. *Miner Electrolyte Metab* 1984; 10:173–177.
30. Levy SB, Talner LB, Coel MN, et al: Renal vasculature in essential hypertension: Racial differences. *Ann Intern Med* 1978; 88:12–16.
31. Mitas JA, Levy SB, Holle R, et al: Urinary kallikrein activity in the hypertension of renal parenchymal disease. *N Engl J Med* 1978; 299:162–165.
32. Berry TD, Hasstedt SJ, Hunt SC, et al: A gene for high urinary kallikrein may protect against hypertension in Utah kindreds. *Hypertension* 1989; 13:3–8.
33. Hollenberg NK, Borucki LJ, Adams DF: The renal vasculature in early essential hypertension: Evidence for a pathogenetic role. *Medicine* 1978; 57:167–178.

34. Kohno M, Yasunari K, Murakawa K-I, et al: Plasma immunoreactive endothelin in essential hypertension. *Am J Med* 1990; 88:614–618.
35. Ku DD: Increase in endothelin contraction in renal arteries but not in aortae of the Dahl 'S' hypertensive rats. *Physiologist* 1990; 33:53.
36. Bolin P, Jaffa AA, Rust PF, et al: Acute and chronic responses of human renal kallikrein and kinins to dietary protein. *Am J Physiol* 1989; 257:718–723.
37. Tobian L: Potassium and sodium in hypertension. *J Hypertension* 1988; 6:12–24.
38. Reaven GM: Role of insulin resistance in human disease. *Diabetes* 1988; 37:1595–1607.
39. Ferrannini E, Defronzo RA: The association of hypertension, diabetes, and obesity: A review. *J Nephrol* 1989; 1:3–15.
40. Landsberg L: Diet, obesity and hypertension: An hypothesis involving insulin, the sympathetic nervous system and adaptive thermogenesis. *Q J Med* 1986; 61:1080–1090.
41. Pollare T, Lithell H, Berne C: Insulin resistance is a characteristic feature of primary hypertension independent of obesity. *Metabolism* 1990; 39:167–174.
42. Falkner B: Differences in blacks and whites with essential hypertension: Biochemistry and endocrine. *Hypertension* 1990; 15:681–686.
43. Advance Data from Vital and Health Statistics, no 130. Hyattsville, Md, Public Health Service, DHHS Publication No 87-1250, pp 1–16.
44. Knowler WC, Pettitt DJ, Saad MF, et al: Diabetes mellitus in the Pima Indians: Incidence, risk factors and pathogenesis. *Diabetes Metab Rev* 1990; 6:1–27.
45. DeFronzo RA, Goldberg M, Agus ZS: The effects of glucose and insulin on renal electrolyte transport. *J Clin Invest* 1976; 58:83–90.
46. Rostand SG, Watkins JB, Clements RS Jr: The effect of insulin and anti-insulin serum on handling of sodium by the isolated, perfused kidney of the streptozotocin-diabetic rat. *Diabetes* 1980; 29:679–685.
47. Moore RD: Effect of insulin upon the sodium pump in frog skeletal muscle. *J Physiol (London)* 1973; 232:23–45.
48. Hall JE, Coleman TG, Mizelle HL, et al: Chronic hyperinsulinemia and blood pressure regulation. *Am J Physiol* 1990; 258:722–731.
49. Messerli FH, DeCarvalho JGR, Christie B, et al: Essential hypertension in black and white subjects: Hemodynamic findings and fluid volume state. *Am J Med* 1979; 67:27–31.
50. Harshfield GA, Alpert BS, Willey ES, et al: Race and gender influence ambulatory blood pressure patterns of adolescents. *Hypertension* 1989; 14:598–603.
51. O'Connor DT, Levine GL, Frigon RP: Homologous radio-immunoassay of human plasma dopamine-B-hydroxylase: Analysis of homospecific activity, circulating plasma pool and intergroup differences based on race, blood pressure and cardiac function. *J Hypertension* 1983; 1:227–233.
52. Fredrickson M: Racial differences in cardiovascular reactivity to mental stress in essential hypertension. *J Hypertension* 1986; 4:325–331.
53. Light KC, Obrist PA, Sherwood A, et al: Effects of race and marginally elevated blood pressure on responses to stress. *Hypertension* 1987; 10:555–563.
54. Murphy JK, Alpert BS, Moes DM, et al: Race and cardiovascular reactivity: A neglected relationship. *Hypertension* 1986; 8:1075–1083.

55. Ekelund L-G, Suchindran CM, Karon JM, et al: Black-white differences in exercise blood pressure: The lipid research clinics program prevalence study. *Circulation* 1990; 31:1568–1574.
56. Dimsdale J, Ziegler M, Graham R: The effect of hypertension, sodium and race on isoproterenol sensitivity. *Clin Exp Hypertens Theory Pract* 1988; 10:747–756.
57. Dimsdale JF, Graham R, Zieger MG, et al: Age, race, diagnosis and sodium effects on the pressor responses to infused norepinephrine. *Hypertension* 1987; 10:564–569.
58. Falkner B, Kushner H: Effect of chronic sodium loading on cardiovascular response in young blacks and whites. *Hypertension* 1990; 15:36–43.
59. Aviv A, Gardner J: Racial differences in ion regulation and their possible links to hypertension in blacks. *Hypertension* 1989; 14:584–589.
60. Canessa M, Spalvins A, Adragna N, et al: Red cell sodium countertransport and cotransport in normotensive and hypertensive blacks. *Hypertension* 1984; 6:344–351.
61. Weder AB, Torretti BA, Julius S: Racial differences in erythrocyte cation transport. *Hypertension* 1984; 6:115–123.
62. Lijnen P, M'Buyamba-Kabangu J-R, Fagard R, et al: Erythrocyte concentrations and transmembrane fluxes of sodium and potassium in essential hypertension: Role of intrinsic and environmental factors. *Cardiovasc Drugs Therapy* 1990; 4:321–333.
63. Persky V, Ostrow D, Langenberg P, et al: Hypertension and sodium transport in 390 healthy adults in Chicago. *J Hypertension* 1990; 8:121–128.
64. Hasstedt SJ, Hunt SC, Wu LL, et al: The inheritance of intraerythrolytic sodium level. *Am J Med Genet* 1988; 29:193–203.
65. Williams RR, Hasstedt SJ, Hunt SC, et al: Genetic studies of cation tests and hypertension. *Hypertension* 1987; 10:37–41.
66. Aalkjaer C: Regulation of intracellular pH and its role in vascular smooth muscle function. *J Hypertension* 1990; 8:197–206.
67. Aviv A: The link between cytosolic Ca2+ and the Na+–H+ antiport: A unifying factor for essential hypertension. *J Hypertension* 1988; 6:685–691.
68. Berk BC, Vallega G, Muslin AJ, et al: Spontaneously hypertensive rat vascular smooth muscle cells in culture exhibit increased growth and Na+/H+ exchange. *J Clin Invest* 1989; 83:822–829.
69. Lifton RP, Hunt SC, Williams RR, et al: Exclusion of the Na+/H+ antiporter as a candidate gene in human hypertension. *Clin Res* 1990; 38:469.
70. Schmouder RL, Weder AB: Platelet sodium-proton exchange is increased in essential hypertension. *J Hypertension* 1989; 1:325–330.
71. Kuriyama S, Hopp L, Tamura H, et al: A higher cellular sodium turnover rate in cultured skin fibroblasts from blacks. *Hypertension* 1988; 11:301–307.
72. Ives HE: Ion transport defects and hypertension: Where is the link? *Hypertension* 1989; 14:590–597.
73. Haddy FJ: Potassium, Na+–K+ pump inhibitor and low renin hypertension. *Clin Invest Med* 1987; 10:547–554.
74. Songu-Mize E, Alpert BS, Willey ES: Race, sex and family history of hypertension and erythrocyte sodium pump [^{3}H[ouabain binding. *Hypertension* 1990; 15:146–151.
75. DeLuise M, Blackburn GL, Flier JS: Reduced activity of red-cell sodium-potassium pump in human obesity. *N Engl J Med* 1980; 303:1017–1022.
76. Stunkard AJ, Harris JR, Pedersen NL, et al: The body-mass index of twins who have been reared apart. *N Engl J Med* 1990; 322:1483–1487.

77. Dustan HP: Obesity and hypertension in blacks. *Cardiovasc Drugs Therapy* 1990; 4:395–402.
78. Akinkugbe OO: World epidemiology of hypertension in blacks, in Hall WD, Sanders E, Shulman NB (eds): *Hypertension in Blacks: Epidemiology, Pathophysiology and Treatment.* Chicago, Year Book Medical Publishers, 1985, pp 3–16.
79. Joseph JG, Prior AM, Salmond CE, et al: Evaluation of systolic and diastolic blood pressure associated with migration: The Tokelau Island migrant study. *J Chronic Dis* 1983; 36:507–516.
80. Langford HG, Watson RL: Potassium and calcium intake, excretion and homeostasis in blacks, and their relation to blood pressure. *Cardiovasc Drugs Therapy* 1990; 4:403–406.
81. Loomis WF: Skin-pigment regulation of vitamin-D biosynthesis in man. *Science* 1967; 157:501–506.
82. Bell NH, Greene A, Epstein A, et al: Evidence for alteration of the vitamin-D endocrine system in blacks. *J Clin Invest* 1985; 76:470–473.
83. Weinstein RS, Bell NH: Diminished rates of bone formation in normal black adults. *N Engl J Med* 1988; 319:1698–1701.
84. McCarron DA: Ca^{2+}, vitamin D, parathyroid hormone and blood pressure: Why should it matter? *J Lab Clin Med* 1987; 110:663–664.
85. Resnick LM, Muller FB, Laragh JH: Calcium-regulating hormones in essential hypertension: Relation to plasma renin activity and sodium metabolism. *Ann Intern Med* 1986; 105:649–654.
86. Kim H, Kalkhoff RK, Costrini NV, et al: Plasma insulin disturbances in primary hyperparathyroidism. *J Clin Invest* 1971; 50:2596–2605.
87. Salahudeen AK, Thomas TH, Sellars L, et al: Hypertension and renal dysfunction in primary hyperparathyroidism: Effect of parathyroidectomy. *Clin Sci* 1989; 76:289–296.
88. Tyroler HA: Socioeconomic status, age and sex in the prevalence and prognosis of hypertension in blacks and whites, in Laragh JH, Brenner BM (eds): *Hypertension: Pathophysiology, Diagnosis and Management.* New York, Raven Press, 1990, pp 159–174.
89. Anderson NB, Myers HF, Pickering T, et al: Hypertension in blacks: Psychosocial and biological perspectives. *J Hypertension* 1989; 7:161–172.
90. Rostand SG, Brown G, Kirk KA, et al: Renal insufficiency in treated essential hypertension. *N Engl J Med* 1989; 320:684–688.
91. Brazy PC, Fitzwilliam JF: Progressive renal disease: Role of race and antihypertensive medications. *Kidney Int* 1990; 37:1113–1119.
92. Ferguson R, Grim CE, Opgenorth TJ: A familial risk of chronic renal failure among blacks on dialysis? *J Clin Epidemiol* 1988; 41:1189–1196.
93. Curtis JJ, Luke RG, Dustan HP, et al: Remission of essential hypertension after renal transplantation. *N Engl J Med* 1983; 309:1009-1115.
94. Curtis JJ, Luke RG, Diethelm AG, et al: Benefits of removal of native kidneys in hypertension after renal transplantation. *Lancet* 1985; 2:739–742.
95. Schrier RW, Harris DCH, Chan L, et al: Tubular hypermetabolism as a factor in the progression of chronic renal failure. *Am J Kidney Dis* 1988; 12:243–249.
96. Tobian L, MacNeill D, Johnson MA, et al: Potassium protection against lesions of the renal tubules, arteries and glomeruli and nephron loss in salt-loaded hypertensive Dahl S rats. *Hypertension* 1984; 6:170–176.
97. Krolewski AS, Canessa M, Warram JH, et al: Predisposition to hypertension

and susceptibility to renal disease in insulin-dependent diabetes mellitus. *N Engl J Med* 1988; 318:140–145.

98. Harris DCH, Hammond WS, Burke TJ, et al: Verapamil protects against progression of experimental chronic renal failure. *Kidney Int* 1987; 31:41–46.
99. Brazy PC, Stead WW, Fitzwilliam JF: Progression of renal insufficiency: Role of blood pressure. *Kidney Int* 1989; 35:670–674.
100. Pettinger WA, Lee HC, Reisch J, et al: Long-term improvement in renal function after short-term blood pressure control in hypertensive nephrosclerosis. *Hypertension* 1989; 13:766–772.

Search for the Gene Responsible for Polycystic Kidney Disease and Its Clinical Consequences

Martijn H. Breuning, M.D. Ph.D.

Department of Human Genetics, State University Leiden, Sylvius Laboratories, Leiden, The Netherlands

Jasper J. Saris

Department of Human Genetics, State University Leiden, Sylvius Laboratories, Leiden, The Netherlands

Johannes G. Dauwerse

Department of Human Genetics, State University Leiden, Sylvius Laboratories, Leiden, The Netherlands

Liesbeth Breslau-Siderius

Department of Clinical Genetics, Academic Hospital Maastricht, Maastricht, The Netherlands

Martin C. Wapenaar

Department of Human Genetics, State University Leiden, Sylvius Laboratories, Leiden, The Netherlands

Gert-Jan B. van Ommen, Ph.D.

Department of Human Genetics, State University Leiden, Sylvius Laboratories, Leiden, The Netherlands

Polycystic kidney disease is an important cause of renal failure. The most frequent form of polycystic kidney disease shows autosomal dominant inheritance.[1] The gene responsible for this type of polycystic kidney disease was mapped to the short arm of chromosome 16 in 1985.[2] The mutation responsible for the disease was proved to be tightly linked to a highly polymorphic marker, the 3′hypervariable region, close to the gene coding for the α chain of hemoglobin.[3] Since that time, an intensive search for the gene has been started. A large number of DNA fragments on the short arm of chromosome 16 was isolated.[4] A physical map around the polycystic kidney disease 1 (PKD1) gene was constructed,[5] and so-called candidate genes are being investigated.

Meanwhile, the DNA fragments close to the mutation responsible for polycystic kidney disease can be used for presymptomatic and prenatal diagnosis of the disease.[6] The use of DNA marker studies in families is particularly helpful when young patients below the age of 30 years wish to know whether or not they have inherited the mutation. Ultrasonography at this young age can give false-negative results[7] of up to 15%. With DNA marker studies, the diagnosis of disease in the family members of a patient can be reinforced. In addition DNA markers are helpful when intrafamilial kidney transplantation is considered. In such cases, absolute certainty on the status of the donor is essential.

However, the adult form of polycystic kidney disease has been shown to be genetically heterogeneous. In some families, the mutation is not linked to markers on the short arm of chromosome 16.[8, 9] In one large family, a suggestion of linkage has been found with a DNA marker on chromosome 2.[10] In this chapter, we will outline the use of DNA markers on chromosome 16 in the clinic. Some of the pitfalls inherent to this approach, such as genetic heterogeneity and nonpaternity, will be outlined.

Materials and Methods

Diagnosis of Polycystic Kidneys

For the diagnosis of cyst formation in the kidneys, ultrasonography is the method of choice.[11] For the number of false-negative results with ultrasound we have used the criteria formulated by J. C. Bear et al.[7]

DNA Studies

Probes for the analysis of the short arm of chromosome 16 have been described in detail elsewhere.[4] Briefly, DNA was isolated from peripheral blood lymphocytes with standard methods[12] and was digested with restriction enzymes under appropriate conditions, run overnight on 0.7% agarose gels, and blotted on filters. The filters were hybridized with probes labeled with ^{32}P with a multiprime labeling kit (Amersham). After washing, the filters were exposed to x-ray films, which were developed after 24 to 48 hours. The names of the probes used for DNA analysis of the families depicted in this paper are given in the figures, as well as the restriction enzymes showing the polymorphism.

Risk Calculation

In families in which this is necessary the risk can be calculated with the computer programs designed for genetic linkage studies from the LINKAGE package.[13]

Results and Discussion

The adult form of polycystic kidney disease is dominantly inherited. By the time the disease is detected, most of the patients have passed on the mutation to their offspring. Questions from the patients regarding the utility of presymptomatic diagnosis in their children and their brothers and sisters can be expected. Since the nephrologist is used to dealing with individual patients suffering from kidney disease, such questions can be difficult to handle. Advantages of early diagnosis, such as early treatment of hyper-

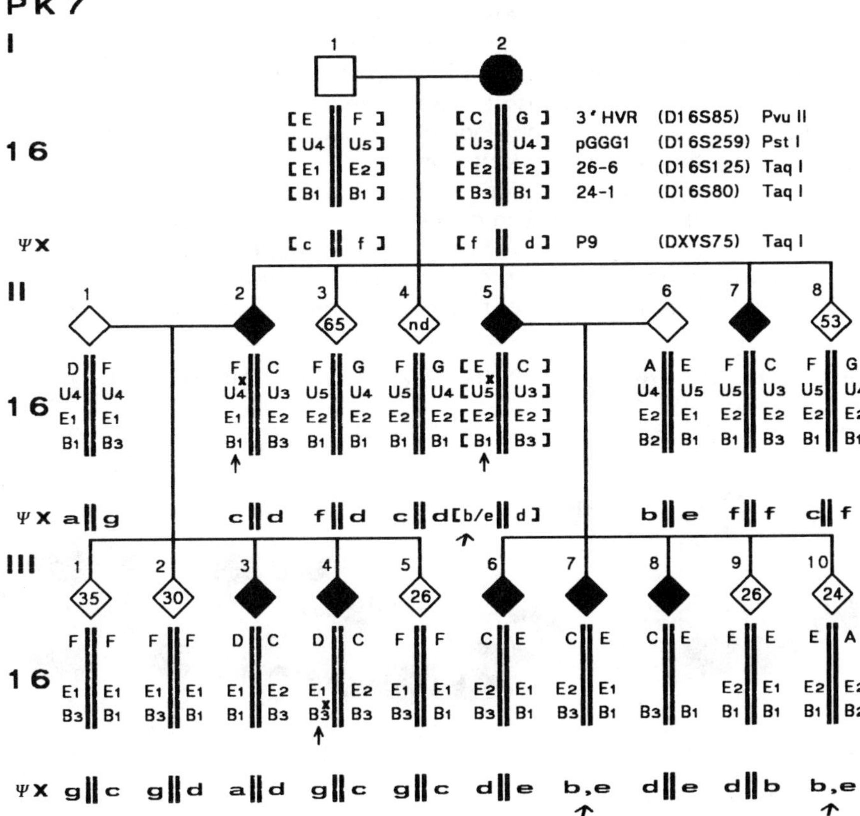

FIG 1.
Family with polycystic kidney disease. Sex of family members not shown, for reasons of privacy. *Filled symbols* = affected; *open symbols* = negative ultrasound at age depicted within; *nd* = no ultrasound done. *Straight arrows* indicate apparent single recombinations, oblique arrows indicate unexpected bands. Inferred typings are given within brackets. The PKD1 mutation maps between pGGG1 (U), and 26-6 (E) on chromosome 16.[4] P9 is a highly polymorphic marker on the chromosomal region shared between the X and Y chromosomes (pseudo-autosomal region).[20]

tension and urinary tract infection, and family planning on an informed basis, as well as disadvantages, such as employment or insurance problems, have to be discussed.

Technically, the family study is performed in three steps: first, counseling of all members of the family wishing to participate; second, laboratory research consisting of ultrasonography and blood sampling of all at-risk family members for DNA studies and evaluation; and third, reporting to the family and counseling affected individuals. Genetic markers are used to follow the inheritance of the mutation through the pedigree. In large families, the chromosome carrying the mutation can be readily recognized, and in the absence of recombination between the mutation and surrounding genetic markers, the predictions are highly accurate.[4] In Figure 1, we show a large family in which the mutation responsible for polycystic kidney disease can be followed with the C,U3,E2,B3 haplotype. If one of the individuals in generation three would wish to have prenatal diagnosis performed, this would be possible with a high degree of accuracy with polymorphic DNA markers on either side of the mutation.

However, on closer inspection, we detect two apparent recombinations between 3′HVR and pGGG1 in generation II (II,2, and II,5). When the filters containing the DNA of this family were hybridized with a highly polymorphic marker on the X and Y chromosomes, the probe P9 (DXYS75) (Fig 2) individual II,5 turned out to have a band (B or E in Fig 1, 2) not

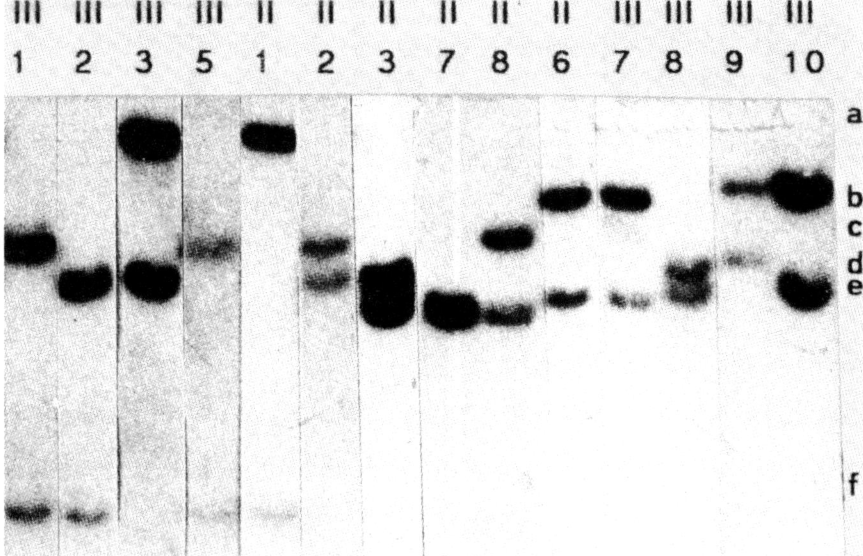

FIG 2.
Filter of DNA from the family in Figure 1 digested with the restriction enzyme Taq I, and hybridized with P9.[20] For clarity, the lanes have been reordered. II,4, III,4, and III,6 not shown.

present among the five siblings. Most likely, this is a case of nonpaternity. This finding is in fact fortuitous, since this identified the mother as the affected parent (consistent with anamnestic information), and shows that errors due to nonpaternity can be prevented even two generations later, after all the individuals concerned are dead. When sufficient polymorphic markers are tested around the mutation, a paternity problem will very rarely lead to a wrong diagnosis, provided the family is of sufficient size to show clearly the linkage phase of the markers under study.

The adult form of polycystic kidney disease has been shown to be genetically heterogeneous.[8, 9] Figure 3 shows a family with independent segregation of the mutation responsible for polycystic kidney disease, and chromosome 16 markers. There is no recombination between 3′HVR, PGP, and the VK5 marker, except in individual II,6, in whom the maternal or paternal chromosome shows a single recombination event between 3′HVR and VK5. The E-1-V1 haplotype is found twice in an unaffected individual and three times in an affected person. The haplotype F-2-V2 is found twice in an affected individual and twice in an unaffected individual. The PDK1 mutation maps in the part of chromosome 16 *between* 3′HVR and VK5.[4] The presence of the same haplotype for markers on both sides of the PKD1 gene in affected and unaffected family members can only be explained by double recombination events (crossover both between 3′HVR and PKD1, and between PKD1 and VK5). The probability of a double recombination between 3′HVR and VK5 is less than 1 in 400. In this family, at least 4 such double recombinants should have occurred if

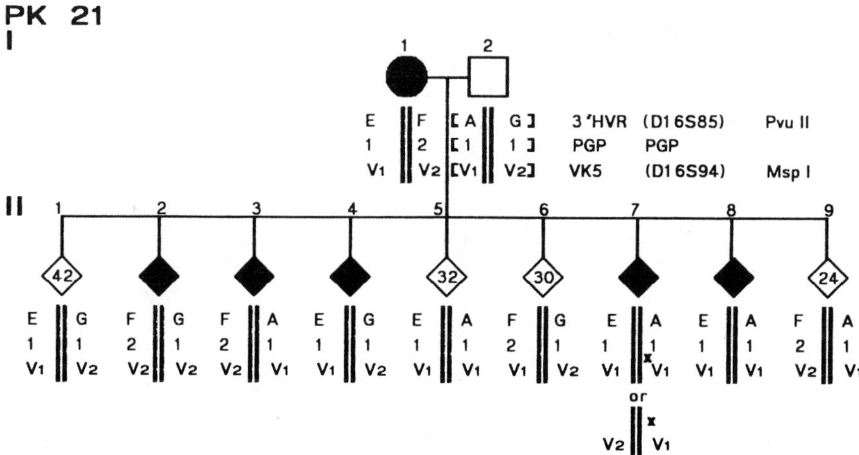

FIG 3.
Family with polycystic kidney disease. Sex of family members not shown for reasons of privacy. *Filled symbols* = affected; *open symbols* = negative ultrasound at age depicted within; *PGP* = phosphoglycolate phosphatase, a protein marker;[21] the localization of PGP relative to PKD1 is not known.[4] PKD1 maps between 3′HVR and VK5.[4]

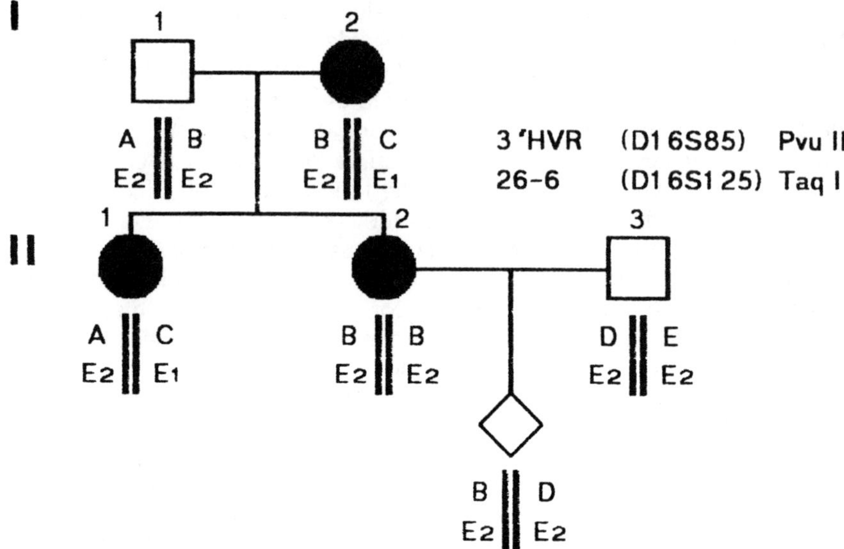

FIG 4.
Family with polycystic kidney disease. PKD1 maps between 3′HVR and 26-6. II,1 and II,2 have inherited different flanking markers from the affected mother.

the mutation responsible for polycystic kidney were at PKD1. A mutation at another locus (PKD2, etc) is the more likely explanation.

In large families, the problems of nonpaternity and nonlinkage can be easily traced, but in small families, a clear indication of nonlinkage can be found sometimes. In Figure 4, a small family is shown in which two siblings have inherited a different haplotype of informative DNA markers around PDK1 from the affected parent. Since a double recombination is extremely rare, this is most likely a case of nonlinkage. Therefore, DNA marker studies will not be helpful for a prenatal diagnosis in the ongoing pregnancy of individual II,2.

DNA marker studies can be useful in presymptomatic diagnosis of the disease. However, both patients and nephrologists find it difficult to ask for cooperation from family members, many of whom are not aware of being at risk for the mutation. For this reason, the clinician would prefer to have a direct test to identify mutations at the PKD1 gene. The hunt for the PKD1 gene is now drawing to a close.[5] Undoubtedly new methods will be developed to diagnose the disease once the mutated gene has been identified. Recent results in other inherited diseases have shown, however, that family studies continue to be necessary in many of the cases. It is at this time difficult to predict whether presymptomatic diagnosis will be performed later on individual family members by direct detection of the mutation, or whether the tracking of the mutation through the family will continue to be needed. For example, with Duchenne's muscular dystrophy, caused by mutations in the short arm of the X chromosome, only 60% of the patients have a deletion, which can be identified directly.[14] In another inherited disease, cystic fibrosis, one and the same mutation accounts for almost all cases in Scandinavia.[15] This so-called δF508 mutation is a deletion of three nucleotides.[16, 17] In southern Europe, however, only approximately 50% of the carriers have the δF508 mutation.[18] In those families in which the mutation cannot be directly identified, carrier detection and prenatal diagnosis are still based on polymorphic markers flanking the affected gene.[19] Until the PKD1 gene and some of its mutations have been characterized, we do not know whether only one, or a few, or many different changes in the structure of the gene are responsible for the disease. We expect, therefore, that the approach to the family with polycystic kidney disease we have described here will continue to be used in the coming years.

References

1. Dalgaard OZ: Bilateral polycystic disease of the kidneys: A follow-up of two hundred and eighty four patients and their families. *Acta Med Scand* 1957; 328:1–255.
2. Reeders ST, Breuning MH, Davies KE, et al: A highly polymorphic DNA marker linked to adult polycystic kidney disease on chromosome 16. *Nature* 1985; 317:542–544.
3. Jarman AP, Nicholls RD, Weatherall DJ, et al: Molecular characterisation of a hypervariable region downstream of the alpha-globin gene cluster. *EMBO J* 1986; 5:1857–1863.
4. Breuning MH, Snijdewint FGM, Brunner H, et al: Map of 16 polymorphic loci on the short arm of chromosome 16 close to the polycystic kidney disease gene (PKD1). *J Med Genet* 1990; 27:603–613.
5. Germino GG, Barton NJ, Lamb J, et al: Identification of a locus which shows no recombination with the autosomal polycystic kidney disease gene on chromosome 16. *Am J Hum Genet* 1990; 46:925–933.
6. Reeders ST, Zerres K, Gal A, et al: Prenatal diagnosis of autosomal dominant polycystic kidney disease using a DNA probe. *Lancet* 1986; 2:7–9.
7. Bear JC, McManamon P, Morgan J, et al: Age at clinical onset and at ultrasonographic detection of adult polycystic kidney disease—data for genetic counseling. *Am J Med Genet* 1984; 18:45–53.
8. Romeo G, Devoto M, Costa G, et al: A second genetic locus for autosomal dominant polycystic kidney disease. *Lancet* 1988; 2:8–10.
9. Kimberling WJ, Fain PR, Kenyon JB, et al: Linkage heterogeneity of autosomal polycystic kidney disease. *N Engl J Med* 1988; 319:913–917.
10. Norby S, Schwartz M: Possible locus for polycystic kidney disease on chromosome 2. *Lancet* 1990; 336:323–324.
11. Hogewind BL, Veltkamp JJ, Koch CW, et al: Genetic counseling for adult polycystic kidney disease. Ultrasound a useful tool in presymptomatic diagnosis? *Clin Genet* 1980; 18:168–172.
12. Breuning MH, Snijdewint FGM, Dauwerse JG, et al: Two step procedure for early diagnosis of polycystic kidney disease with polymorphic DNA markers on both sides of the gene. *J Med Genet* 1990; 27:614–617.

13. Lathrop GM, Lalouel JM: Easy calculations of lod scores and genetic risks on small computers. *Am J Hum Genet* 1984; 36:460–465.
14. den Dunnen JT, Grootscholten PM, Bakker E, et al: Topography of the Duchenne muscular dystrophy (DMD) gene: FIGE and cDNA analysis of 194 cases reveals 115 deletions and 13 duplications. *Am J Hum Genet* 1989; 45:835–847.
15. Schwartz M, Johansen HK, Koch C, et al: Frequency of the delta F508 mutation on cystic fibrosis chromosomes in Denmark. *Hum Genet* 1990; 85:427–428.
16. Kerem BS, Rommens JM, Buchanan JA, et al: Identification of the cystic fibrosis gene: Genetic analysis. *Science* 1989; 245:1073–1080.
17. Riordan JR, Rommens JM, Kerem BS, et al: Identification of the cystic fibrosis gene: Cloning and characterization of complementary DNA. *Science* 1989; 245:1066–1072.
18. European Working Group on CF Genetics: Gradient of distribution in Europe of the major CF mutation and of its associated haplotype. *Hum Genet* 1990; 85:436–445.
19. Bakker E, Kneppers ALJ, Voorhoeve E, et al: Advances and pitfalls in prenatal diagnosis: Five year DNA-analysis for Duchenne and Becker muscular dystrophy and hemophilia, in Angelini C (ed): *Proceedings of a Satellite Symposium on Muscular Dystrophy Research: Molecular Diagnosis Towards Therapy.* Elsevier, Amsterdam, 1990.
20. Wapenaar MC, Pearson PL, van Ommen GJB: P9 (DXYS75) detects a VNTR-type RFLP in the pseudoautosomal region (abstract). *Nucleic Acids Res* 1990; 18:384.
21. Reeders ST, Breuning MH, Corney G, et al: Two genetic markers closely linked to adult polycystic kidney disease on chromosome 16. *Br Med J* 1986; 292:851–853.

Autosomal Dominant Polycystic Kidney Disease: Cellular and Molecular Mechanisms of Cyst Formation

Patricia D. Wilson, Ph.D.

Associate Professor, Department of Physiology and Biophysics, University of Medicine and Dentistry of New Jersey, Robert Wood Johnson Medical School at Rutgers, Piscataway, New Jersey

Christopher R. Burrow, M.D.

Assistant Professor, Division of Nephrology, The Johns Hopkins University School of Medicine, Baltimore, Maryland

Autosomal dominant polycystic kidney disease (ADPKD) is one of the most common purely genetic disorders in humans with an estimated 5 million individuals at risk worldwide.[1] The primary target organ for the phenotypic expression of this gene abnormality is the kidney in which certain populations of renal tubules enlarge progressively until renal function is compromised, typically in the third or fourth decade of life. At present no therapy has been proven to retard the expansion of cysts, and end-stage renal failure ensues and is treated with dialysis or transplantation. Although the ADPKD-1 gene, linked to the hypervariable α-globin locus on the short arm of chromosome 16[2] is thought to have 100% penetrance, there is a wide variation in both the age of appearance of cysts and in the rapidity of progression to renal failure. This could be explained partially by the expression of a different, non-chromosome 16 linked gene (ADPKD-2) in a subgroup of approximately 10% of patients,[3] but might also suggest additional environmental or genetic factors involved in the regulation of cyst enlargement. Gabow et al.[4] have clearly demonstrated that the ADPKD gene(s) has pleiotropic effects including the generation of cysts in the liver, intestinal diverticulae, intracranial aneurysms, and mitral valve prolapse.

Although renal cyst formation is a multiple and asynchronous event that can apparently result from the enlargement of any segment of the nephron,[5] the end result is consistent and results in the formation of a distended, fluid-filled sac lined by a layer of structurally simplified, but polarized epithelial cells. To achieve this condition, at least two processes must occur in each individual cyst: abnormal epithelial cell proliferation to account for the growth of the cyst lining[6] and fluid accumulation to account for the distension. Several cellular and molecular mechanisms have been shown to control and influence epithelial cell proliferation in a variety of cell systems in vivo and in vitro, including the nature of the basement membrane and extracellular matrix on which the epithelial cells rest and the mitogenic effects of specific peptide growth factors. In addition, it is well known that the vectorial transport of fluid across renal epithelia is the result of electrochemical and osmotic gradients established by the activity and polarized membrane location of the NaK-ATPase (sodium pump) enzyme.

The aim of our studies has been to identify any alterations in proliferative or transport control mechanisms that operate in human ADPKD and might contribute to cyst formation. Our approach has been to microdissect and compare human cystic and normal segmental renal tubule epithelia in fully defined monolayer cultures,[7–9] with the ultimate goal to identify the primary gene product(s) responsible for cyst expansion and thereby to devise strategies to inhibit or reverse this destructive process. Biochemical and morphologic characterization studies have demonstrated that primary cultures derived from individually microdissected normal human renal proximal convoluted tubules (PCT), proximal straight tubules (PST), collecting tubules (CT), thick ascending limbs of Henle's loop (TAL), and from ADPKD cyst linings retain similar levels of expression of differentiated structure and function as the epithelium of origin prior to culture.[8, 9] This has been effected by the use of fully defined, segment-specific, serum-free, transferrin and growth factor-supplemented culture media and explantation onto collagen-coated tissue culture substrates.[7, 10]

Proliferation and Growth Control of ADPKD Epithelia

Primary cultures of renal tubule epithelia of normal and ADPKD origin show the following similar overall stages of growth: an initial lag phase, during which no cell division takes place; a period of rapid exponential proliferation; and a maintenance phase, during which cell division has ceased but differentiated properties are expressed.[8] Finally, cell death ensues unless the monolayers are passaged. Plating of equal numbers of epithelial cells from normal human renal tubules and ADPKD cyst linings in parallel suggest an innate proliferative abnormality in ADPKD epithelia, in that they undergo approximately three times more rounds of cell division and can be maintained in a stationary but fully functional state for longer periods of time in primary culture (Fig 1). In addition, ADPKD epithelia can be passaged up to 15 times, while normal renal epithelia survive only 5 passages.

Influence of Extracellular Matrix on Growth

The basement membrane lining ADPKD cysts in pathologic specimens often shows thickening and abnormalities in structure and density.[9] Culture

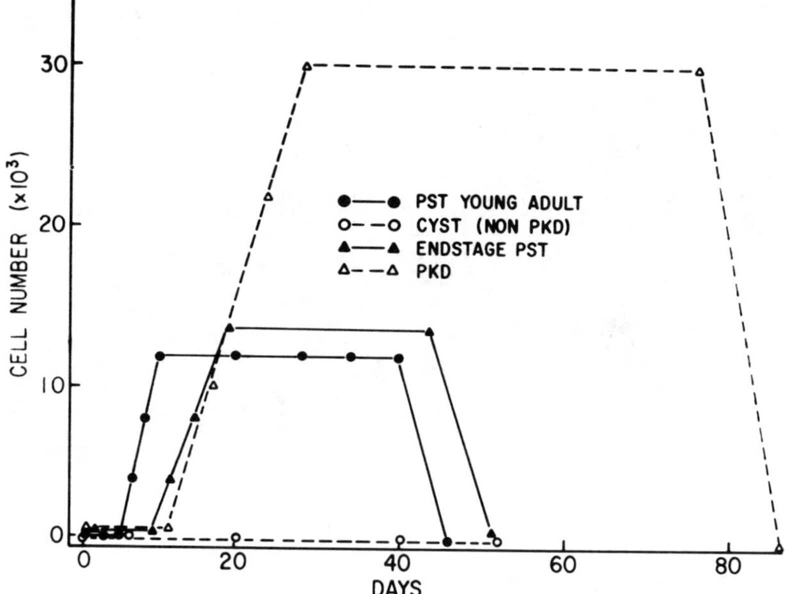

FIG 1.
Growth kinetics of normal, diseased, and PKD epithelia in primary culture. Equal numbers of cells (10^4) were plated on collagen-coated plastic in Hepes buffered, Click-RPMI media containing human transferrin (5 μg/mL), dexamethasone (5×10^{-8}M) insulin (5 μg/mL) and 3% heat-inactivated fetal bovine serum. Normal PST and PST derived from end-stage, non-ADPKD kidneys showed identical growth kinetics, while in ADPKD epithelia, more rounds of cell division and longer maintenance were seen. Cells lining simple renal cysts did not proliferate under these conditions.

of ADPKD epithelia in vitro also showed significant alterations in basement membrane structure by comparison to cultures of normal renal tubules. Instead of the characteristic thin, contiguous layer of electron dense material secreted at the basal surface of normal renal tubule monolayers, ADPKD cultures showed basal secretion of a thickened, discontinuous layer of protein in the form of spheroids that stained with ruthenium red (Fig 2). Since this staining suggested a proteoglycan component in the abnormal basement membrane, studies were conducted to measure the uptake and secretion of ^{35}S-labeled inorganic sulfate into basement membrane extracts from confluent cultures of ADPKD and normal PST epithelia.[11] Incorporation of $H_2{}^{35}SO_4$ (200 μCi/mL) was increased tenfold in ADPKD monolayers over a 24-hour period (85.9×10^4 vs. 8.5×10^4 cpm/μg protein, respectively). This suggests a more rapid turnover of sulfated proteoglycans in ADPKD basement membranes and work is in progress to determine whether this is related to a defect in proteolytic processing.

Immunostaining has been used to demonstrate the location of laminin, type IV collagen, and heparan sulfate proteoglycan in tissue sections from

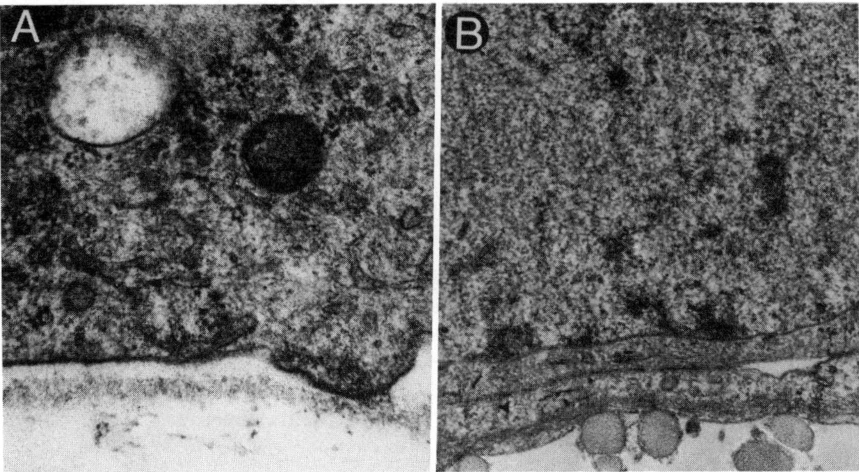

FIG 2.
Electron micrographs of normal vs. ADPKD confluent monolayers, showing the basement membrane region. **A,** normal PST show a thin, continuous layer of electron dense material closely apposed to the basal cell surface (X 128,000). **B,** ADPKD epithelia show a discontinuous, wide basement membrane region containing numerous proteinaceous spheroids with small electron dense deposits of ruthenium red, indicative of proteoglycan content (X 128,000).

normal and end-stage ADPKD kidneys. In each case, staining was polarized and confined to the basement membrane regions lining glomeruli and tubules in normal kidneys and lining cysts in ADPKD kidneys. Type I collagen was localized in the interstitium of all kidneys. In vitro, differences were seen in the ability of extracellular matrix components to stimulate epithelial cell proliferation (Table 1). Mitogenic assays showed that the incorporation of ^{3}H-thymidine into 90% confluent monolayer cultures was increased fourfold in ADPKD epithelia by comparison to normal PST epithelia when tissue culture plates were precoated with type IV collagen and twofold when grown on type I collagen. However, no differences were seen when laminin or fibronectin was the exogenous matrix protein.

Influence of Growth Factors on Epithelial Proliferation

Modifications in the proliferation of renal tubule epithelia to generate cysts in ADPKD might be caused by altered response to soluble growth factors. Mitogenic assays were conducted on parallel series of cultures derived from normal renal tubules and ADPKD epithelia.[12] In cultures of normal proximal tubules (PST) plated on type I collagen, maximal incorporation of ^{3}H-thymidine was mediated by serum-free culture media supplemented with dexamethasone (5×10^{-8} M) and insulin (5 μg/mL). ADPKD epithelia grown under identical conditions showed a significant increase in incorporation (Fig 3). This suggests that endocrine growth factors may elicit an

TABLE 1.
Effects of Extracellular Matrix Components on Epithelial Proliferation*

Matrix	PST	ADPKD
Type I collagen	31 ± 8	72 ± 10†
Type IV collagen	14 ± 4	65 ± 8†
Laminin	20 ± 8	26 ± 4

*Equal numbers (10^4) cells were plated on tissue culture plastic ($1 cm^2$) precoated with extracellular matrix and grown to 80% confluence in Hepes-buffered Click-RPMI media supplemented with human transferrin (5 μg/mL), dexamethasone (5×10^{-8} M) and insulin (5 μg/mL). ^{3}H-thymidine (10 μCi/mL) was added to the medium for 4 hours, the cells washed five times for 5 minutes each in cold phosphate buffered saline (PBS), dissolved in 1N NaOH and cellular incorporation of ^{3}H measured by liquid scintillation.
†$P < .01$, $n = 10$.

increased proliferative response from ADPKD epithelia and this may play a role in cyst formation.

In a survey of mitogenic effects of a wide range of growth factors, it was shown that epidermal growth factor (EGF) was the most potent mitogen for ADPKD epithelia and that its mitogenic stimulation was significantly increased over that in normal renal tubule epithelia (see Fig 3). Since EGF immunoreactivity was detected in ADPKD cyst-lining epithelial cells, in cyst fluid, and in conditioned media of ADPKD cells, this implicates EGF as an autocrine regulator of ADPKD epithelial proliferation. This notion is further supported by the highly mitogenic activity of cyst fluid and ADPKD-conditioned media on normal and ADPKD epithelial cultures (Fig 4). The mechanisms involved in this hypersensitivity include increase in number of high affinity EGF receptors in ADPKD membrane vesicle preparations by comparison to those prepared from normal age-matched kidneys and the location of some of those receptors in the apical membrane fractions. High affinity EGF receptors were located only on the basal membranes from normal kidneys. This alteration in polarized membrane location of ADPKD EGF receptors was also demonstrated by EGF receptor immunostaining localized on the apical membranes of some cyst lining epithelia in vivo and with specific ^{125}I-EGF binding to the apical cell surfaces of confluent ADPKD epithelia grown in vitro on dual compartment, permeable membranes.[12, 13] These changes in EGF receptor number and

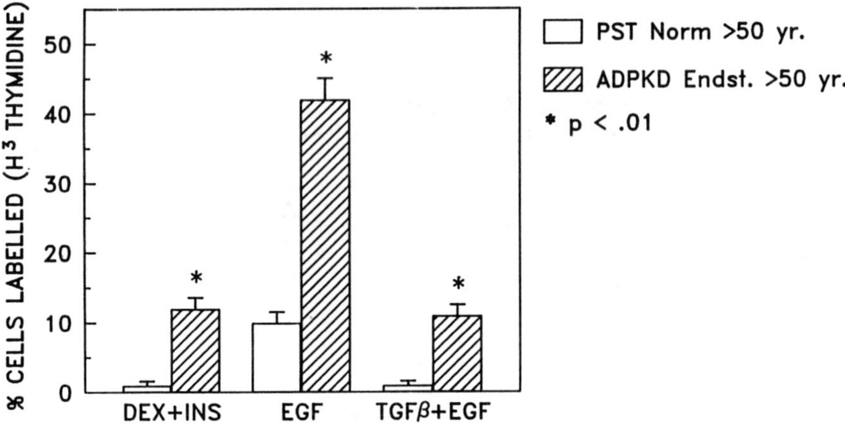

FIG 3.
Mitogenic effect of growth factors on epithelial monolayer cultures of normal PST and end-stage ADPKD. Cultures grown to 90% confluence were rendered quiescent by incubation for 2 days in Click-RPMI media containing transferrin but no growth factors. No ^{3}H-thymidine incorporation was observed in cultures maintained in this media. After 2 days of growth factor deprivation, such quiescent normal PST and ADPKD cultures were incubated in media containing one or more of the following growth factors: dexamethasone (5×10^{-8}M), insulin (5 μg/mL), EGF (5 ng/mL), and TGFβ 20 ng/mL. ^{3}H-thymidine (1 μCi/mL) was added to the media for the final 24 hours, monolayers were washed, fixed, and subjected to autoradiography. Labeled nuclei were counted and expressed as percent of total cells in the culture. *Open bar* = PST normal more than 50 years; *hatched bar* = ADPKD endstage more than 50 years; $^*P < .01$.

polarity occur during the early stages of the disease, before the onset of renal failure.

Changes were also seen in the intracellular protein calpactin II (lipocortin I), which is one of the major substrates phosphorylated by the EGF receptor tyrosine kinase after ligand binding. Calpactin II is one of the five overabundant proteins characterized in ADPKD extracts by sodium dodecyl sulfate (SDS)-polyacrylamide gel electrophoresis and Western analysis.[14] These studies suggest that hypersensitivity to EGF may also in part be the result of increased substrate levels in ADPKD epithelia.

Additional significant alterations in growth factor sensitivity of ADPKD cultures included a loss of complete inhibition of mitogenesis by transforming growth factor β(TGFβ) (see Fig 3). Since TGFβ immunoreactivity was also detected in cyst lining epithelia and in the collecting duct system of normal kidneys, this may have relevance for loss of growth inhibition in vivo in cyst formation. Fibroblast proliferation in the interstitium of ADPKD kidneys is also marked and mitogenic assays carried out on co-cultures of ADPKD epithelia and fibroblasts showed that platelet-derived growth factor (PDGF) was a specific mitogen for fibroblasts but not epithelia. Since

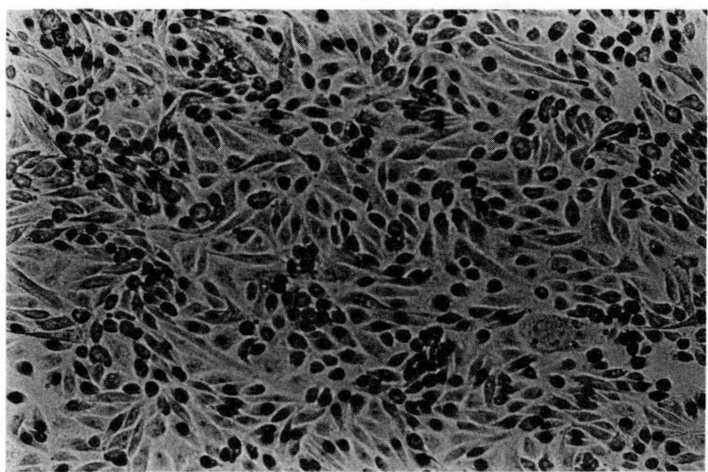

FIG 4.
Autoradiograph of mitogenic activity of ADPKD conditioned media. ADPKD epithelia were grown to 90% confluence, rendered quiescent as described in Figure 3 and incubated for 2 days with conditioned media collected and concentrated twentyfold from ADPKD confluent cultures. ^{3}H-thymidine (1 μCi/mL) was added to the media for the final 24 hours and cells washed, fixed, and autoradiographed. Numerous black labeled nuclei are seen (X 100).

PDGF immunoreactivity was detected only in the cyst lining epithelia in ADPKD kidneys, this suggests a paracrine mechanism of fibroblast growth regulation.

Factors Controlling Fluid Accumulation in ADPKD

NaK-ATPase

The Na^+ ion is the major osmotic determinant in the kidney, and the activity and polarized membrane location of the NaK-ATPase enzyme, which actively pumps sodium out of cells, is ultimately responsible for the generation of electrochemical and osmotic gradients necessary for fluid reabsorption. Widely divergent NaK-ATPase activities are found in different renal tubule segments and these reflect differences in numbers of enzyme molecules.[15] The net vectorial movement across normal renal epithelia is from apical to basal compartments, transporting Na^+ ions from tubule lumen into the blood, and this is always associated with a basolateral membrane location of the NaK-ATPase pump.

The NaK-ATPase molecule is thought to be a heterodimeric complex of α and β subunits. The α subunit (Mr 100,000) has the molecular structure of a typical membrane transport protein with seven hydrophobic, membrane-spanning domains and bears the catalytically important phosphorylation, ATP- and ouabain-binding sites. The β subunit (Mr 55,000) is a glycosylated protein that spans the membrane only once and whose interaction with α subunits is essential for correct membrane insertion and for expression of activity.[16]

Biochemical assays of the catalytic activity of NaK-ATPase in whole tissue homogenates showed a significantly increased specific activity in ADPKD vs. age-matched normal kidneys (Table 2). In particular, activity was induced sixfold in early stage ADPKD, suggesting this may be an important change associated with the onset of cyst formation. With ^{32}P-labeled cDNA probes for α and β subunits of NaK-ATPase for Northern analysis, it was suggested that induction at the transcriptional level alone may not be sufficient to account for the observed activity increase.[10] With comparative densitometric scans of Northern blots, preliminary results, however, suggested possible increased relative expression of β subunit in ADPKD compared to normal age-matched kidneys (J.T. Norman, personal communication, 1990).

A major difference between the membrane location of NaK-ATPase in ADPKD and normal tissues was detected by enzyme cytochemical techniques and also by immunostaining using antibodies against the α subunit of NaK-ATPase (graciously donated by Dr. W. J. Nelson). Both in vivo and in vitro, NaK-ATPase reactivity was confined to the apical membranes of cyst lining epithelia. This was the complete reverse of the basolateral membrane staining in normal renal tubule epithelia (Fig 5). The apparent complete reversal of polarity of NaK-ATPase was further confirmed by specific binding of ^{3}H-ouabain exclusively to apical membrane vesicle preparations from ADPKD kidneys and to basolateral membrane vesicles from normal kidneys.[10] The functional significance of this change was demonstrated in confluent cultures of ADPKD epithelia grown of permeable membranes with separate access to media compartments bathing api-

TABLE 2.
Specific Activity of NaK-ATPase

Condition	Activity*
Normal (n = 10)	1.91 ± 0.5
Early stage ADPKD (n = 5)	6.00 ± 0.9
End-stage ADPKD (n = 10)	4.25 ± 1.9

*Activity was expressed as μmol adenosine diphosphate (ADP)/30 min/mg protein in homogenate; all samples were from donors 32 to 36 years old.

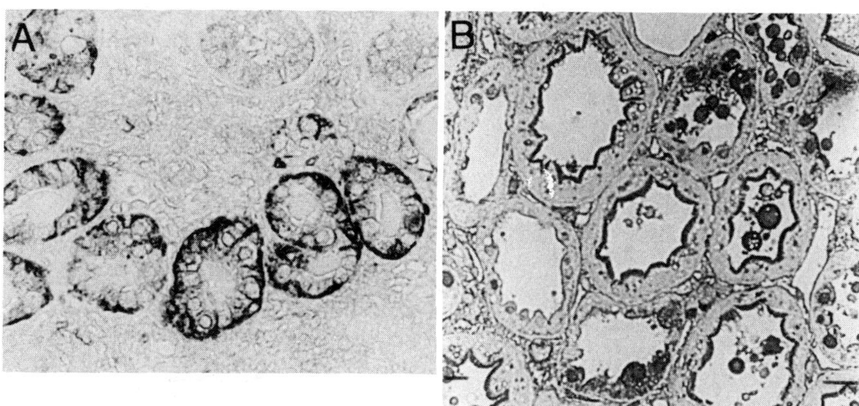

FIG 5.
Avidin-biotin immunoperoxidase staining of NaK-ATPase α subunit antibody 1:100 on 4% paraformaldehyde fixed tissue sections. **A,** staining of basolateral epithelial cell membranes of proximal and distal tubules in a normal human kidney, 45 years (X 155). **B,** staining restricted to apical plasma membranes of minimally expanded cystic tubules in a kidney with early stage ADPKD, 43 years (X 120). This suggests that the altered polarity of NaK-ATPase occurs as an early effect of cystic enlargement.

cal and basal cell surfaces. Vectorial transport of ^{22}NaCl was monitored using liquid scintillation measurements of media samples. The net movement of ^{22}Na added to the basal media compartments of tight ADPKD monolayers was into the apical media compartment and this movement could be inhibited by the apical application of ouabain, but not by ouabain added in the basal media. The reverse was the case in cultures of normal cortical collecting tubules (CCT) since net vectorial transport of ^{22}NaCl was from apical to basal media compartments and basal ouabain addition inhibited movement (Fig 6).

Inhibitor studies showed that in ADPKD epithelia, furosemide and bumetanide inhibited basal uptake of ^{22}NaCl, while amiloride inhibited apical ^{22}Na uptake. This allowed us to construct the model for transporters present in ADPKD epithelia shown in Figure 7, suggesting apically located Na/H antiporters and basally located Na^+,K^+,$2Cl^-$ transporters. It is of importance to emphasize that studies concerning the localization of a number of membrane proteins in ADPKD have failed to demonstrate a general loss or reversal of polarity, since the polarized location of several matrix and integral membrane and transport proteins is quite normal. Examples include the basal location of laminin, fibronectin, type IV collagen, heparan sulfate proteoglycan and the band 3 transporter; and the apical location of the microvillar associated proteins of GP330, α95kD and alkaline phosphatase. This suggests that the altered polarity of NaK-ATPase to the apical membranes of ADPKD cyst epithelia is a specific event, resulting from altered sorting signals at the molecular level.

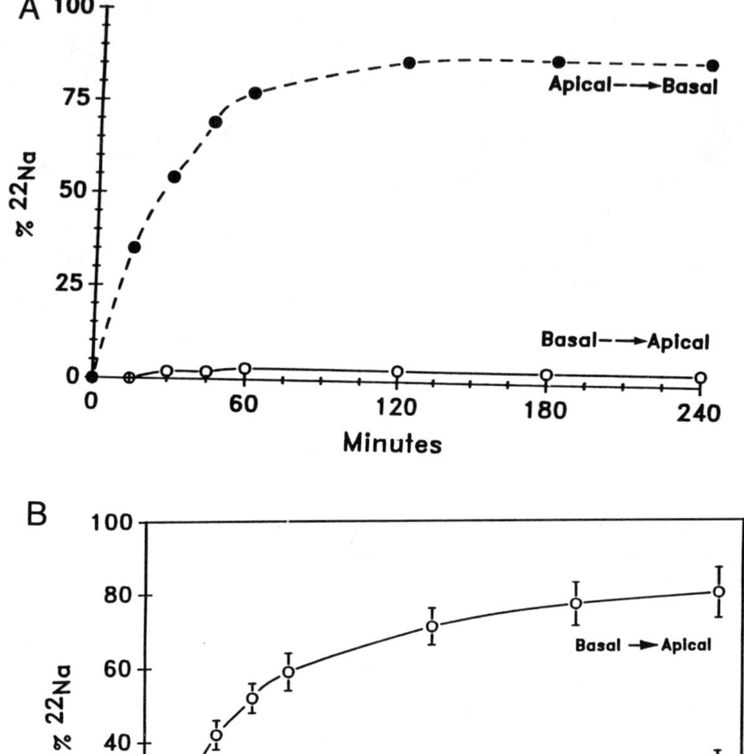

FIG 6.
^{22}Na transport across confluent epithelial monolayers grown on permeable membranes with independent access to apical and basal media compartments. Prior to experimentation, monolayers were judged as tight if they generated an electrical resistance and did not allow passage of ^{14}C-inulin. ^{22}NaCl (1 μCi/mL) was then added either to the apical or the basal media compartment and the appearance of ^{22}Na measured with time by sampling of the media in the contralateral compartment and liquid scintillation counting. **A,** in normal CCT cultures, ^{22}Na was transported only from the apical to basal media. There was no basal to apical movement. **B,** in ADPKD epithelial cultures, the net movement of ^{22}Na was from basal to apical media compartments (80%), whereas only 20% of ^{22}Na was transported from apical to basal compartments. This shows that there is reversal of net vectorial movement of ^{22}Na in ADPKD epithelia.

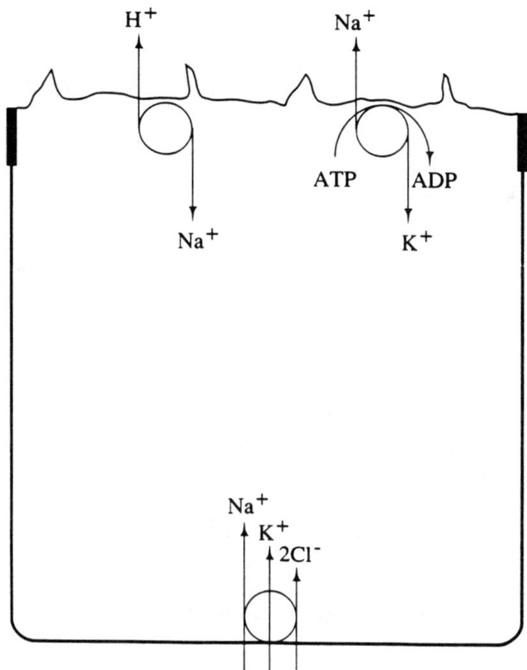

FIG 7.
A schematic model of sodium transporters in ADPKD epithelia. Inhibitor studies suggest that the apical plasma membranes of cyst-lining epithelia contain the ouabain-sensitive sodium pump enzyme, NaK-ATPase, which drives sodium out at a rate which exceeds that of its uptake by the apically located amiloride-sensitive Na/H antiporter. Basal uptake of ^{22}Na is effected by a bumetanide and furosemide-sensitive $Na^{+}K^{+}2Cl^{-}$ cotransporter.

Potential mechanisms involved in this alteration in NaK-ATPase polarity in ADPKD epithelia include a mutation at the transcriptional level resulting in the production of faulty message for one or both of the NaK-ATPase subunits. The β subunit may be considered a good potential candidate since it is involved with antibody complex assembly and membrane insertion. NaK-ATPase subunits are encoded by a multigene family and to date, 3 α and 2 β isoforms have been cloned and sequenced from several species, including human.[17–20] Although there is extensive homology between subunit isoforms in different species, the pattern of isoform expression is clearly tissue specific and developmentally regulated. With the use of cDNA probes it has been shown that the α1 isoform is most commonly expressed in kidney tissue, α2 is expressed mainly in brain, and α3 expression has been reported in a variety of tissues including brain, kidney, and fetal tissues.[21, 22] The β1 and β2 isoforms have also been detected in sev-

```
a1 SENSE :        5'-GAT TAC AAC GGC TGA TAG-3'
a1 ANTISENSE:     5'-TTG GAC GTG ATA AGT ATG-3'


a3 SENSE:         5'-GAA-AAG AAG GTG ATG TTC-3'
a3 ANTISENSE:     5'-GAC AAG AAA GAT GAC AAG-3'


b1 SENSE:         5'-TTC ATC TGG AAC TCA GAG-3'
b1 ANTISENSE:     5'-TCA AGC TTG AAT CTG CAG-3'


b2 SENSE:         5'-AGA CTG AGA ACC TTG ATG-3'
b2 ANTISENSE:     5'-ATG CGA CAT TCT ACA TTC-3'
```

FIG 8.
Sense and antisense oligonucleotide probes for human NaK-ATPase α1, α3, β1, and β2 subunits.

eral tissues, including kidney.[18, 19, 23] Experiments were designed to analyze the expression of α and β isoforms in defined epithelia dissected and cultured from early and end-stage ADPKD and age-matched normal renal tubules. The polymerase chain reaction (PCR) was utilized to amplify message from small numbers of cells. Total RNA was isolated from confluent cultures and reverse transcribed to cDNA by random hexamer priming. Sense and anti-sense primer pairs, each 18-nucleotides in length, were constructed for the amplification of human α1, α3, β1 and β2 NaK-ATPase isoforms, delineating 409, 701, 419 and 529-mers, respectively (Fig 8). Since the N-terminal regions of the proteins are the most divergent,[20] the sense primer was positioned towards the 5′ end of the coding region. PCR analysis, using each primer pair, showed that only α1 and β1 products could be amplified from defined epithelial cultures of normal human CCT and TAL, early stage and end-stage ADPKD cysts (Fig 9). Studies are in progress to determine whether the isoforms expressed in normal and ADPKD cells differ in sequence.

Cytoskeletal Changes

Cytoskeletal proteins play a major structural role in cells and the actin-based membrane skeleton has been implicated in normal sorting and anchoring of membrane proteins in polarized renal epithelia.[24] In ADPKD kidneys, one- and two-dimensional Western blot analysis not only demonstrated that actin was a major protein, significantly more abundant than in extracts from normal kidneys, but also that novel, acidic isoforms occur in ADPKD.[25] Since actin can interact with ankyrin and fodrin to anchor NaK-ATPase and other membrane proteins, their role in ADPKD has been studied with immunofluorescence and some colocalization of staining with the apically mistargetted NaK-ATPase demonstrated (Fig 10). No information is available to determine whether these cytoskeletal abnormalities are primary or secondary to the NaK-ATPase defect.

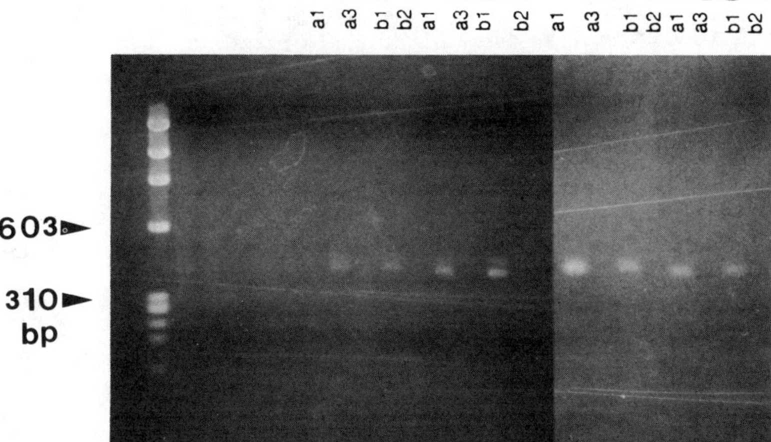

FIG 9.
Amplification of NaK-ATPase α1, α3, β1, and β2 isoform fragments in cDNA reverse transcribed from RNA isolated from cultures of normal human adult collecting tubules *(CCT),* thick ascending limbs of Henle *(TAL),* early stage ADPKD *(E)* and end-stage ADPKD *(ES)* cyst epithelia. Products of α1 and β1 are seen and are of the predicted sizes 410 and 418 bp, respectively. Samples of 100 μL contained standard buffer, 200 nM each dNTP, 30 pM each primer, 1 ng cDNA, and 1 U Taq polymerase and were subjected to 30 cycles of 94° C 45 sec, 55° C 10 sec, and 72° C 60 sec.

Additional cytoskeletal modulations have been described and relate to an increased abundance of the calcium-phospholipid actin binding protein, calpactin II (lipocortin I), which is also a major substrate for the tyrosine kinase activity of the EGF receptor. It is also of interest that in ADPKD, calpactin I was shifted from Triton insoluble to soluble fractions, which may further implicate some role for cytoskeletal proteins in the sorting and targeting defects of ADPKD cells.

Membrane Phospholipid Changes

Since calpactin II is thought to inhibit phospholipase A2 activity by binding to and sequestering membrane phospholipid, alterations in arachidonic acid metabolites have been studied. In assays designed to examine arachidonic acid release in vitro, ADPKD cultures not only showed lower levels of unstimulated release than cultures of normal renal tubule epithelia, but the majority was released into apical compartments instead of into basal media compartments.[14, 25] Studies are in progress to delineate the effects of EGF stimulation on arachidonic acid release in ADPKD and normal epithelia and to determine whether there are gross differences in phospholipid composition in ADPKD cell membranes compared to normal epithelia.

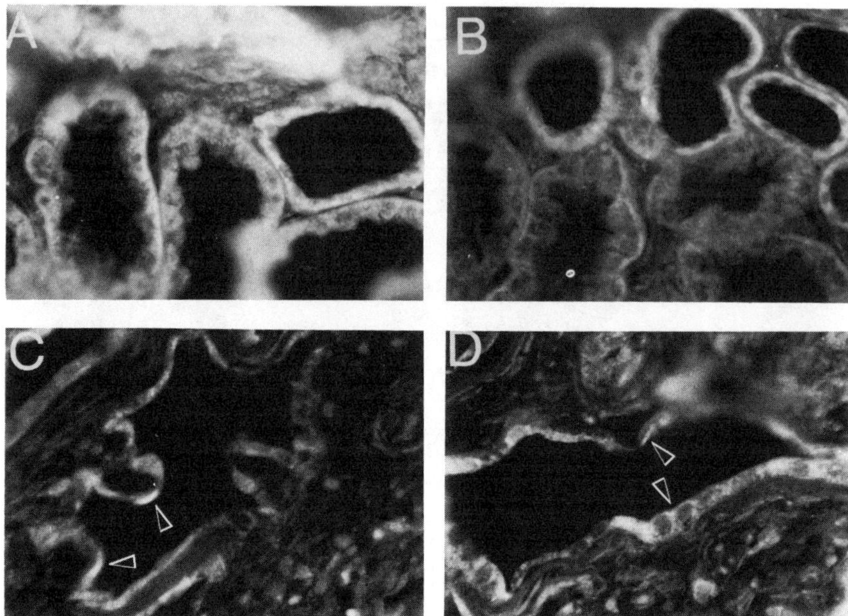

FIG 10.
Immunofluorescence staining of ankyrin and fodrin antibodies in normal and ADPKD kidneys. **A,** ankyrin staining in basolateral membranes of a normal distal tubule (X 100). **B,** fodrin staining in basolateral membranes of a normal distal tubule (X 100). **C,** ankyrin staining associated with apical membranes *(arrows)* in ADPKD cyst lining epithelia (X 100). **D,** fodrin staining in ADPKD cyst lining epithelia (X 100).

Discussion and Perspectives

In the past, several theories have been proposed to account for cystic enlargement of tubules in polycystic kidney disease, including obstruction, increased basement membrane compliance, secretion and hyperplasia. However, none of these properties has been shown to be the primary cause of cystic expansion. It is clear from our own studies described above and from those of others that the ADPKD mutant gene product elicits wide-ranging and pleiotropic effects. To elucidate the prime determining factor(s) leading to the onset of cyst formation, it is necessary to examine those changes that occur at the earliest stages of expression of the disease in vivo or to study active, cyst forming cells in vitro. Using such cellular approaches, we conclude that there are at least two fundamental modifications in ADPKD epithelial cells related to their ability to form cysts: an increased capacity to proliferate and reversed membrane polarity of NaK-ATPase, since both of these properties have been demonstrated in kidneys derived from early stage ADPKD kidneys, prior to the onset of renal malfunction. However, at present, no information is available as to which, if either of these changes is the primary event leading to cystic expansion.

In vitro, the increased proliferative capacity of ADPKD epithelia can be seen in response to specific extracellular matrix proteins and to soluble growth factors, notably EGF. The potential importance of EGF in autocrine regulation of increased proliferation in ADPKD kidneys in vivo is emphasized by the existence of increased receptor numbers and translocation of a population of high-affinity receptors to the apical membranes of ADPKD epithelia in early stages of the disease. Although analogies may be drawn between the proliferative defect clearly apparent in ADPKD and those seen in hyperplasia and tumor formation,[26, 27] there are also notable differences. In ADPKD, there is not a complete loss of growth control. Cysts enlarge, but at some point in time cease to do so, and although a small percentage of cysts produce hyperplastic nodules, the majority of cysts are lined by a single layer of epithelium, rather than the formation of solid balls of cells as would be the case in tumorigenesis. This limited proliferative defect is also evident in vitro. Although microdissected ADPKD epithelia can be cultured through more passages than similarly treated normal renal epithelia, they do not produce immortal cell lines, pile up or grow in soft agar, as would be expected in neoplastically transformed cells. This may explain why the search for significant increase or novel protooncogene expression in the early stages of ADPKD has proved disappointing in our hands. To date the only alteration documented has been an elevation in the constitutively expressed c-*myc* in the murine (cpk) model of recessive PKD.[28] Since these studies were conducted in animals late in the course of cyst formation a casual role could not be determined. Intriguing findings in transgenic mice harboring the early region of the SV40 chromosome which contains T-antigen coding sequences showed production of choroid plexus tumors, glomerulosclerosis, and renal cysts.[29, 30] This could suggest a link between oncogene expression, tumor and cyst formation or may simply reflect renal cyst formation as a common response to trauma. This might be analagous to renal cysts induced by age, dialysis, or drugs. Although it cannot be ruled out that the proliferative changes seen in ADPKD might be akin to a preneoplastic type of condition, future studies should also consider the possibility of reversion to the proliferative condition seen during renal development, since the ADPKD gene is naturally present at this stage. Our working hypothesis is that the ADPKD gene could encode a regulatory element, transiently expressed during development and involved in the establishment of epithelial cell polarity.

This would be consistent with our findings of a major reversal of polarity of the NaK-ATPase protein inserted into the apical membranes of a subset of renal tubules destined to expand and become cysts, but the normal basolateral location of NaK-ATPase in renal tubules with normal morphology. Later in the progression of the disease, the proliferative nature of the cystic epithelia with apical NaK-ATPase would cause expansion and physically squeeze out the normal tubules and lead to renal failure. The actual mutation might be as simple as an alteration in NaK-ATPase sequence with resultant effects on complex assembly, sorting in the Golgi, sorting vesicle or cytoskeletal interactions, or insertion into specific plasma membrane domains. However, the demonstration of additional alterations in membrane polarity in the distribution of EGF receptors and apical secretion of ^{35}S-methionine-labeled proteins and arachidonic acid seem to suggest a more basic defect in the signaling machinery responsible for polarized sorting in epithelial cells. The absence of major disturbances in polarity of the majority of polarized membrane proteins, however, also suggests that the mutation cannot be so fundamental as to destroy all sorting signals. Indeed, such a mutation would surely be lethal. Rather, it would seem likely to reside in a signal responsible for the polarized sorting of a particular subset of proteins and lipids.

In summary, although much progress has been made toward understanding the cellular changes associated with cyst formation in ADPKD, the question remains as to the nature of the ADPKD gene product, and how this is expressed. Once we fully understand which of the many cellular defects is the primary event which triggers the rapid expansion of cysts, the final goal may be achieved to prevent cystic expansion in those patients carrying the ADPKD gene.

Acknowledgments

This work was supported by National Institutes of Health grants R01DK40698 and P01DK34039, and tissue was supplied by the Cooperative Human Tissue Network and Institute for the Advancement of Medicine.

Reference

1. Polycystic Kidney Research Foundation Report, Kansas, Mo, 1988.
2. Reeders ST, Breuning MH, Davies KE, et al: A highly polymorphic DNA marker linked to adult polycystic kidney disease on chromosome 16. *Nature* 1985; 317:542–544.
3. Kimberling WJ, Fain PR, Kenyon JB, et al: Linkage heterogeneity of autosomal dominant polycystic kidney disease. *N Engl J Med* 1988; 319:913–918.
4. Gabow PA, Ikle DW, Holmes LH: Polycystic kidney disease. Progressive analysis of nonazotemic patients and family members. *Ann Intern Med* 1984; 101:238–247.
5. Grantham JJ: Polycystic kidney disease: A predominance of giant nephrons. *Am J Physiol* 1983; 244:3–10.
6. Welling LW, Welling D: Theoretical models of cyst formation and growth. *Scan Microsc* 1988; 2:1097–1102.
7. Wilson PD, Anderson RJ, Breckon RD, et al: Retention of differentiated characteristics by cultures of defined rabbit kidney epithelia. *J Cell Physiol* 1987; 130:245–254.
8. Wilson PD, Dillingham MA, Breckon RD, et al: Defined human renal tubular

epithelia in culture: Growth characterization and hormonal response. *Am J Physiol* 1985; 248:436–443.
9. Wilson PD, Schrier RW, Breckon RD, et al: A new method for studying polycystic kidney disease epithelia in culture. *Kidney Int* 1986; 30:371–378.
10. Wilson PD, Sherwood AC, Palla K, et al: Reversed polarity of $Na+K^+$-ATPase: Mislocation to apical plasma membranes in polycystic kidney disease epithelia. *Am J Physiol,* in press.
11. Wilson PD, Hreniuk D, Gabow PA: Relationship between abnormal extracellular matrix and excessive growth of human adult polycystic kidney disease epithelia. *J Cell Physiol,* in press.
12. Wilson PD, Du J, Norman JT: Autocrine, endocrine and paracrine regulation of growth abnormalities in autosomal dominant polycystic kidney disease. *Eur J Cell Biol,* in press.
13. Du J, Wilson PD: Mislocation of high affinity epidermal growth factor receptors in human autosomal dominant polycystic kidney disease (abstract). *J Am Soc Nephrol* 1990; 1:627.
14. Sherwood AC, Wilson PD: Actin cytoskeleton in autosomal dominant polycystic kidney disease epithelial cells (abstract). *Kidney Int* 1990; 37:229.
15. Katz AI, Doucet A, Morel F: Na,K-ATPase activity along the rabbit, rat and mouse nephron. *Am J Physiol* 1979; 237:114–120.
16. McDonough AA, Geering K, Farley RA: The sodium pump needs its β subunit. *Faseb J* 1990; 4:1598–1605.
17. Kawakami K, Ohta T, Nojima H, et al: Primary structure of the a-subunit of human Na,K-ATPase deduced from cDNA sequence. *J Biochem* 1986; 100:389–397.
18. Kawakami K, Nojima H, Ohta T, et al: Molecular cloning and sequence analysis of human Na,K-ATPase b-subunit. *Nucleic Acid Res* 1986; 14:2833–2844.
19. Martin-Vasallo P, Dackowski W, Emanuel JR, et al: Identification of a putative isoform of the Na,K-ATPase b subunit. Primary structure and tissue specific expression. *J Biol Chem* 1989; 264:4613–4618.
20. Shull MM, Lingrel JB: Multiple genes encode the human Na+K+-ATPase catalytic subunit. *Proc Natl Acad Sci* 1987; 84:4039–4043.
21. Shull GE, Greeb J, Lingrel JB: Molecular cloning of three distinct forms of the $Na+K^+$-ATPase a-subunit from rat brain. *Biochemistry* 1986; 25:8125–8132.
22. Sverdlov ED, Akopyanz NS, Petrukhin KE, et al: Na+,K+-ATPase: Tissue specific expression of genes coding for α-subunit in diverse human tissues. *FEBS Lett* 1988; 239:65–68.
23. Young RM, Shull GE, Lingrel JB: Multiple mRNAs from rat kidney and brain encode a single Na^+,K^+,-ATPase β subunit protein. *J Biol Chem* 1987; 262:4905–4910.
24. Nelson WJ, Hammerton RW: A membrane-cytoskeletal complex containing $Na+K^+$-ATPase, ankyrin and fodrin in Madin-Darby canine kidney (MDCK) cells. Implications for the biogenesis of epithelial cell polarity. *J Cell Biol* 1989; 108:893–902.
25. Sherwood AC, Wilson PD: Membrane phospholipid-protein interactions in autosomal dominant polycystic kidney disease (abstract). *J Am Soc Nephrol* 1990; 1:642.
26. Bernstein J, Evan, AP, Gardner KD: Epithelial hyperplasia in human polycystic kidney diseases. *Am J Pathol* 1987; 129:92–101.
27. Grantham JJ, Geiser JL, Evan AP: Cyst formation and growth in autosomal

dominant polycystic kidney disease. *Kidney Int* 1987; 31:1145–1152.
28. Cowley BD, Smardo FL, Grantham JJ, et al: Elevated c-myc protooncogene expression in autosomal recessive polycystic kidney disease. *Proc Natl Acad Sci* 1987; 84:8394–8398.
29. Brinster RL, Chen HY, Messing A, et al: Transgenic mice harboring SV40 T-antigen genes develop characteristic brain tumors. *Cell* 1984; 37:367–379.
30. Mackay K, Striker LJ, Pinkert CA, et al: Glomerulosclerosis and renal cysts in mice transgenic for the early region of SV40. *Kidney Int* 1987; 32:827–837.

Ophthalmologic Involvement in Inherited Renal Disease

Jean-Louis Dufier, M.D.

Department of Ophthalmology, Hôpital Necker, Hôpital des Enfants-Malades, Paris, France

Ocular involvement is a common feature in many hereditary nephropathies such as cystinosis, nephronophtisis, Alport's syndrome, Lowe's syndorme, and lecithine cholesterol acyl transferase (LCAT) deficit. All ocular tissues may be involved: the cornea, the lens, and the retina. In some renal diseases such as Alport's syndrome, Fabry's disease, and LCAT deficit, the main interest of the ophthalmologic examination is its contribution to diagnosis of the disease.

In X-linked diseases, female carriers can be detected with slit lamp examination of the cornea in Fabry's disease and of the lens in Lowe's syndrome. In other diseases, such as cystinosis nephronophtisis and Lowe's syndrome, determining the severity of visual impairment participates in the prognosis of idiopathic renal disease. In all cases, routine fundus examination is an essential factor in the follow-up of renal insufficiency leading to retinopathy caused by high blood pressure.

Two Diseases Affecting the Cornea: Fabry's Disease and LCAT

Fabry's Disease

Fabry's disease is a lysozomal X-linked disease caused by α-galactosidase deficit. This deficit leads to accumulation of dihexoside and trihexoside ceramides in all tissues, particularly in the kidneys, skin, blood vessels, and the corneal epithelium. In males, the disease appears in childhood as pain in the hands and feet, associated with myalgia, polyarthralgia (which may be confused with articular acute rheumatism or Raynaud's syndrome). It associates with cutaneous thin telangiectasias called angiokeratomes that are deposited in the genital region and the hips.

During adolescence, renal function deteriorates, leading to hypertensive renal insufficiency and uremia by about the third or fourth decades unless this interval is shorted by cardiac or cerebral vascular accident.[1] In female carriers, episodes of pain in the extremities may be observed as well as moderately elevated blood pressure and sweating disorders.

Given the disparate symptoms, misdiagnosis in young boys and false screening results in women carriers would be common were it not for a constant and very evocative early corneal anomaly: the verticillated cornea.[2] The whirling aspect of the verticillated cornea is easily identified with slit lamp examination. The opacities are bilateral, more or less symmetric, and always located in the corneal epithelium, without change in vision. They resemble the corneal overcharge observed after intoxication by amiodarone, indomethacine, or synthetic anti-paludian (Fig 1).

Deduve and Liber's work shows that the verticillated cornea has the same mechanism as that for lysozomal stockage. Theories as to the formation of the verticillate feature (intracorneal fluid current, palpebral rhythmic blinking, magnetic field effect) do not appear to be of interest.

Other ocular symptoms have been described, especially microaneurysms of conjunctival vessels, which appear as cutaneous angiokeratomes, and nonspecific linear opacities of the posterior capsule of the lens. There is no sign of overcharge at fundus examination.

With regard to the cornea, Jules François has found osmophilic inclusions in all layers of the epithelium, especially the basal layer; the rest of the cornea (stroma, endothelium) is normal.

Weingeist and Blodi observed a series of crests compounded by two elements, the first formed by splitting of the epithelial basement membrane and the second formed by amorphous material situated between the epi-

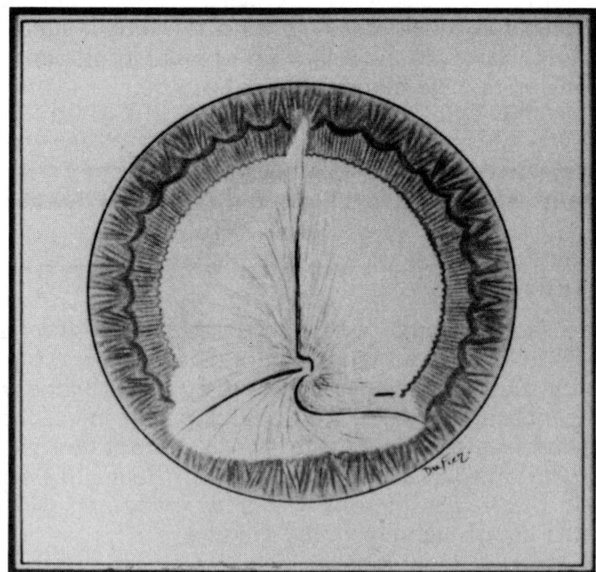

FIG 1.
Fabry's disease: verticillated cornea.

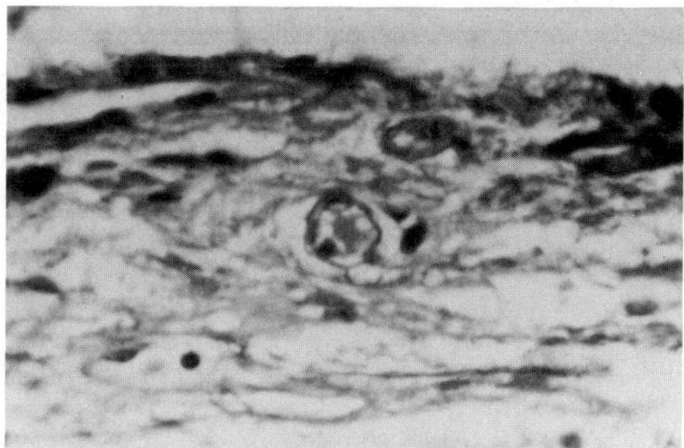

FIG 2.
Fabry's disease: conjunctival biopsy, lipid storage at vessel level.

thelial basement and Bowman's capsule. It is possible that these subepithelial crests are responsible for the verticillate feature. This overcharge is composed of ceramide dihexosides and trihexosides.

In subjects with normal blood pressure, some tortuous retinal vessels are observed.

To complete the ophthalmologic evaluation, two laboratory examinations, enzymatic analysis of tears and conjunctival biopsy, may be necessary. In hemizygote patients, α-galactosidosic activity in tears is reduced up to 80% or 90% and in heterozygote female carriers, by about 50%. This observation reflects the difference in clinical findings according to sex.

Black Sudan staining of conjunctival biopsy material shows lipid deposits in the epithelium and vessels (Fig 2). The inclusions are dense, osmiophilic corpuscles showing alternate light and dark laminas with a 40 A frequency.

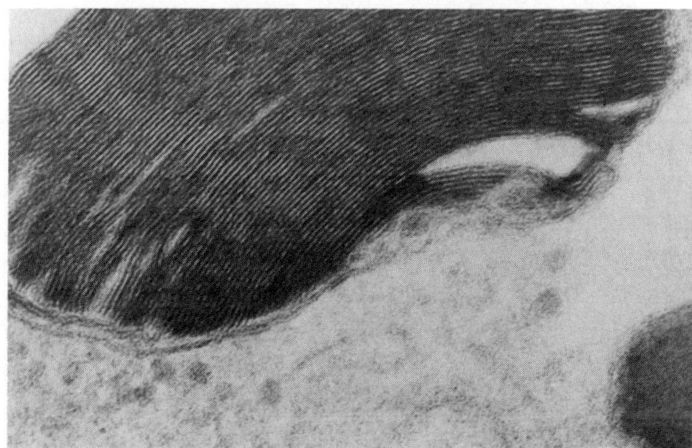

FIG 3.
Fabry's disease: lamelated bodies (transmission electron microscopy).

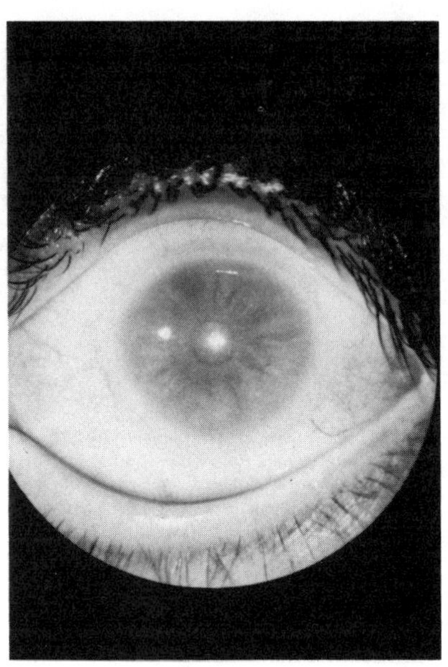

FIG 4.
LCAT deficit: limbal corneal ring.

They are surrounded by a unique membrane probably corresponding to a lysozomial membrane (Fig 3).

LCAT

LCAT deficit is a rare lipidic metabolism defect with recessive autosomal transmission, affecting young adults. Complications such as early arteriosclerosis, renal insufficiency, and clear elevation of blood pressure make it severe.[3] The first sign of the disease is corneal impairment or damage manifest as bilateral arcus cornealis associated with greyish stromacal opacities (Fig 4).[4]

Two Affections Exclusively Involving the Crystalline Lens

Alport's Syndrome

Alport's syndrome is a hereditary hematuric glomerular nephropathy, more frequent and more severe in males than in females. Deafness is associated in 85% of patients and ocular impairment is less frequent, occurring in 10% cases.[5, 6] The lenticonus-specific lens alteration is usually bilateral and anterior and leads to decreased visual acuity, amblyopia, nystagmus, and monocular diplopia.[7] Posterior lenticonus and lenti-eyeball are more rare. Lens opacities due to lenticonus can be observed.

A macular anomaly, a yellowish-white stippling of the macular area with no effect on visual acuity, is particularly suggestive of the disorder (Fig 5).[8, 9] The pathogenesis of these lens and macular laterations is unknown.

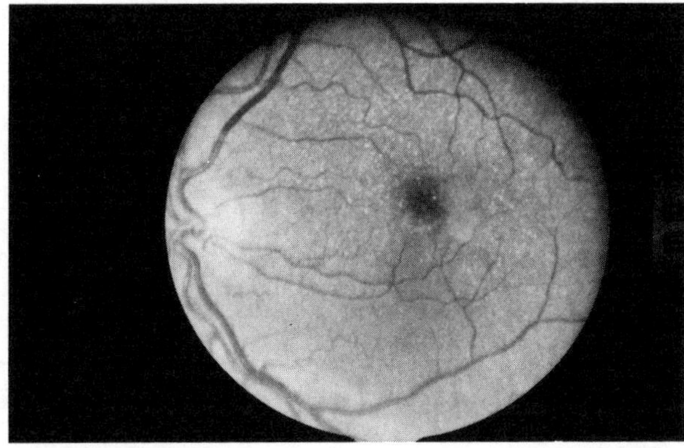

FIG 5.
Alport's syndrome: wide, yellowish, punctated maculopathy.

In a personal series of 28 patients, anterior lenticonus was observed in 6 cases. It was always bilateral and caused severe changes in visual acuity. In 1 case, nystagmus due to amblyopia was observed.

Macular retinopathy was observed in 13 cases. In 11, there was yellowish-white, thin perimacular stippling without consequence on visual acuity, color vision, or fluorescence angiography. In only 1 case was macular reflect absent, and angiography showed atrophy of pigmented epithelium and electroretinogram showed minimal photopic alteration. In another case, irregular retinal pigmentation was observed, and the amplitude of the electroretinogram was slight; however, visual acuity was 7/10.

Lowe's Syndrome

Lowe's syndrome, also called oculocerebrorenal syndrome, is a rare hereditary X-linked disease that manifests in male newborns by cranio-facial dysmorphia with cataract and/or glaucoma.[10] Later in childhood, the picture includes mental retardation, tubular nephropathy, and hyperamnioaciduria.

The cataract is present in 90% of cases, always complete and bilateral, usually observed at birth, and recognized early by blind behavior and Franceschetti's digito-ocular sign. Partial forms (nuclear, zonular, and posterieur polar) as well as some degrees of microphakia are possible.

Bilateral glaucoma is present in 50% of cases in association with cataract. It is rare without unilateral or bilateral cataract. Its type depends on its precociousness, either congenital glaucoma (buphthalmia) or, after the age of 3 years, infantile glaucoma marked by chronic ocular hypertension justifing ophthalmologic follow-up.

The rare pathologic ocular examinations that have been performed suggest that the disorder is a classic dysgenetic glaucoma related to abnormal development of the anterior segment of the eye, especially in the irido-corneal angle.

During follow-up of a couple at risk who already were parents of a young boy carrier of Lowe's syndrome, antenatal amniocentesis diagnosis with determination of sex was positive, and therapeutic abortion was decided by the parents.[11] Histologic examination of the eyes of the fetus showed congenital cataract and persistence of hyaloid vessels, with anomaly in angle and anterior chamber formation, showing that the fetus was indeed a carrier of the disease. In genetic counseling, routine ophthalmologic examination of female carriers is essential to seek the clinical genetic marker of congenital lens microopacity without loss of vision.

Two Nephropathies Involving Both Cornea and Retina: Cystinosis and Nephrosialidosis

Cystinosis

Cystinosis is a rare metabolic disease with autosomal recessive inheritance that occurs in three clinical forms.[12] The infantile form is characterized by severe renal failure, which is generally lethal prior to puberty. There is a rare juvenile form with milder nephropathy, and a totally benign adult form.

All three forms can be diagnosed with the slit lamp appearance of golden cystine crystals in the cornea.[13] Burki[14] described this corneal involvement in 1941. It has been observed in all subsequently reported cases and is considered to be pathognomonic for cystinosis.[15]

In addition, the infantile form includes a retinopathy that causes progressive and rather late loss of vision.

Since 1959, a group of 25 patients with cystinosis consisting of 15 men and 10 women, ranging in ages from 1 to 26 years, has been followed up in the Necker Enfants Malades Hôpital.

Corneal Involvement

In these patients, slit lamp examination revealed gold-colored and needle-shaped cystine crystals dispersed throughout the cornea. They were found consistently after patients reached 1 year of age (Fig 6).

Initially, the epithelium was affected, then at 3 to 4 years of age, the endothelium, and after 7 years, the whole thickness of the cornea was infiltrated in all cases. When the whole endothelium was infiltrated, superficial stippled keratopathy appeared, including photophobia and watering.

Later, nonspecific calcifications were observed in the peripheral cornea of children receiving hemodialysis. In the latest stages, 2 of the 3 blind patients (20 and 21 years old) had bilateral band keratopathy and bilateral tight myosis. Extensive corneal vascularization appeared in the cornea of another patient who had been followed up over 26 years.

Retinopathy

Characteristic retinopathy was observed as early as 3 years of age and was constantly present at 7 years of age. It consisted of juxtaposition of patch

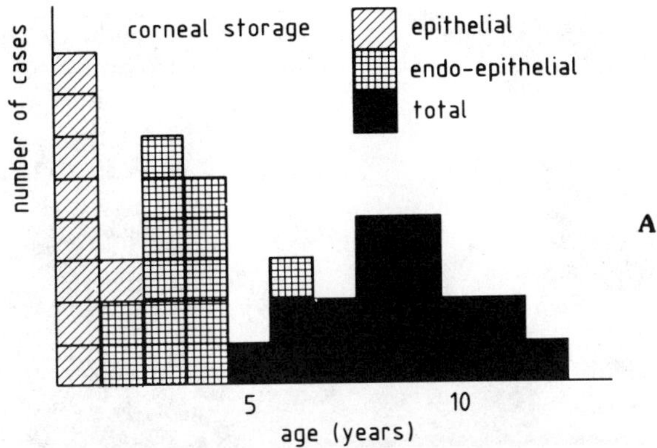

A

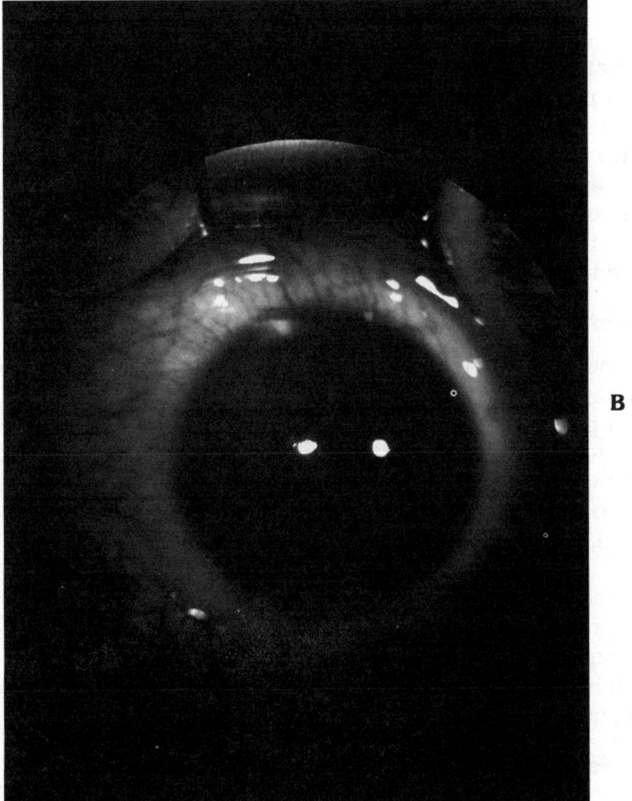

B

FIG 6.
A, Involvement of cornea related to age in infantile cytinosis. **B,** Gold-colored and needle-shaped cystine crystals throughout cornea.

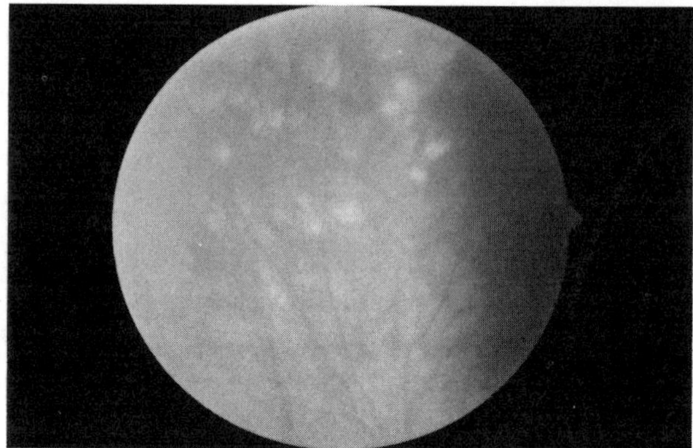

FIG 7.
Cystinosis: peripheral retinopathy.

depigmentation of the periphery (Fig 7), which was due to degeneration and loss of pigment epithelium, mainly in the temporal quadrant of the retina. Obvious worsening of the retinopathy was observed in 3 patients after a follow-up of 16, 20, and 21 years. In these blind patients, total retinopathy with severe depigmentation and cystine infiltration was observed, and small yellowish granules were present at their maculae.

Papilledema was observed in a 22-year-old woman affected by hydrocephalus and cerebral atrophy.

Electroretinogram

Electroretinograms (ERGs) were obtained in 20 patients. Results were normal in 6 cases, supranormal in 3 cases, and flat in 3 others. A photopic defect was present in 8 cases. When the ERG results were compared with the most recent measurement of visual acuity (VA), a correlation was observed between retinopathy and visual defect (Fig 8). In all cases of the first group of seven children under 10 years of age, sight remained within a good range, and ERGs were normal in four cases and hypernormal in 3 cases.

In the second group of children ranging in age between 10 and 16 years, progressive loss of sight occurred, and all who were examined had an abnormal ERG with a photopic defect.

In the third group of individuals, those over 16 years of age, the three blind patients had diffuse retinopathy and a flat ERG.

Histologic Findings

Cornea.—Polarized light microscopy showed birefringent crystals in corneal epithelial cells that mainly appeared in the basement layer.

Conjunctiva.—On light microscopy, there were many crystals, particu larly in the subconjunctival tissue. On electron microscopy, these

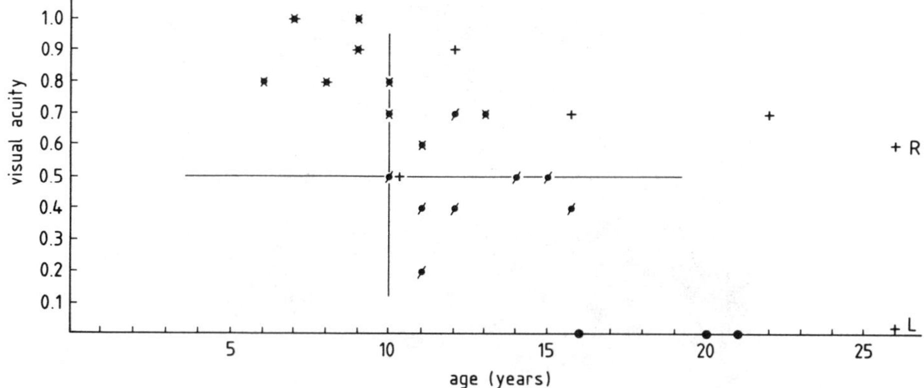

FIG 8.
Most recently measured visual acuity related to findings of ERGs in 25 patients with infantile cystinosis. *R* = right eye, *L* = left eye (in same patient); X = normal; * = hypernormal; *barred full point* = photopic defect; *full point* = flat; + = not investigated.

crystalline deposits were invariably intracellular in conjunctival fibroblasts (Fig 9).

Uvea, sclera.—Cystine deposits were abundant in the ciliary body, the choroid, the iris, and the sclera (Fig 10).

Retina.—Few crystals were observed in the retina. They may have been dissolved during tissue processing in aqueous solution. The retinal pigment epithelium was destroyed and occasionally there was pigment migration into the inner layer of the retina. It was rather similar to the lesions of retinitis pigmentosa.

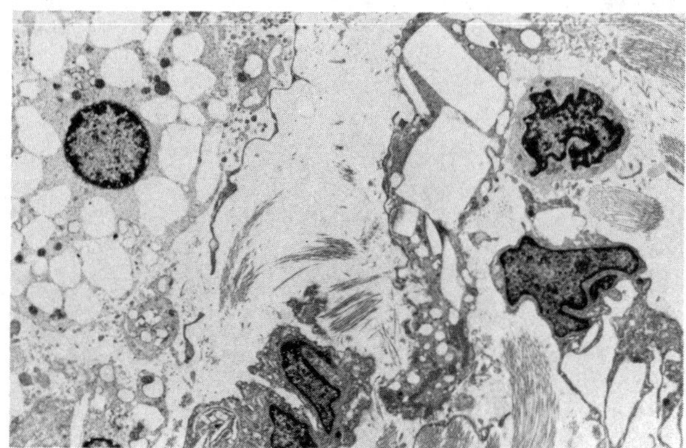

FIG 9.
Cystinosis: cystin crystals in the conjunctival fibroblasts (transmission electron microscopy).

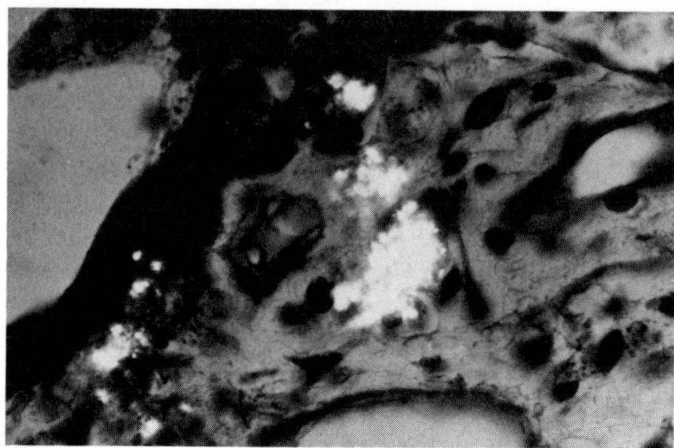

FIG 10.
Cystin crystal deposits in ciliary body.

Treatment

No significant decrease in ocular deposits was observed after hemodialysis, renal transplantation, or cysteamine treatment. Photophobia decreased in a patient treated with topic cysteamine, but storage remained the same.

Nephrosialidosis

The term nephrosialidosis was proposed to describe a variety of oligosaccharidosis in which glomerular nephropathy develops and causes death in the early years of life. Clinical and x-ray features of this disease are facial dysmorphia, visceral storage, early and severe mental retardation, and skeletal involvement, consistently described in this group of diseases. Spumous cells are present in the bone marrow. The disease is caused by an α-2-6 neuraminidase deficit transmitted as an autosomic recessive trait. We

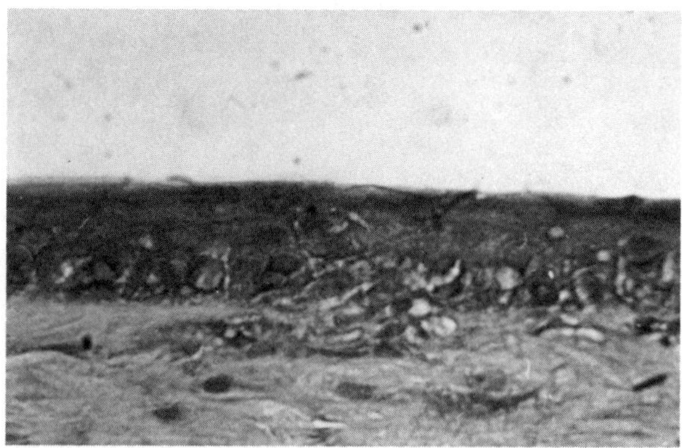

FIG 11.
Nephrosialidosis: corneal epithelium infiltration (blue Alsyan staining).

have observed two cases in the ophthalmologic department of Necker hospital.[16]

Besides epicanthus and hypertelorism, which are part of the dysmorphia, we noted corneal signs of mucopolysaccharidosis (thinly cloudy and granular infiltrations of the corneas) and retinal signs of sphingolipidosis (brown and rather thick aspect of the maculae with pallor of the optic disk). Histologic electron microscopy was possible after death in a 5-year-old child.

Cornea

Confirming clinical observations, the cornea showed spumous alcyan blue positive cells, especially in the epithelium and anterior stroma, but also in all stroma and the endothelium (Fig 11). The same alcyan blue positive cells were found in the sclera, iris stroma, trabeculum, and the choroid. Choroidal thickness was due to plumped histiocytes, stained with periodic acid-Schiff (PAS), and especially with alcyan blue, but not with luxol fast blue.

These abnormal cells were observed with the electron microscope in all tissues, especially in the iris stroma where large vacuoles appeared full of mucopolysaccharide acid material.

Retina

We noted swelling of the ganglion cells in the retina, which were stained with PAS, luxol fast blue, and Sudan black (Fig 12). This staining confirmed glycolipid storage, also observed in gangliosidosis disease. Electron microscopy confirmed the presence of lamelled membraneous bodies surrounded by a membrane in the cytoplasm of ganglion cells.

The Optic Nerve

The optic nerve was atrophic, the fibers were demyelinated, and vacuolized histiocytes were present in the septa.

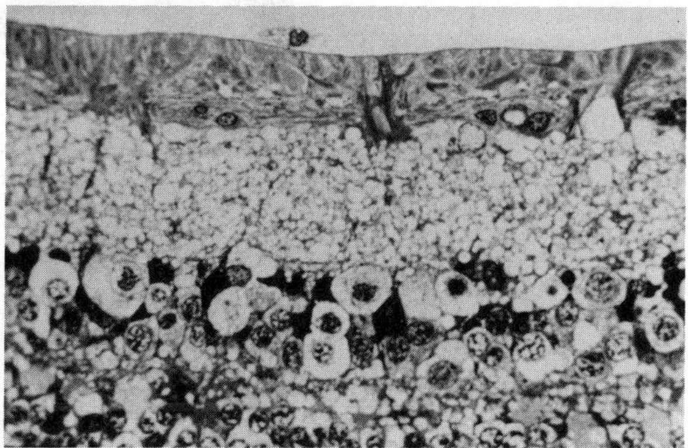

FIG 12.
Nephrosialidosis: plumped ganglion cells.

Nephronophtisis, a Disorder Comprising a Severe Retinal Deficit

Nephronophtisis is a familial chronic tubulointerstitial autosomal recessive nephropathy and may be associated with tapeto-retinal degeneration and occasionally with skeletal abnormalities, cerebellar ataxia, and liver fibrosis.[17–19]

Chorioretinal degeneration was initially reported in 1960 by Contreras and Espinoza[20] and later by Senior[21] and Loken.[22] It consists of a very early type of retinitis pigmentosa with a sensory deficit varying from amblyopia to blindness, and flat ERG and fundus alterations: thread arteries and modifications of the retinal pigmentation even attaining constitution of bone spicule pigmented dots (Fig 13).

A series of 51 patients was divided into three groups with different degrees of visual alteration.[23]

The first group consisted of 18 children (5 girls, 13 boys) less then 10 years old having evident retinopathy with severe sensorial deficit (Fig 14).

In 12 cases (10 boys), the association of the retinopathy and nephronophtisis was identical to Senior and Loken's description. In the 6 other cases, extraoculorenal anomaly was also observed. The retinopathy was detected anterior to the nephropathy in 6 cases and during investigation of nephronophtisis in 5 cases. One boy progressively became blind by the age of 8, although nephronophtisis had been regularly followed up since the age of 3. There was no dissociation between the renal and the ocular involvements in the other family members. In one family, a girl presented

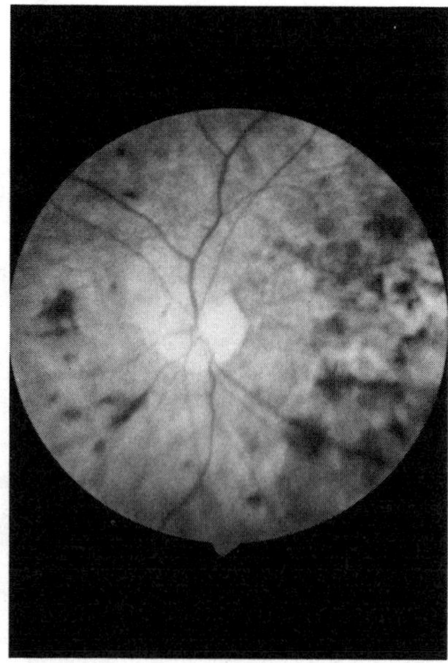

FIG 13.
Nephronophthisis: retinitis pigmentosa.

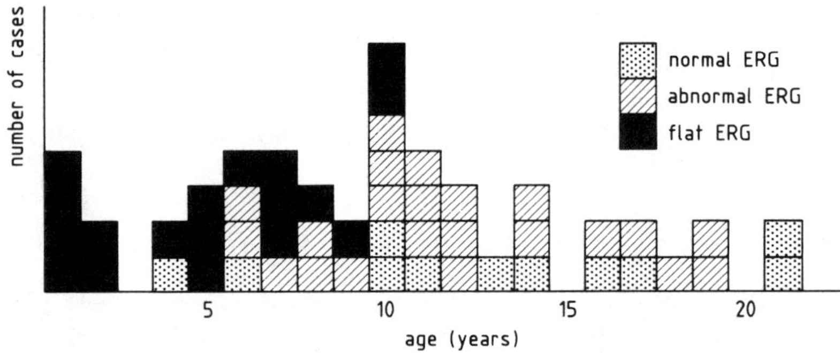

FIG 14.
ERG findings in 51 patients with nephronophthisis related to age.

an authentic syndrome of Senior and Loken; her brother, affected by Leber's congenital amaurosis, was also found to have acquired nephronophtisis.

In the second group of 11 children (4 girls, 7 boys) with normal clinical and electrophysiological findings, aged from 10 to 21, there were 5 cases from 3 consanguineous families.

In the third group of 22 children (14 girls, 8 boys), the clinical findings were normal but ERGs presented variable abnormalities. The range in age was from 6 to 19 years old. ERG abnormalities were of two types, photopic ERG and subnormal tracings. Abnormal scotopic ERG indicating the onset of pigmentary retinopathy was never noted.

Long follow-up is essential in cases with ERG abnormalities. This follow-up consisted of 12 consecutive years in 10 cases and no aggravation or fundus abnormality was noted.

Conclusion

Ophthalmologic examination contributes to the diagnosis of hereditary nephropathies and provides accurate information for genetic counseling.

In addition, concerning the general concepts of these disorders, with the exception of Alport's syndrome and nephronophtisis, it appears that most involve the renal tubule epithelium in a fashion similar to their involvement of the cornea, the conjunctiva, and the pigment of the retinal epithelium.

References

1. Hamburger J, Crosnier J, Grunfeld JP: L'atteinte rénale au cours de la maladie de Fabry, in *Nephrologie Flammarion,* vol 1. Paris, 1979, p 732.
2. Dufier JL, Gubler MC, Dhermy P, et al: La maladie de Fabry et ses manifestations ophthalmologiques. *J Fr Ophthalmol* 1980; 11:625–630.
3. Gjone E, Norum KR: Familial serum cholesterol ester deficiency. Clinical study of a patient with a new syndrome. *Acta Med Scand* 1968; 183:107–112.

4. Frise P: *Manifestations ophtalmologiques du déficit héréditaire en lécithine cholestérol actyl transférase. A propos de deux cas.* These Med Paris, 1988.
5. Gubler MC, Levy M, Broyer M: Alport's syndrome. A report of 58 cases and a review of the literature. *Am J Med* 1981; 70:493–505.
6. Purriel P, Drests M: Familial hereditary nephropathy (Alport's syndrome). *Am J Med* 1970; 49:753–773.
7. Nielson CE: Lenticonus anterior and Alport's syndrome. *Acta Ophthalmol* 1978; 56:518–529.
8. Perrin D, Jungers P, Grunfeld JP: Perimacular changes in Alport's syndrome. *Clin Nephrol* 1980; 13:163–167.
9. Polak BC, Hogewind BL: Macular lesions in Alport's disease. *Am J Ophthalmol* 1977; 84:532–535.
10. Lowe A, Terry M, McLachlan EA: Organic aciduria, decreased renal ammonia production, hydrophtalmos and mental retardation. *Am J Dis Child* 1962; 1:164–185.
11. Dufier JL, Dhermy P, Farriaux JP, et al: Contribution au diagnostic anténatal d'un syndrome de Lowe par l'examenhistologique des yeux du foetus. *J Fr Ophthalmol* 1986; 5:361–366.
12. Broyer M, Guillot M, Gubler MC, et al: Infantile cystinosis: A reappraisal of early and late symptoms. *Adv Nephrol* 1981; 10:137–166.
13. Dufier JL, Dhermy P, Gubler MC, et al: Ocular changes in long term evolution of infantile cystinosis. *Ophthalmol Paediatr Gen* 1987; 8:131–137.
14. Burki E: Uber die Cystinkrankheit im Kleinkindesalter unter besonderer Berücksichtigung des Augenbefundes. Ophthalmologica 1941; 101:257–262.
15. Francois J, Hanssens H, Coppieters R, et al: Cystinose (étude clinique et histopathologique). *Bull Soc Belg Ophthalmol* 1971; 57:354–360.
16. Dufier JL, Dhermy P, Limons S, et al: Manifestations oculaires d'une forme particulière de mucolipidose: La néphrosialidose. *J Fr Ophthalmol* 1980; 4:247–256.
17. Mainzer F, Saldino RM, Ozonoff MB, et al: Familial nephropathy associated with retinotis pigmentosa, cerebellar ataxia and skeletal abnormalities. *Am J Med* 1964; 49:556–562.
18. Proesmans W, Van Damme B, Macken J: Nephronophthisis and tapeto-retinal degeneration associated with liver fibrosis. *Clin Nephrol* 1975; 3:160–164.
19. Saldino RM, Mainzer F: Cone shaped epiphyses in siblings with hereditary renal disease and retinitis pigmentosa. *Radiology* 1971; 98:39–45.
20. Contreras CB, Espinoza JS: Discussion clinica y anatomo pathologica de enfermos que presentaron un problema diagnostico. *Pediatrica* 1960; 3:271–282.
21. Senior B, Friedman A, Braudo JL: Nephropathy with tapeto-retinal degeneration. *Am J Ophthalmol* 1961; 52:624–633.
22. Loken AC, Hanssen O, Halvorsen S, et al: Hereditary renal dysplasia and blindness. *Acta Pediatr Scand* 1961; 50:177–184.
23. Dufier JL, Orssaud Ch, Dhermy P, et al: Ocular changes in some progressive hereditary nephropathies. *Pediatr Nephrol* 1987; 1:525–530.

Part II

Renal Physiology and Pharmacology

Glomerular Permselectivity in Healthy and Nephrotic Humans

John D. Scandling, M.D.

Associate Professor of Medicine, Division of Nephrology, Department of Medicine, University of Rochester School of Medicine and Dentistry, Rochester, New York

Virginia M. Black, B.S.

Life Science Research Assistant, Division of Nephrology, Department of Medicine, Stanford University School of Medicine, Stanford University Medical Center, Stanford, California

William M. Deen, Ph.D.

Professor of Chemical Engineering, Department of Chemical Engineering, Massachusetts Institute of Technology, Cambridge, Massachusetts

Bryan D. Myers, M.D.

Professor of Medicine, Division of Nephrology, Department of Medicine, Stanford University School of Medicine, Stanford University Medical Center, Stanford, California

Albumin is the most abundant protein in plasma and comprises more than 80% of the protein excreted in urine of patients with the nephrotic syndrome. Because of its predominance, albuminuria is often equated inadvertently with total proteinuria, and the physicochemical properties of albumin have been used widely to formulate hypotheses to explain the barrier dysfunction that underlies proteinuria. A widely espoused hypothesis holds that abundant, anionic matrix components confer the properties of a negatively-charged electrostatic barrier on the glomerular capillary wall.[1, 2] Based on the Bowman's space-to-plasma concentration ratio of neutral dextrans of broad-size distribution, the functional pores that perforate the glomerular capillary wall have been estimated to have radii larger than the molecular radius of albumin (50 to 57 Å vs. 36 Å). It has been proposed, therefore, that depletion of its anionic components could impair electrostatic retardation of albumin by a glomerular capillary wall that is normal with respect to its size-selective properties.[3, 4]

Immunoglobulin G (IgG) is the second most abundant protein of plasma and is also lost in large amounts in the urine of patients with nephrotic syndrome.[5–7] Consideration of its physicochemical properties makes it unlikely that impairment of barrier charge-selectivity can be invoked to explain immunoglobulinuria, however. A majority of IgG species excreted in nephrotic urine are neutral or cationic.[6, 8] Furthermore, the molecular radius of IgG is 55 Å and is independent of its molecular charge.[9] According to pore theory, therefore, IgG is too large to permeate the restrictive pores that perforate the normal glomerular capillary wall. Thus, enlargement of at least a subset of such pores, and hence impairment of barrier size, rather than charge-selectivity, appears to be necessary to account for immunoglobulinuria in the nephrotic syndrome.

Early studies used the differential clearance of discrete proteins to explore the nature of barrier dysfunction in the nephrotic syndrome.[10–12] Because IgG clearance was grossly elevated, it was inferred that barrier size-selectivity had become impaired, permitting IgG to escape across the glomerular capillary wall. However, the IgG-to-albumin clearance ratio (also known as the proteinuria selectivity index) revealed that IgG was invariably cleared into the urine less readily than albumin. This finding was interpreted to indicate that although disrupted, the size-selective barrier continued to discriminate between larger IgG and smaller albumin molecules.

The fundamental quantity that allows definition of the membrane-pore structure of the glomerular capillary wall is the sieving coefficient (Θ), which is the Bowman's space fluid-to-plasma concentration ratio of a given macromolecule. From a biologic standpoint, protein macromolecules would be the obvious probes with which to characterize glomerular membrane-pore structure. However, Bowman's space fluid is inaccessible and final urine is not an adequate substitute because a variable fraction of filtered protein undergoes reabsorption in the proximal tubule.[13, 14] Another confounding factor is that proteins are heterogeneous with respect to both size and charge, thus presenting the investigator with two variables when attempting to infer membrane-pore structure from the differential urinary clearance of endogenous proteins.

To circumvent these limitations of proteins, investigators have used nonreabsorbable polymers of uniform charge to probe the intrinsic selectivity of the glomerular filtration barrier. The preparation that we have selected for this purpose is dextran 40 (Rheomacrodex, Pharmacia Fine Chemicals, Uppsala, Sweden). It has the requisite properties of an ideal marker for this purpose. First, its component molecules have a broad distribution of molecular radii, ranging from those small enough to be freely filtered (20 Å) to those that are sufficiently large to be impermeant (70 Å). Second, dextran 40 is uncharged, thereby permitting exclusive evaluation of the size-selective properties of glomerular capillary walls. Finally, dextran is neither reabsorbed nor secreted by tubular cells.[15, 16] Dividing its clearance by that of inulin thus corrects for water reabsorption along the nephron, so that the fractional urinary clearance of dextran is equal to Θ (the Bowman's space fluid-to-plasma concentration ratio). Knowledge of the Θ of dextrans of graded size, in turn, allows the walls of filtering glomerular capillaries to be represented as a heteroporous membrane with the use of a hydrodynamic theory of solute transport through pores.[17]

Methods

Patient Population

During the past 6 years we have used dextran sieving to evaluate nephrotic range proteinuria in 110 adult patients with one of six categories of discrete glomerular disease. A clinical diagnosis of diabetic glomerulopathy (DG, N = 39) was made on the basis of coexistent proliferative retinopathy in a subject with long-standing insulin-dependent diabetes mellitus. The remaining categories were based on the histopathologic appearance of glomeruli in a needle biopsy specimen of renal tissue. They included minimal change nephropathy (MCN, N = 8), membranous glomerulopathy (MG, N = 18), focal-segmental glomerulosclerosis (FSGS, N = 14), diffuse proliferative lupus nephritis (DPLN, N = 23), and diffuse proliferative seronegative nephritis (DPSN, N = 8), where seronegativity refers to the absence of diagnostic titers of antinuclear antibodies.

Twenty-one healthy volunteers were examined during the same period with identical physiologic techniques and provide a control range for the glomerular functional quantities of interest. They spanned an age range of 18 to 54 years (vs. 15 to 71 years) and exhibited a gender distribution similar to that encountered in the nephrotic population. They had no history of renal disease, hypertension, or diabetes mellitus. At the time of evaluation, each was found to be normotensive and normoglycemic and to have a negative dipstick test for urinary protein.

Physiologic Determinations

Each patient and volunteer was studied in a clinical research center after giving informed consent to a protocol that had been approved previously by the Institutional Review Board at Stanford University. Differential solute clearances were performed during water diuresis between 1 and 7 days after antihypertensive and diuretic agents had been withdrawn in patients receiving such therapy. The glomerular filtration rate (GFR) was estimated from the clearance of inulin, renal plasma flow (RPF) from the clearance of para-aminohippuric acid and plasma oncotic pressure (π_A) was measured with membrane osmometry. Each of the pertinent laboratory methods has been described in detail elsewhere.[5–8]

The fractional clearances (relative to freely permeant inulin) of endogenous albumin and IgG, and of exogenous uncharged dextrans of broad size distribution, were used to evaluate the glomerular barrier function. Concentrations of albumin and IgG in serum and urine were determined with radial immunodiffusion. When the concentration of either protein fell below the detection limits of the low level plates used for assay of urine (50 and 20 μg/mL, respectively), we used a sensitive enzyme-linked immunosorbent assay (ELISA), the lower detection limit of which is only 3 ng/mL.[6, 8] The renal handling of anionic vs. cationic IgG molecules was evaluated in 24 subjects with nephrotic syndrome by flat bed electrofocussing, as described previously.[6, 8] In brief, two fractions of IgG, respectively between pI 4.5 to 5.0 and pI 8.5 to 9.0, were eluted from an ampholyte-containing, granulated gel after electrophoresis, and the concentration of IgG in each fraction was determined with ELISA. Concentrations of dextran were assayed with anthrone after deproteinized plasma and urine had been separated into narrow 2 Å fractions with gel permeation chromatography, using Ultragel ACA 44 (LKB, Pleasant Hill, Calif.) as the column bed.[5–8]

Analysis of Intrinsic Glomerular Membrane-Pore Structure

To characterize the size-selective properties of the glomerular filtration barrier, we applied the fractional clearances of dextrans in the 28- to 60-Å radius interval to a heteroporous membrane model that has been described in detail previously.[17] In this model, the major portion of the capillary wall is assumed to be perforated by restrictive, cylindrical pores of identical radius (r_0). The model assumes that there exists in addition a parallel shunt pathway that does not discriminate on the basis of dextran size (up to 60 Å radius), and through which passes a small fraction of the filtrate volume. The shunt pathway is characterized by a parameter, ω_0, which governs the fraction of the total filtrate volume passing through this nonrestrictive portion of the membrane. Specifically, ω_0 is the fraction of the filtrate volume that would pass through the nonselective pores in the absence of a transmembrane oncotic pressure difference. The actual fraction of the filtrate volume passing through these pores, $<\omega>$, is calculated to slightly exceed ω_0, because while fluid movement through the small pores is retarded by the capillary oncotic pressure, that through the large pores is not.[17] Since oncotic pressure varies with position along a capillary, $<\omega>$ denotes the average value along a capillary. This isoporous with shunt model has been shown to provide a more satisfactory representation of fractional dextran clearances in humans than an isoporous model or several other alternative heteroporous models. According to this model, the membrane barrier to filtration of water and uncharged macromolecules is characterized fully by the values of r_0, ω_0, and K_f, where K_f is the product of effective hydraulic permeability and total glomerular capillary surface area (for two kidneys). An additional membrane parameter that can be derived from this analysis is the ratio of effective pore area-to-pore length (S'/l). To the extent that r_0 and pore length are likely to remain nearly constant, changes in S'/l are proportional to and closely reflect the total number of restrictive pores in the two kidneys.[18, 19] The approach used for calculating these intrinsic membrane parameters separates their effects on fractional dextran clearance from those of purely hemodynamic changes.

Statistical Analysis

Student's *t* test was used to examine the significance of differences between fractional dextran clearances in each nephrotic category and corresponding values in the control group. Differences between groups for the remaining findings were evaluated with analysis of variance (ANOVA) and Duncan's test for multiple comparisons with the CLINFO system. Because of the wide range of glomerular injury observed, we also used univariate linear regression analysis to explore associations between the measured variables. The distribution of protein excretion rates, fractional protein clearances, and membrane parameters (other than r_0) was skewed, and these values were log transformed before analysis. All results are presented as the mean ±1 standard error.

Results

Renal Handling of Protein

The excretion rate of albumin was massively elevated to between 4792 ± 651 μg/min and 9918 ± 1462 μg/min in each category of nephrotic injury (Table 1). A parallel increase in the IgG excretion rate was also massive. However, immunoglobulinuria tended to be less marked in MCN (293 ± 110 μg/min) than in the remaining five nephrotic categories (418 ± 63 to 678 ± 104 μg/min). These massive urinary protein losses were associated with an approximate 50% depression of the circulating level of each protein, with two exceptions. Serum albumin was only slightly lowered and serum IgG concentration was unaffected in DG. Although DPLN was accompanied by severe hypoalbuminemia, the serum IgG level remained similar to that in control subjects (see Table 1).

At the massive filtered loads predicted from the protein excretion rate in each nephrotic group, fractional protein reabsorption should be minor.[13, 14] Accordingly, the fractional clearance should underestimate only slightly the Bowman's space-to-plasma concentration ratio (or sieving coefficient) of a given protein. This relatively sensitive expression of glomerular permeability to protein serves to isolate the glomerular injury in MCN as the mildest among those examined (Table 1). The fractional albumin clearance in MCN was 2 to 5 times lower than that in the remaining nephrotic disorders (469 ± 115 vs. 951 ± 261 to 2214 ± 1,000 × 10^{-5}), and significantly lower than corresponding values in DPSN and FSGS. The disparity was even more striking for fractional IgG clearance, which was 7 to 22 times lower in MCN than in the remaining nephrotic categories (66 ± 32 vs. 459 ± 173 to 1,452 ± 1,133 × 10^{-5}). In keeping with earlier observations, MCN exhibited the most marked selectivity of proteinuria.[10–12] The IgG-to-albumin clearance ratio (selectivity index) was substantially lower than that in other nephrotic categories, 0.15 ± 0.006 vs. 0.25 ± 0.04 to 0.41 ± 0.03, respectively (seeTable 1). Of interest, the highest ratio observed was in DG, sug-

TABLE 1.
Renal Protein Handling*

	Control	MCN	MG	DPLN	DPSN	FSGS	DG
Excretion rate (μg/min)							
Albumin	13.0^{a}	$5{,}776^{b,c}$	$9{,}918^{d}$	$4{,}792^{b}$	$9{,}084^{c,d}$	$6{,}292^{b,c,d}$	$5{,}471^{b,c}$
	± 3.0	± 1,268	± 1,462	± 651	± 2,363	± 805	± 649
IgG	1.7^{a}	293^{b}	$645^{b,c}$	$418^{b,c}$	$511^{b,c}$	$478^{b,c}$	678^{c}
	± 0.3	± 110	± 167	± 63	± 124	± 139	± 104
Serum concentration (mg/dL)							
Albumin	$3{,}860^{a}$	$1{,}832^{b}$	$2{,}030^{b}$	$2{,}221^{b}$	$1{,}722^{b}$	$1{,}740^{b}$	$3{,}090^{c}$
	± 91	± 273	± 189	± 130	± 269	± 307	± 115
IgG	946^{a}	$607^{b,c,d}$	$544^{c,d}$	$769^{a,b,c}$	424^{d}	382^{d}	$912^{a,b}$
	± 74	± 137	± 102	± 122	± 117	± 88	± 53
Fractional clearance ($\times 10^{-5}$)							
Albumin	0.40^{a}	469^{b}	$1{,}207^{b,c}$	$951^{b,c}$	$2{,}214^{c}$	$1{,}999^{c}$	$964^{b,c}$
	± 0.10	± 145	± 324	± 261	± 1,000	± 562	± 192
IgG	0.10^{a}	66^{b}	459^{c}	473^{c}	$1{,}452^{c}$	818^{c}	475^{c}
	± 0.03	± 32	± 173	± 178	± 1,133	± 268	± 112
Selectivity index	-----	0.15^{a}	$0.25^{a,b}$	0.34^{b}	0.40^{b}	0.35^{b}	0.41^{b}
		± 0.06	± 0.04	± 0.04	± 0.12	± 0.03	± 0.03

*Means that are not different from one another by Duncan's multiple comparison test are designated with the same letter.

gesting that the injured filtration barrier discriminates least well between albumin and IgG in this disorder.

The charge-selectivity of renal IgG handling is illustrated in Figure 1. Twenty-four patients, representing each nephrotic category, were arbitrarily selected on the basis of sufficiently heavy immunoglobulinuria (>300 μg/min) to permit the urinary concentration of anionic species of IgG (which comprise only between 1% and 4% of total IgG) to be accurately determined with ELISA. On average, the fractional clearance of anionic IgG did not differ significantly from that of cationic IgG, 668 ± 227 vs. 782 ± 264 $\times 10^{-5}$. However, careful inspection of Figure 1 suggests that discrimination on the basis of molecular charge varies with the actual level of fractional IgG clearance. At lower levels ($<10^{-3}$), the fractional clearance of anionic IgG exceeds that of cationic IgG in 10 of 11 instances. At higher levels of fractional IgG clearance ($>10^{-3}$), the difference disappears; the remaining 13 data points in this range are evenly distributed on either side of the identity line. Of note, neither enhanced nor similar transglomerular passage of anionic relative to cationic IgG is consistent with an association between IgG permeable pores and a negatively charged electrostatic barrier.

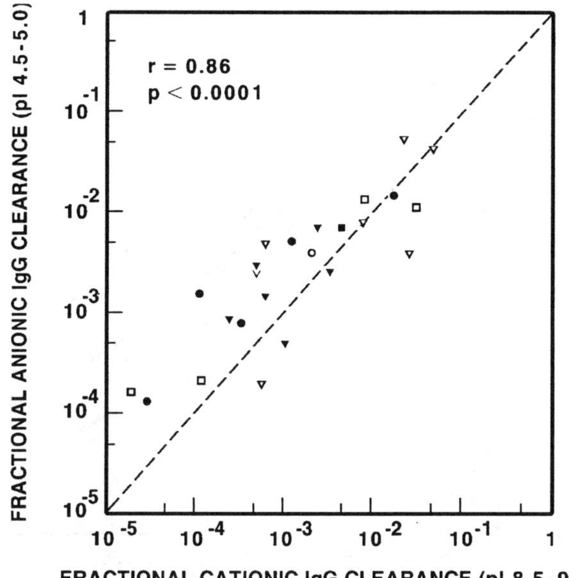

FIG 1.
Relationship between fractional clearances of anionic (pI 4.5 to 5.0) and cationic (pI 8.5 to 9.0) IgG species in 24 patients with nephrotic syndrome. The *dashed line* is the line of identity. categories of nephrotic injury are: *Open circle* = MCN; *filled circle* = MG; *open square* = DPLN; *filled square* = DPSN; *open triangle* = FSGS; *filled triangle* = DG.

Barrier Size-Selectivity

The profile of mean sieving coefficients for dextrans of broad size distribution in each nephrotic category are compared to the control sieving profile in Figures 2, 3, and 4. The configuration of the sieving profile was similarly altered from normal in each nephrotic category. Sieving coefficients of relatively permeant dextrans at the low radius end of the profile were significantly depressed in all six nephrotic categories. Each nephrotic profile then intersected the control profile. The intersection occurred at 58 and 50 Å in MCN and MG, respectively, the two nonproliferative immune injuries illustrated in Figure 2. Intersection of the control profile occurred earlier (46 to 48 A) in the two proliferative glomerulonephritides illustrated in Figure 3 and in the two sclerosing glomerulopathies illustrated in Figure 4. Beyond the intersection, the passage of large, nearly impermeant dextrans was enhanced in each nephrotic category. With the exception of MCN, the elevation of sieving coefficients beyond the intersection reached statistical significance for three or more of the largest dextrans examined. Selective elevation of the sieving coefficients of larger, nearly impermeant dextrans points to a membrane with a less sharp cutoff in nephrotic groups than in control

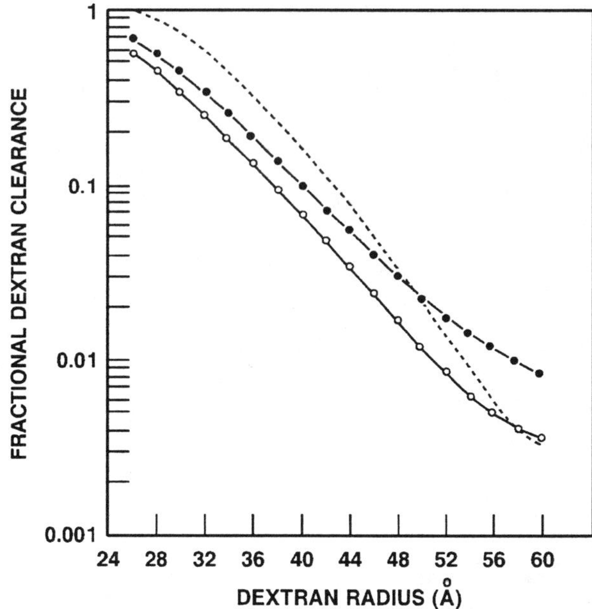

FIG 2.
Fractional dextran clearance profiles in healthy control subjects *(broken line)* and in patients with nephrotic syndrome with MCN *(open circle)* or MG *(filled circle)*. Sieving coefficients differ from those for control subjects at the $P < .05$ level over the dextran radius interval 26 to 54 Å in MCN and 26 to 46 plus 54 to 60 Å in MG.

subjects, and hence to a defect of barrier size-selectivity in each category of nephrotic injury.

Filtration Dynamics

On average, the GFR was significantly depressed below the control value in each nephrotic category (Table 2). In keeping with a more modest glomerular injury suggested by milder barrier dysfunction, the GFR was less depressed in MCN than in the remaining nephrotic categories. In contrast to GFR, RPF was similar to control values in each nephrotic group with the exception of DG, in which it was significantly depressed. A uniform lowering of the filtration fraction in each disorder points to a selective, or at least a disproportionate, depression of GFR (see Table 2).

Reflecting profound hypoalbuminemia (see Table 1), afferent oncotic pressure (π_A) was uniformly depressed by between 2.4 and 10.5 mm Hg on average in each nephrotic category (see Table 2). A curve fitting technique, which has been described elsewhere,[20, 21] was used to approximate the transmembrane hydraulic pressure gradient (ΔP) for each nephrotic group from the low radius end of the corresponding mean dextran sieving

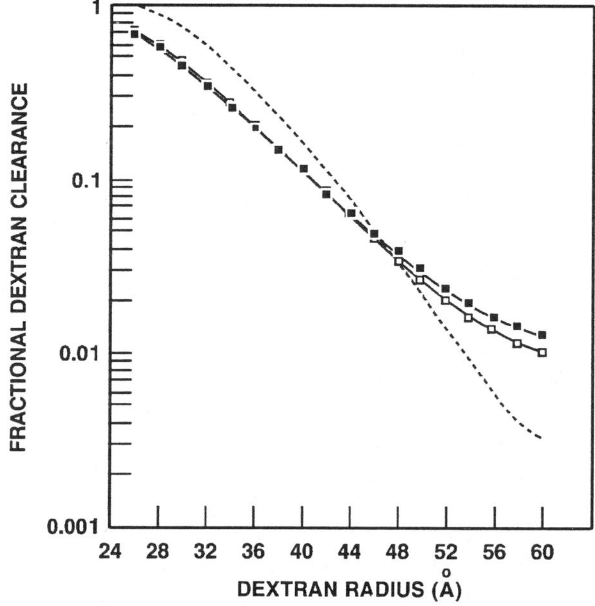

FIG 3.
Fractional dextran clearance profiles in healthy control subjects *(broken line)* and in patients with nephrotic syndrome with DPLN *(open square)* of DPSN *(filled square)*. Sieving coefficients differ from those for control subjects at the $P < .05$ level over the dextran radius interval 26 to 42 plus 50 to 60 Å in DPLN and 26 to 40 plus 56 to 60 Å in DPSN.

profile. The best fit value for ΔP at 5 mm Hg intervals over a 30 to 45 mm Hg range was 35 in control subjects, MCN, DPLN, and DPSN, and 40 mm Hg in MG, FSGS, and DG. In accordance with the probability that ΔP was not depressed in any nephrotic group is the finding of significant arterial hypertension in each category of glomerular injury (see Table 2). Thus, neither the pressure driving (ΔP) nor opposing (π_A) filtrate formation appears to account for the hypofiltration observed in the nephrotic syndrome. This suggests that hypofiltration is a consequence of reductions in the number of functioning glomeruli and/or changes in the properties of the walls of glomerular capillaries that remain perfused.

Membrane-Pore Structure

The dextran sieving profile of each individual subject, along with GFR and its hemodynamic determinants, was applied to the isoporous plus shunt membrane model to compute membrane parameters for the glomerular capillary wall. The computations are summarized in Table 3. They reveal a similar alteration of intrinsic membrane properties in all categories of the nephrotic syndrome. Judged by severe depression of K_f (by between 70% and 90% below control values), there was a marked reduction of ultrafil-

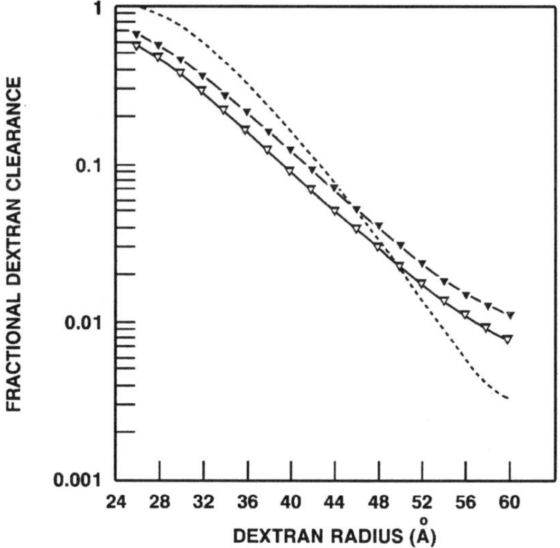

FIG 4.
Fractional dextran clearance profiles in healthy control subjects *(broken line)* and in patients with nephrotic syndrome with FSGS *(open triangle)* or DG *(filled triangle)*. Sieving coefficients differ from those for control subjects at the $P < .05$ level over the dextran radius interval 26 to 60 Å in FSGS and 26 to 42 plus 48 to 60 Å in DG.

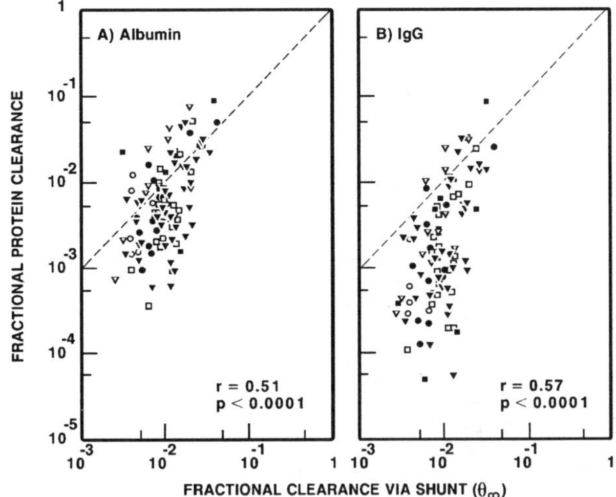

FIG 5.
Relationship in patients with nephrotic syndrome between the fractional urinary clearances of albumin *(left)* and IgG *(right)*, and the corresponding fractional clearances attributable to the shunt pathway (θ_∞). The *dashed lines* are the lines of identity. *Open circle* = MCN; *filled circle* = MG; *open square* = DPLN; *filled square* = DPSN; *open triangle* = FSGS; *filled triangle* = DG.

tration capacity in each disorder. S'/l, an approximate measure of the number of restrictive pores, was reduced in parallel (by between 63% and 87%). Restrictive pore radius was diminished, so that computed r_0 was below the control value by between 1 and 5 Å in each nephrotic category. Together, these three alterations are predicted to increase resistance to transmembrane water flow and to account for the hypofiltration observed in patients with nephrotic syndrome (see Table 2). In contrast, the prominence of the shunt pathway was increased in each nephrotic group so that ω_0 was larger than that in control subjects (0.0013 ± 0.0001) by between 3.2-fold and 10.2-fold (0.0041 ± 0.007 to 0.0132 ± 0.0070). In keeping with milder hypofiltration and relatively modest enhancement of fractional protein clearances, the values of K_f, S'/l, and ω_0 in MCN were intermediate between values in control subjects and corresponding values in the remaining categories of nephrotic injury (see Table 3).

Based on the filtration data in Table 2 and the membrane parameters in Table 3, we can calculate the expected contribution of the shunt pathway to the fractional clearance of a given macromolecule. Intraluminal concentration of a retained macromolecule will increase with distance along the glomerular capillaries as water is removed by ultrafiltration. As a result, the fractional clearance attributable to the shunt (denoted by Θ_∞ and neglecting tubule reabsorption) slightly exceeds $<\omega>$, the fraction of filtrate volume calculated to pass through the shunt. The relationship between Θ_∞ and fractional clearances of albumin or IgG in patients with nephrotic syndrome is illustrated in Figure 5. The two quantities are related (*r* value of .51 and .57, respectively). Especially noteworthy is that the value for Θ_∞ is similar to or in excess of the corresponding fractional IgG clearance in al-

TABLE 2.
Filtration Dynamics*

	Control	MCN	MG	DPLN	DPSN	FSGS	DG
GFR (mL/min/1.73m²)	108[a] ± 3	86[b] ± 9	62[c] ± 7	51[c,d] ± 8	46[c,d] ± 11	39[d] ± 6	36[d] ± 4
RPF (mL/min/1.73 m²)	582[a,b] ± 24	678[a] ± 65	718[a] ± 120	567[a,b] ± 61	364[b,c] ± 72	375[b,c] ± 71	317[c] ± 32
Filtration fraction	0.19[a] ± 0.01	0.13[b,c] ± 0.01	0.13[b,c] ± 0.02	0.09[c] ± 0.01	0.13[b] ± 0.02	0.12[b,c] ± 0.01	0.12[b,c] ± 0.01
π_A (mm Hg)	23.0[a] ± 0.4	14.9[b] ± 1.8	14.9[b] ± 0.9	14.7[b] ± 0.8	12.5[b] ± 1.1	12.8[b] ± 1.4	20.6[a] ± 0.7
Best fit ΔP (mm Hg)	35	35	40	35	35	40	40
Mean arterial pressure (mm Hg)	85[a] ± 2	98[b] ± 4	108[b] ± 2	104[b] ± 3	102[b] ± 6	104[b] ± 4	107[b] ± 2

*Means that are not different from one another by Duncan's test are designated with the same letter.

TABLE 3.
Membrane Parameters*

	Control	MCN	MG	DPLN	DPSN	FSGS	DG
K_f (mL/min · mm Hg/ 1.73 m^2)	16.2[a] ± 2.0	4.9[b] ± 0.9	2.7[c] ± 0.4	3.4[c] ± 0.8	2.5[c] ± 0.7	1.7[c] ± 0.4	2.2[c] ± 0.3
S'/l (km)	349[a] ± 43	128[b] ± 22	66[c] ± 9	77[c] ± 17	56[c] ± 14	44[c] ± 11	51[c] ± 6
r_0 (A)	56.9[a] ± 0.2	51.5[b] ± 0.9	54.3[c,d] ± 0.6	55.9[a,d] ± 0.4	55.2[a,c,d] ± 1.0	53.6[c] ± 0.9	56.0[a,d] ± 0.4
ω_0	0.0013[a] ± 0.0001	0.0041[b] ± 0.0010	0.0093[c] ± 0.0018	0.0104[c] ± 0.0013	0.0132[c] ± 0.0045	0.0099[c] ± 0.0015	0.0089[c] ± 0.0011

*Means that are not different from one another by Duncan's test are designated with the same letter.

most all instances. This indicates that the fraction of shunted filtrate can largely account for the amount of IgG cleared into urine of the patients with nephrotic syndrome in the present study. In contrast, fractional albumin clearance exceeded Θ_∞ in a substantial minority of cases (see Figure 5). Thus, in addition to the shunt-like pores that are freely permeable to dextrans of 60 Å radius, there must be yet another subset of albumin-permeable pores in many instances of the nephrotic syndrome.

Discussion

Our analysis of membrane-pore structure suggests that all glomerular diseases associated with nephrotic range proteinuria evoke a common and nonspecific injury to the glomerular capillary wall. Regardless of the etiology or histopathologic appearance of the underlying glomerulopathy, this response is characterized by a simultaneous loss of ultrafiltration capacity and impairment of barrier size-selectivity. Furthermore, the extent to which ultrafiltration capacity is impaired appears to be related to the magnitude of the defect in barrier size-selectivity.

Our analysis also suggests that, if anything, net pressure for ultrafiltration is elevated in the presence of a nephrotic syndrome (see Table 2) and that depression of K_f is uniquely responsible for the hypofiltration that usually attends this disorder. Inasmuch as effective pore length is unlikely to be greatly increased, if at all, a parallel reduction of S'/l (see Table 3) points to a predominant loss of filtration surface area rather than to diminished hydraulic conductivity of the glomerular capillary wall.[6, 22] This suggests that the number of functional, water-filled pores is substantially reduced in the nephrotic syndrome. Furthermore, as illustrated in Figure 6, a strong inverse relationship between S'/l and ω_0 suggests that as the density of pores becomes reduced, their size distribution is shifted toward pores of larger radius.

The possibility that insufficiency of the glomerular capillary wall as a negatively charged electrostatic barrier can account for proteinuria (and particularly albuminuria) stems largely from the finding that passage of anionic dextran sulfate molecules of intermediate size distribution (20 to 42 Å radius) is enhanced in proteinuric glomerular injuries in the rat, whereas the corresponding passage of uncharged dextrans is restricted.[23–25] In keeping with more recent studies in rodent analogues of the human glomerular injuries under consideration,[26–29] our study demonstrates that when dextrans of broader size distribution are used (up to 60 Å radius), a defect in barrier size-selectivity is invariably revealed (see Figs 2–4). This is manifest by a selective enhancement of the passage of large, nearly impermeant dextrans, a finding that points to the presence in the nephrotic glomerular capillary wall of a subset of pores which, although few in number, are nondiscriminatory toward large dextrans. It is important to emphasize that even though passage of large dextrans (>56 Å radius) is not significantly increased in MCN (see Fig 2), the failure of the barrier to restrict the latter,

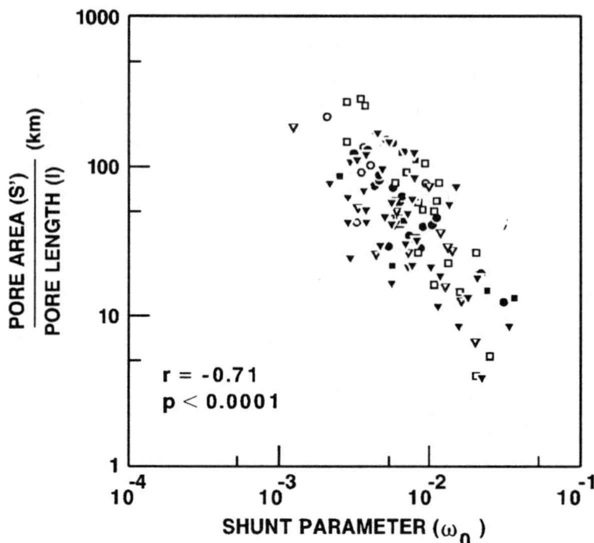

FIG 6.
Relationship between S'/l (effective pore area-to-pore length) and ω_0 (membrane shunt parameter) in patients with nephrotic syndrome. *Open circle* = MCN; *filled circle* = MG; *open square* = DPLN; *filled square* = DPSN; *open triangle* = FSGS; *filled triangle* = DG.

while substantially hindering dextrans of smaller radius (<50 Å radius), is also consistent with the presence in this disorder of a subpopulation of large, nonrestrictive pores.

In interpreting the sieving behavior of glomeruli toward dextrans, we have chosen to represent the glomerular capillary wall as a heteroporous membrane, one perforated by two parallel but discrete pore populations of widely varying size. The larger pores in the upper distribution are characterized by their failure to discriminate among dextrans of up to 60 Å radius. The amount of plasma permeating this shunt-like region of the membrane is computed to be large enough to account fully for the immunoglobulinuria, and for most, but not all, of the albuminuria observed in our patients with nephrotic syndrome (see Fig 5).

It appears to be an expansion of this shunt-like component of the membrane that constitutes the defect in barrier size-selectivity that attends the nephrotic syndrome. That transmembrane shunting through nondiscriminatory pores likely accounts for the bulk of nephrotic range proteinuria becomes likely when differences in configuration between dextran and proteins are taken into account. Passage of dextrans has been shown to be considerably enhanced during transglomerular permeation when compared to that of more rigid, spherical protein molecules of equivalent gel chromatographic radius.[30] Whereas the sieving coefficient of a neutral 28 Å radius dextran is in excess of 0.5 (see Figs 2–4), the corresponding value for neutral 28 Å horseradish peroxidase has been shown in the rat to be only 0.068.[30] Thus, restrictive pores that present an effective radius to neutral dextrans of 51 to 56 Å (see Table 3) are likely to be completely impermeable to IgG and only modestly permeable to 36 Å albumin. The importance of the contribution to proteinuria of a defect in size-selectivity has already been noted in connection with Figure 5. In the theoretical calculations, the most direct manifestation of impaired size-selectivity is an increase in Θ_∞, the fractional clearance of any large nonreabsorbed molecule that can be attributed to the postulated shunts. Whereas Θ_∞ is large enough to account fully for the observed fractional IgG clearance in virtually all patients with nephrotic syndrome, the fractional albumin clearance is in excess of Θ_∞ in a substantial minority of our nephrotic population (see Fig 5). This raises the possibility that a portion of the filtered albumin load gains access to Bowman's space fluid via restrictive pores, presumably as a consequence of depletion of negatively charged membrane sites.

There are at least two mechanisms by which a loss of negatively charged sites from the glomerular capillary wall could contribute to proteinuria in the nephrotic syndromes. As previously suggested, the first is a loss of electrostatic retardation of anionic albumin by the restrictive pores of the membrane, thereby explaining the excess of fractional albumin clearance over Θ_∞ in some patients with nephrotic syndrome. In keeping with a loss of barrier charge-selectivity by at least the nondiscriminatory pores of the shunt pathway is the observed similarity between the fractional clearances of highly anionic and cationic species of IgG (see Fig 1). The trend toward enhanced clearance of anionic over cationic species at lower levels of fractional IgG clearance is inconsistent with a negatively charged electrostatic barrier. A more likely basis for the disparity is the finding that proteins bind to the anionic glycocalyx of proximal tubular brush border in proportion to their isoelectric points.[31–33] Facilitated tubular reabsorption of cationic IgG with preferential escape of anionic IgG into urine could thus explain the trend to higher urinary clearance of the latter, notwithstanding equality of glomerular sieving coefficients for each species. That the trend is only discernable at lower filtered IgG loads is consistent with the saturable nature of the tubular protein transport process.[33]

A second mechanism by which a reduction in negatively charged membrane sites could contribute to nephrotic range proteinuria is more indirect. Infusion of the polycation hexadimethrine in experimental animals, partially neutralizing fixed anionic groups in the glomerular capillary wall, has been found to result in immunoglobulinuria[34–36] and in enhanced passage of large, neutral dextrans.[35] Thus, it is likely that the charged groups of the glomerular capillary wall are integral to maintenance of its structural integrity, and that depletion of these groups results in impairment of size selectivity.

In accordance with the hypothesis proposed by those who formulated the proteinuria selectivity index more than two decades ago,[10–12] we interpret our findings to indicate that impairment of barrier size-selectivity likely provides the major basis for proteinuria in the nephrotic syndrome. A novel insight to emerge from our study of sieving behavior of the nephrotic glomerular capillary wall toward uncharged dextrans is that impaired barrier size-selectivity is related inversely to ultrafiltration capacity. The fewer the overall number of functional glomerular pores in a given glomerular injury, the larger is the fraction of pores that behave as nondiscriminatory shunts. It remains to be elucidated whether depletion of negatively charged membrane sites in the nephrotic syndrome plays a causal role in this striking alteration of membrane-pore structure, and whether such charge depletion also contributes more directly to albuminuria by impairing charge-selectivity of the major, restrictive component of the membrane.

Acknowledgments

This study was supported by grants DK-29985, DK-20368, DK-40800, and M0)1-RR00070 from the National Institutes of Health.

References

1. Deen WM, Bridges CR, Brenner BM: Biophysical basis of glomerular permselectivity. *J Membr Biol* 1983; 71:1–10.
2. Venkatachalam MA, Rennke HG: The structural and molecular basis of glomerular filtration. *Circ Res* 1978; 43:337–347.
3. Cotran RS, Rennke HG: Anionic sites and the mechanisms of proteinuria. *N Engl J Med* 1983; 309:1050–1052.
4. Levin M, Gascoine P, Turner MW, et al: A highly cationic protein in plasma and urine of children with steroid-responsive nephrotic syndrome. *Kidney Int* 1989; 36:867–877.
5. Chagnac A, Kiberd BA, Fariñas MC, et al: Outcome of the acute glomerular injury in proliferative lupus nephritis. *J Clin Invest* 1989; 84:922–930.
6. Nakamura Y, Myers BD: Charge-selectivity of proteinuria in diabetic glomerulopathy. *Diabetes* 1988; 37:1202–1211.
7. Shemesh O, Ross JC, Deen WM, et al: Nature of the glomerular capillary injury in human membranous glomerulopathy. *J Clin Invest* 1986; 77:868–877.
8. Golbetz H, Black V, Shemesh O, et al: Mechanisms of the antiproteinuric effect of indomethacin in nephrotic humans. *Am J Physiol* 1989; 256:44–51.
9. Burton DR, Gregory L, Jefferis R: Aspects of the molecular structure of IgG subclasses. *Monogr Allergy* 1986; 19:7–35.
10. Blainey JD, Brewer DB, Hardwicke J, et al: The nephrotic syndrome. Diagnosis by renal biopsy and biochemical and immunological analyses related to the response to steroid therapy. *Q J Med* 1960; 29:235–255.
11. Cameron JS, Blandford G: The simple assessment of selectivity in heavy proteinuria. *Lancet* 1966; 2:242–247.
12. Joachim GR, Cameron JS, Schwartz M, et al: Selectivity of protein excretion in patients with the nephrotic syndrome. *J Clin Invest* 1964; 43:2332–2346.
13. Baldamus CA, Galaske R, Eisenbach GM, et al: Glomerular protein filtration in normal and nephritic rats. *Contrib Nephrol* 1975; 1:37–49.
14. Oken DE, Kirschbaum BB, Landwehr DM: Micropuncture studies of the

mechanisms of normal and pathological albuminuria. *Contrib Nephrol* 1981; 24:1–7.

15. Chang RLS, Deen WM, Robertson CR, et al: Permselectivity of the glomerular capillary wall. Studies of experimental glomerulonephritis in the rat using neutral dextran. *J Clin Invest* 1976; 57:1272–1286.
16. Chang RLS, Ueki IF, Troy JL, et al: Permselectivity of the glomerular capillary wall to macromolecules. II. Experimental studies in rats using neutral dextran. *Biophys J* 1975; 15:887–906.
17. Deen WM, Bridges CR, Brenner BM, et al: A heteroporous model of size-selectivity. Application to normal and nephrotic humans. *Am J Physiol* 1985; 249:374–389.
18. Chang RLS, Robertson CR, Deen WM, et al: Permselectivity of the glomerular capillary wall to macromolecules. I. Theoretical considerations. *Biophys J* 1975; 15:861–886.
19. Winetz JA, Robertson CR, Golbetz HV, et al: The nature of the glomerular injury in minimal change and focal sclerosing glomerulopathies. *Am J Kidney Dis* 1981; 1:91–98.
20. Chan AYM, Cheng ML, Keil LC, et al: Functional response of healthy and diseased glomeruli to a large, protein-rich meal. *J Clin Invest* 1988; 81: 245–254.
21. Myers BD, Peterson C, Molina C, et al: Role of cardiac atria in the human renal response to changing plasma volume. *Am J Physiol* 1988; 254:562–573.
22. Deen WM, Robertson CR, Brenner BM: A model of glomerular ultrafiltration in the rat. *Am J Physiol* 1972; 223:1178–1183.
23. Bennett CM, Glassock RJ, Chang RLS, et al: Permselectivity of the glomerular capillary wall. Studies of experimental glomerulonephritis in the rat using dextran sulfate. *J Clin Invest* 1976; 57:1287–1294.
24. Bohrer MP, Baylis C, Robertson CR, et al: Mechanisms of the puromycin-induced defects in the transglomerular passage of water and macromolecules. *J Clin Invest* 1977; 60:152–161.
25. Deen WM, Satvat V: Determination of the glomerular filtration of proteins. *Am J Physiol* 1981; 241:162–170.
26. Alfino PA, Neugarten J, Schacht RG, et al: Glomerular size-selective barrier dysfunction in nephrotoxic serum nephritis. *Kidney Int* 1988; 34:151–155.
27. Olson JL, Hostetter TH, Rennke HG, et al: Altered glomerular permselectivity and progressive sclerosis following extreme ablation of renal mass. *Kidney Int* 1982; 22:112–126.
28. Weening JJ, Rennke HG: Glomerular permeability and polyanion in adriamycin nephrosis in the rat. *Kidney Int* 1983; 24:152–159.
29. Yoshioka T, Rennke HG, Salant DJ, et al: Role of abnormally high transmural pressure in the permselectivity defect of glomerular capillary wall. A study in early passive Heymann nephritis. *Circ Res* 1987; 61:531–538.
30. Rennke HG, Venkatachalam MA: Glomerular permeability of macromolecules. Effect of molecular configuration on the fractional clearance of uncharged dextran and neutral horseradish peroxide in the rat. *J Clin Invest* 1979; 63:713–717.
31. Christensen EI, Carone FA, Rennke HG: Effect of molecular charge on endocytic uptake of ferritin in renal proximal tubule cells. *Lab Invest* 1981; 44:351–358.
32. Christensen EI, Rennke HG, Carone FA: Renal tubular uptake of protein. Effect of molecular charge. *Am J Physiol* 1983; 244:436–441.

33. Sumpio BE, Maack T: Kinetics, competition, and selectivity of tubular absorption of proteins. *Am J Physiol* 1982; 243:379–392.
34. Bertolatus JA, Abuyouseff M, Hunsicker LG: Glomerular sieving of high molecular weight proteins in proteinuric rats. *Kidney Int* 1987; 31:1257–1266.
35. Bridges CR, Rennke HG, Deen WM, et al: Reversible polycation-induced proteinuria (abstract). *Kidney Int* 1983; 23:201.
36. Hunsicker LG, Shearer TP, Shaffer SJ: Acute reversible proteinuria induced by infusion of the polycation hexadimethrine. *Kidney Int* 1981; 20:7–17.

Endothelins: Renal and Cardiovascular Actions

Michael S. Simonson, B.S.

Department of Medicine, Case Western Reserve University School of Medicine, Cleveland, Ohio

Mark Kester, Ph.D.

Departments of Medicine and Physiology/Biophysics, Case Western Reserve University School of Medicine, Cleveland, Ohio

Elisabetta Baldi, Ph.D.

Department of Pathophysiology, University of Florence, Florence, Italy

Tomohiro Osanai, M.D.

Second Department of Internal Medicine, Hirosaki University, Hirosaki City, Japan

Christie P. Thomas, M.D.

Department of Medicine, Case Western Reserve University School of Medicine, Cleveland, Ohio

Paolo Menè, M.D.

Cattedra di Ne Frologia Medica, University of Rome, Rome, Italy

Michael J. Dunn, M.D.

Hanna Payne Professor of Medicine, Director, Division of Nephrology, Departments of Medicine and Physiology/Biophysics, Case Western Reserve University School of Medicine, Cleveland, Ohio

The Discovery of Endothelin

The recent discovery of endothelins by Yanagisawa et al. in 1988 has triggered immense interest in the field of endothelin and endothelial regulation of vasomotor tone.[1] Masaki et al. purified the 21-amino acid peptide endothelin, sequenced the peptide, cloned and sequenced the complementary DNA (cDNA) encoding the preproendothelin, and documented the potent biologic effects of endothelin, particularly on blood pressure. This work built on the earlier observations of other investigators who had demonstrated an endothelial origin of a contracting factor, which was stimulated by a variety of chemical and physical stimuli as well as by hypoxia.[2–4]

Structure and Synthesis of Endothelin Isopeptides

Endothelins constitute a family of 21-amino acid peptides with four isoforms discovered to date. ET-1 (formerly human and porcine endothelin), ET-2, ET-3 (formerly rat endothelin), and endothelin beta or vasoactive intestinal contractor (VIC) have been characterized.[5–8] As illustrated in Figure 1, the endothelin (ET) isopeptides have significant homology including two disulfide bonds, a cluster of polar-charged side chains on the hairpin loop, and a hydrophobic C terminus. Endothelin peptides also share significant sequence homology with the poisonous venom, sarafotoxin, of the

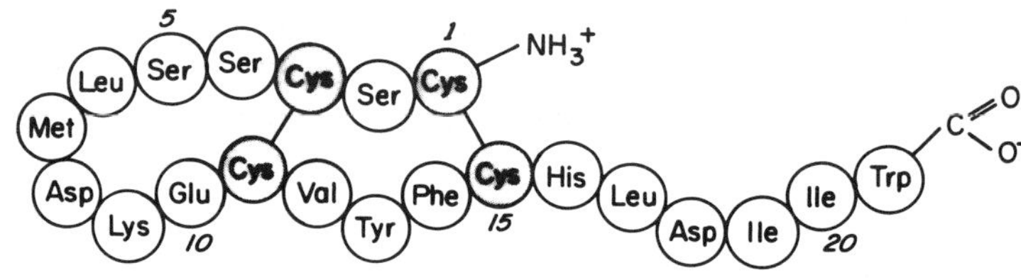

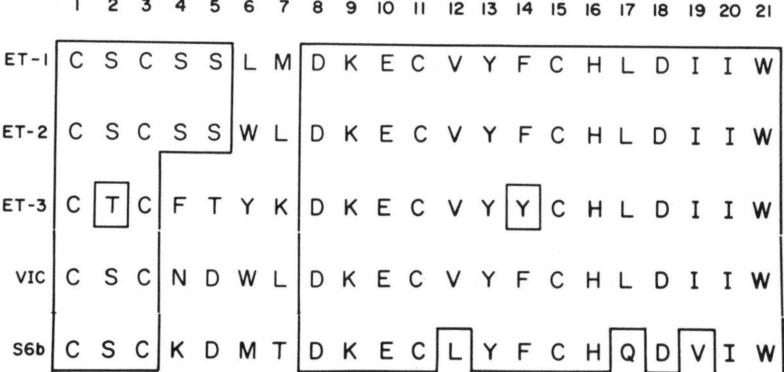

	1	2	3	4	5	6	7	8	9	10	11	12	13	14	15	16	17	18	19	20	21
ET-1	C	S	C	S	S	L	M	D	K	E	C	V	Y	F	C	H	L	D	I	I	W
ET-2	C	S	C	S	S	W	L	D	K	E	C	V	Y	F	C	H	L	D	I	I	W
ET-3	C	T	C	F	T	Y	K	D	K	E	C	V	Y	Y	C	H	L	D	I	I	W
VIC	C	S	C	N	D	W	L	D	K	E	C	V	Y	F	C	H	L	D	I	I	W
S6b	C	S	C	K	D	M	T	D	K	E	C	L	Y	F	C	H	Q	D	V	I	W

FIG 1.
Structure and sequence homology of ET isopeptides. At the top of the figure, the amino acid sequence and structural confirmation of the mature 21-amino acid peptide ET-1 is shown. At the bottom of the figure, the amino acid sequences and the sequence homologies (denoted by the enclosures) are shown for the endothelins, vasoactive intestinal contractor *(VIC)*, and sarafotoxin *(S6B)*. (From Simonson MS, Dunn MJ: *FASEB J* 1990; 4:2989–3000. Used by permission.)

Egyptian burrowing asp.[9] This snake kills its victim by coronary vasoconstriction undoubtedly because the sarafotoxin activates and occupies endothelin receptors on the coronary vasculature.

Analogous to other peptide hormones, ET isopeptides result from proteolytic processing of isopeptide-specific prohormones. The amino acid sequences of the prepropeptides have been predicted by sequencing cDNA clones isolated from porcine aortic endothelial cell and human placenta cDNA libraries.[5–8] The prepro-ETs are large polypeptides of about 200 amino acids that are proteolytically cleaved to form a 38- or 39-amino acid proET-1. Endothelin-converting enzyme, an enzyme that has not been purified or well characterized, converts the proET-1 to the mature 21-amino acid ET-1. This conversion of proET-1 to ET-1 is essential for bioactivity as the proform of the peptide has no significant biologic actions.[10]

Sites of Endothelin Synthesis

The name endothelin or the earlier name, endothelial-derived contracting factor, connoted an endothelial cell origin for the contractile peptide. The vascular endothelium of both arteries and veins is a major site of endothelin synthesis, but it is quite clear that other cells and tissues also contain the ET gene or secrete the mature peptide.[10] Table 1 shows a summary of the currently described sites of endothelin synthesis.[1, 7, 11–13] Although it was originally believed that only the large vessels such as the aorta synthesized endothelin, it is now documented that the microvascular as well as the macrovascular endothelium is capable of ET synthesis. In the central nervous system, major sites for ET synthesis exist in the hypothalamus and in the posterior pituitary and there is a growing belief that ET is an important neurotransmitter. Bronchial and intestinal epithelium can synthesize one or more forms of the ET isoform and this site of synthesis suggests a paracrine

TABLE 1.
Sites of Endothelin Synthesis

Sites of Endothelin Synthesis
Vascular endothelium
Central nervous system
Bronchial epithelium
Intestinal epithelium
Placenta
Glomerular mesangial cells
Collecting duct epithelium
Medullary vasa recta

action to regulate bronchial tone and intestinal contractions. Placental synthesis of endothelin raises the provocative possibility for a role of endothelin in placental ischemia and eclampsia. Within the kidney, endothelin synthesis occurs in the vascular endothelium, glomerular mesangial cells, collecting tubule epithelium, and the medullary vasa recta.[14–18] Some of these conclusions are based both on Northern analysis of prepro-ET mRNA transcripts and in situ hybridization on fresh tissues and some on synthesis of assayable ET with cultured cells. It seems likely that other cellular sites of synthesis will be uncovered and that regulation of both transcriptional and translational events will elucidate the biologic control of the synthetic rates of the peptides.

Stimuli of ET Synthesis

Diverse stimuli for endothelin synthesis have been characterized with either vascular strips with an intact endothelium or endothelial cells in culture.[10, 19] Very little is known about in vivo stimulation of ET transcription and/or translation. Table 2 shows a summary of these stimuli. It is difficult to develop a logical picture of endothelin regulation. What is the biologic meaning of increased synthesis of this vasoconstrictor endothelial peptide stimulated by the autacoid, thromboxane A_2, or the hormone, angiotensin II, which themselves are potent constrictors? Do any of these stimuli exert major regulatory control in healthy states or do these in vitro studies point toward pathophysiologic pathways? Phorbol esters, which are potent stimuli of protein kinase C, increase endothelin synthesis and perhaps angiotensin, vasopressin, epinephrine, thromboxane, and thrombin all work through a common pathway, namely phospholipase C stimulation and the release of diacylglycerol in the activation of protein kinase C, thereby inducing endothelin synthesis.

TABLE 2.
Stimuli of Endothelin Synthesis

Mechanical: shear stress, pressure, hypoxia
Hormonal: angiotensin, vasopressin, epinephrine
Autacoids: thromboxane A_2, thrombin, transforming growth factor β ($TGF_β$)
Miscellaneous: Ca^{2+} ionophores, phorbol esters, endotoxin, cyclosporine

Endothelin Receptors

ET receptors have been localized in vivo with radiolabeled ET and autoradiography (Table 3).[13, 20–23] Saturable and specific binding sites with a dissociation constant of approximately 0.5 nM have been found in fetal and adult organs including kidney, lung, heart, intestine, adrenal glands, eye, brain, and vasculature. Within the kidney, ET receptors are present in glomeruli, medullary vasa recta, and medullary and papillary collecting tubules. A word of caution is in order since in vivo receptor mapping with the radioligand does yield some false-negative results, and it is highly likely that additional receptor sites in the kidney and elsewhere will be discovered. Certainly, endothelin acts in many cell types and in most, if not all, organs. In many tissues, the ET binding sites and the cellular site of synthesis of ET suggests that the ET peptide probably acts as a local hormone that communicates in a paracrine fashion with nearby smooth muscle cells, pericytes, or fibroblasts. It is unlikely that endothelin is a circulating hormone or that endothelin synthesis in one organ will influence endothelin responses in a distant organ. An exception may be hypothalamic-pituitary ET. Injected endothelin has a very short half-life (1 to 2 minutes) and lung, liver, and kidney are major sites of endothelin uptake. The short half-life is the result of receptor-mediated uptake of ET and not of ET degradation.

ET binding sites have been biochemically characterized with in vitro techniques. High affinity saturable binding sites for ^{125}I-ET isopeptides have been characterized in intact cells as well as in membrane preparations from vascular and nonvascular smooth muscle, 3T3 fibroblasts, and glomerular mesangial cells.[24–30] Both saturation and competitive displacement binding studies have characterized multiple classes of ET receptors with differing affinities for the ET isopeptides and sarafotoxins. The disso-

TABLE 3.
Endothelin Receptor Mapping

Kidney: glomeruli and inner medulla
Lung: bronchi
Heart: coronary arteries, atria, and ventricles
Intestine: mucosa or smooth muscle
Adrenals: zona glomerulosa > medulla
Brain: widespread
Eye: iris, choroid, retina, and endothelial layer of cornea
General: most vascular smooth muscle

ciation constants for these receptors range from 0.1 to 10nM and, in many tissues, investigators describe a high-affinity and a low-affinity receptor. We have evaluated ^{125}I-ET-1 binding to cultured rat glomerular mesangial cells and have found, as did Badr and coworkers, two classes of ET binding sites.[31, 32] With competition binding studies between ^{125}I-ET-1 and the different isopeptides, ET-1, ET-2, ET-3, and sarafotoxin, the heterologous competition curves with ET-1, ET-2, ET-3, and sarafotoxin were consistent with a two-site model. Combining the saturation analysis with Scatchard transformation and the competition experiments, we concluded that the high-affinity site has a dissociation constant of approximately 30pM whereas the low-affinity site has a dissociation constant of 40nM. Nonradioactive ET-1 or acid washes of these cells dissociated only 20% to 30% of the bound ^{125}I ET-1, pointing to a very strong ET-receptor affinity. Preincubation of mesangial cells with ET-1 induced a 95% decrease in ET-receptor number without a change in receptor affinity or dissociation constant.[32]

Postreceptor Signals Triggered by Endothelins

Phospholipase C.—ET activates phospholipase C in diverse cell types including vascular smooth muscle cells, fibroblasts, and glomerular mesangial cells.[10, 33] In our experiments with cultured rat glomerular mesangial cells labelled with ^{3}H-myoinositol, ET-1 activated phospholipase C, releasing inositol 1,4,5 P_3 as well as other water-soluble inositol phosphate isomers. The threshold concentration for activation of phospholipase C with the release of inositol phosphates was between 1×10^{-10} and 1×10^{-9} M whereas much lower concentrations, in the range of 1×10^{-12} M, trigger an increase in cytosolic calcium[34] (see later). As would be expected after the phosphodiesteric hydrolysis of phosphatidylinositol bisphosphate, diacylglycerol increases rapidly with the inositol phosphates and there is a sustained diacylglycerol peak. This release of diacylglycerol may result not only from the action of phospholipase C and phosphatidylinositol bisphosphate but also phospholipase C-mediated breakdown of phosphatidylcholine (Baldi, Kester, and Dunn, unpublished data). The ET receptor is linked to phospholipase C by a pertussis toxin-inhibitable guanosine triphosphate (GTP) binding protein (G protein) in glomerular mesangial cells. We have demonstrated not only pertussis toxin inhibition (approximately 50%) of ET-stimulated inositol phosphate release but also a potentiating effect of GTPγS on ET-stimulated phospholipase C.[35] Other workers using different cell types have been unable to characterize the endothelin-linked G protein as pertussis toxin-inhibitable. It is possible that ET receptors utilize different G proteins in different tissues and that different G proteins may couple ET to different signaling mechanisms.

Cytosolic calcium.—ET activation of ET receptors and phospholipase C causes a rapid spike increment of cytosolic calcium attributable to mobilization of calcium from the endoplasmic reticulum as a result of inositol

1,4,5 P_3 release. In our studies of glomerular mesangial cells from rats and humans, ET-1 and ET-2 are substantially more potent than sarafotoxin, which is more potent than ET-3 to increase cytosolic calcium.[36, 37] The cytosolic calcium response, in addition to a dependence on intracellular calcium mobilization, also results from augmented calcium entry. ET-stimulated calcium influx in the mesangial cells is not inhibited by calcium channel blocking agents, which block voltage-gated calcium channels. The ET receptor-operated calcium entry channel is opened by very low concentrations of ET (1×10^{-12} M), and calcium entry accounts for increments of cytosolic calcium at concentrations of ET below that necessary to stimulate phospholipase C.[34] At higher concentrations of ET, above 0.1 to 1nM, increased cytosolic calcium in response to ET represents both intracellular mobilization and substantial calcium influx. The sustained calcium increase in the cytosol, which can last for 15 minutes, is entirely dependent on persistent calcium influx and is absent in calcium-free solutions. Figure 2 shows a comparison of the ET-1 responses in cultured rat glomerular mesangial cells at low and high dose of ET with and without extracellular calcium. The calcium responses show extensive homologous desensitization with prior exposure to any of the ET isoforms, subsequently reducing the calcium responses to either the same or to a different ET isopeptide.

In mesangial cells from rat and humans, we have found an important

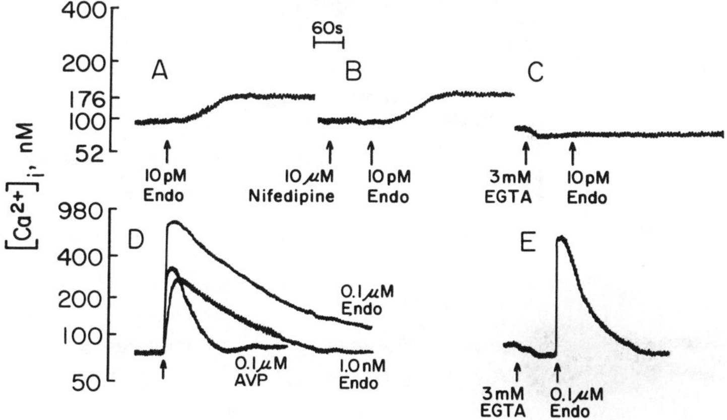

FIG 2.
The effects of endothelin on cytosolic calcium ($[Ca^{2+}]_i$). Low concentrations of endothelin *(endo)* 10 pM slowly increased $[Ca^{2+}]_i$ *(A)*, and this increment was not blocked by nifedipine *(B)* but was dependent on the presence of extracellular calcium *(C)*. Larger concentrations of endothelin from 1 nM to 0.1 μM induced dramatic and rapid increments of $[Ca^{2+}]_i$ with a very sustained elevation of intracellular calcium *(D)*. The effects of arginine vasopressin *(AVP)* are shown for comparison. Removal of extracellular calcium attenuates the prolonged phase of calcium increase but has little effect on the spike increment after addition of endothelin *(E)*. (From Simonson MS, Wann S, Mene' P, et al: *J Cardiovasc Pharmacol* 1989; 13:S80–S83. Used by permission.)

regulatory role of protein kinase C on calcium signaling. Acute activation of protein kinase C downregulates or diminishes ET-induced calcium increments. Inactivation of protein kinase C has the opposite effect and increases calcium responses to ET.[36, 37] The effects of protein kinase C to inhibit calcium signaling induced by ET may be due to phosphorylation of the phospholipase C enzyme, activation of calcium pumps to remove calcium from the cytosol, or stimulation of a phosphatase to degrade inositol 1,4,5 P_3. Figure 3 shows the effects of two stimuli of protein kinase C, the phorbol ester 12-tetradecanoyl phorbal 13-acetate (TPA) or the synthetic diacylglycerol diC8, to significantly inhibit ET-stimulated calcium signaling. Figure 3 also shows that chronic protein kinase C (PKC) depletion by preincubation with TPA upregulates the responses, yielding a greater peak of

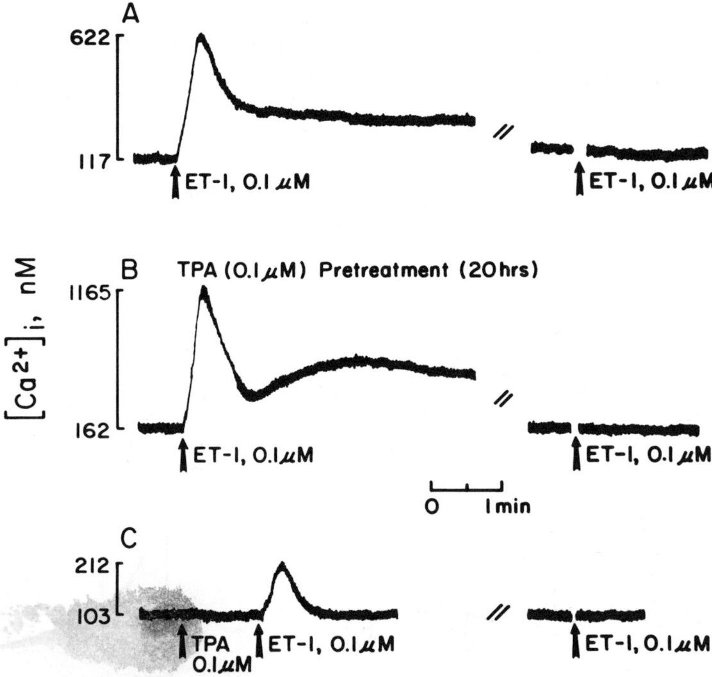

FIG 3.
Homologous downregulation of ET-1 responses and the role of protein kinase C. Cultured rat glomerular mesangial cells were exposed briefly to ET-1 0.1 μM, the cells washed and then reexposed to the same concentration of ET-1 *(A)*. This type of downregulation was also seen if ET-2 or ET-3 were used. Chronic exposure of the cells to the phorbol ester TPA downregulates the protein kinase C activity and potentiates the calcium responses to ET-1 but does not affect the homologous downregulation of the response *(B)*. Acute stimulation of protein kinase C with TPA significantly reduces ET-simulated calcium responses but does not affect the homologous desensitization *(C)*. (From Simonson MS, Dunn MJ: *Exp Cell Res* 1991; 192:148—156. Used by permisison.)

cytosolic calcium and some elevation of the sustained phase after ET stimulation.

Sodium-Hydrogen Exchange.—Activation of sodium-hydrogen antiport (sodium influx and H^+ efflux) across the plasma membrane will alkalinize the intracellular pH in bicarbonate-free buffers. This cytosolic alkalinization may play a role, perhaps a permissive one, in the mitogenic response of cells to growth factors. We have studied mesangial cells loaded with BCECF, a pH-sensitive probe, to evaluate possible changes of pH_i induced by ET. ET, 10 to 100nM, induced transient and rapid acidification that quickly yielded a net alkalinization 5 minutes after addition of the peptide. This alkalinization lasted for at least 15 minutes (Fig 4). The initial transient acidification may have been a result of a large increase in cytosolic calcium with subsequent calcium-hydrogen exchange. The alkalinization of the cytosol was due to a sodium-hydrogen antiporter as amiloride inhibited the hydrogen extrusion as did sodium-free media.

Phospholipase A_2 and Adenylate Cyclase: Potential Cross-Talk—Numerous in vivo and in vitro studies show that endothelin can stimulate the synthesis of eicosanoids, especially PGI_2 and PGE_2. We have

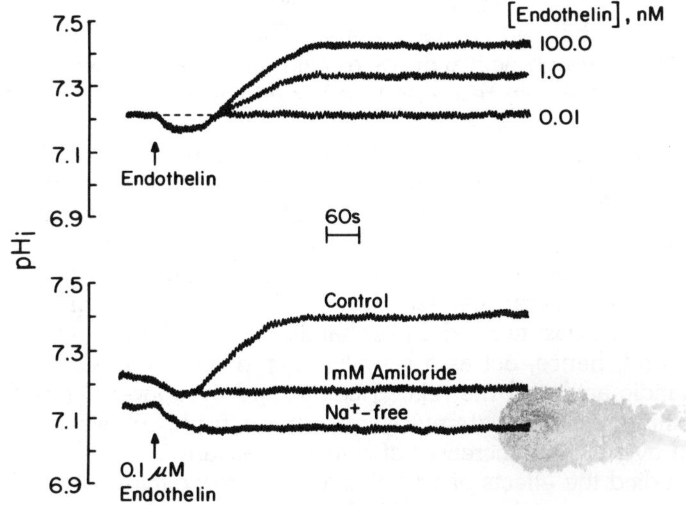

FIG 4.
The effects of endothelin on cytosolic pH (pH_i) in cultured rat glomerular mesangial cells. Mesangial cells were loaded with BCECF, a hydrogen-sensitive fluorescent probe. After the addition of various concentrations of endothelin, there was a transient cytosolic acidification followed by a sustained alkalinization with concentrations of endothelin of 1 nM and greater. We attribute this cytosolic alkalinization to activation of sodium-hydrogen exchange since sodium-free solutions block the response and the inhibitory diuretic, amiloride, also negated the endothelin-induced alkalinization. (From Simonson MS, Wann S, Mene' P, et al: *J Clin Invest* 1989; 83:708–712. Used by permission.)

evaluated the in vitro effects of ET-1 on arachidonic acid release and prostaglandin synthesis in cultured rat glomerular mesangial cells.[38] ET evoked a time-dependent increase in [^{3}H]arachidonic acid release, which peaked 5 to 10 minutes after the addition of the stimulus and was quite similar to the arachidonate release induced by vasopressin. This was accompanied by rapid increases in prostaglandin synthesis which, in rat mesangial cells, were primarily PGE_2 and $PGF_{2\alpha}$. Since endothelin stimulates contraction in these cultured mesangial cells (measured by changes of planar surface area and rearrangements of actin microfilaments), we wondered whether ET-stimulated PGE_2 was a negative feedback loop to downregulate the contractile (and perhaps other) responses of the mesangial cell. ET-1 augmented isoproterenol-induced cyclic adenosine monophosphate (cAMP) accumulation in cultured rat mesangial cells. This response, which would be expected to relax the cells, was PGE_2-dependent since indomethacin blocked the ET potentiation of cAMP and PGE_2 reconstituted the response.[38] We concluded that phospholipase A_2 activation by ET acts as a negative feedback or modulatory pathway to regulate the contractile and perhaps mitogenic actions of ET. The prostaglandins released, whether PGE_2 or PGI_2, could act directly to stimulate adenylate cyclase or to potentiate adenylate cyclase to other stimuli such as beta adrenergic agonists. The resultant increase in intracellular cAMP, through activation of protein kinase A, relaxes the cells and reduces mitogenesis in response to other growth factors such as serum or PDGF.

Phospholipase D.—Studies in hepatocytes by Exton and coworkers and in neutrophils by Siegal and coworkers have drawn attention to phospholipase D.[39, 40] This enzyme converts phospholipid substrates, especially phosphatidylcholine, directly to phosphatidic acid. Stimuli of phospholipase D include vasopressin in hepatocytes and diverse leukocyte activators in polymorphonuclear leukocytes. The importance of phosphatidic acid may be at least twofold. Phosphatidic acid can be converted to diacyglycerol and, hence, act as a stimulus of protein kinase C. Furthermore, phosphatidic acid and the related compound, lysophosphatidic acid, can apparently directly activate mitogenesis through phospholipase C stimulation and evoke rapid increases of cytosolic calcium.[41]

We studied the effects of endothelin on phospholipase D in cultured rat glomerular mesangial cells. Endothelin rapidly and potently stimulates phospholipase D. The stimulation may be both direct, through a receptor G protein linkage to phospholipase D, and indirect, through the ET receptor phospholipase C linkage and protein kinase C activation.[42] It is unknown which of these signaling pathways plays the dominant role to trigger endothelin's cellular effects. We believe that both pathways are important and that acute increments of cytosolic calcium are phospholipase C-dependent whereas more chronic effects of endothelin on mitogenesis or to cause sustained smooth muscle contraction may depend on both protein kinase C and phospholipase D.

Physiologic Actions of Endothelin

Table 4 lists the renal, cardiovascular, and endocrine actions that are prominent after endothelin infusions in many animal species.[10, 19] The renal vascular bed is exquisitely sensitive to endothelin, and systemic infusions of ET-1 cause greater renal and mesenteric vasoconstriction than is seen in other organs. In the kidney, ET-1 constricts the interlobular arteries as well as the afferent and efferent arterioles. Some studies show greater efferent than afferent arteriolar resistance. The increased renal vascular resistance is accompanied by a decrement in glomerular filtration rate, which results both from the decreased plasma flow rate and a decrease of the glomerular ultrafiltration coefficient, presumably secondary to mesangial contraction.[43–47] After cessation of endothelin infusions, renal plasma flow and glomerular filtration rate may remain suppressed for periods exceeding 60 to 90 minutes. Figure 5 shows the sustained renal vasoconstriction after intrarenal infusion of ET-1 in the dog.[44] The actions of ET-1 on the kidney are either unaffected or only attenuated by calcium channel blockers. The effects of endothelin on sodium reabsorption and sodium excretion are complex. If renal blood flow and glomerular filtration rate fall, sodium excretion and urine volume decrease.[46] Endothelin inhibits sodium reabsorp-

TABLE 4.
Physiologic Actions

Renal
Increases vascular resistance
Decreases renal blood flow and glomerular filtration rate
Decreases glomerular ultrafiltration coefficient
Increases/decreases Na reabsorption
Decreases AVP-stimulated H_2O reabsorption
Cardiovascular
Transient depressor response
Long-lived pressor response, i.e., vasoconstriction
Coronary vasoconstriction
Positive inotropic effect
Endocrine
Increases atrial natriuretic factor secretion
Increases plasma renin and catecholamines
Increases aldosterone secretion

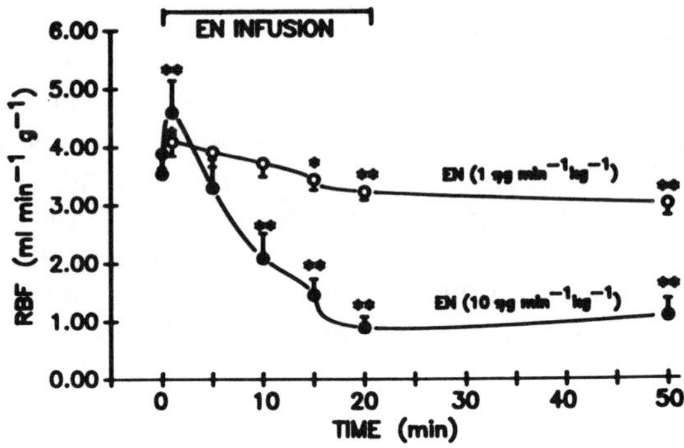

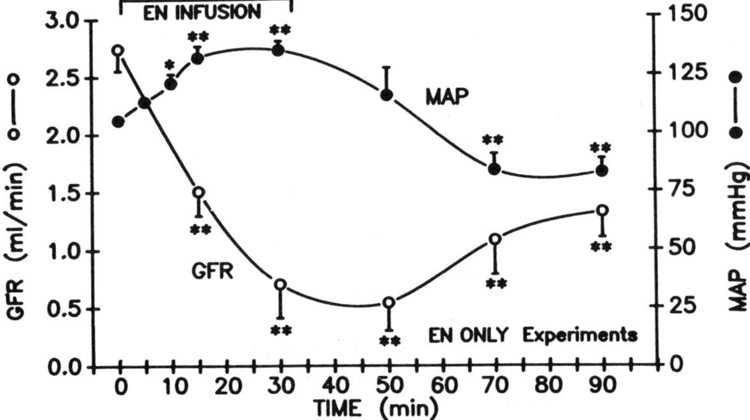

FIG 5.
The effects of endothelin on renal blood flow *(RBF)* and glomerular filtration rate *(GFR)* in the dog and rat. *Upper:* infusion of ET-1 at 1 and 10 ng/min/kg into the renal artery of the dog reduced renal blood flow not only during the ET-1 infusion but for 30 minutes after cessation of the infusion. *Lower:* Infusion of ET-1 0.1 μg/min/kg intravenously in the rat for 30 minutes dramatically reduced GFR and increased mean arterial pressure *(MAP)*. The decrement of GFR persisted during 60 minutes of recovery after cessation of ET-1 infusion. (*) $P < .05$ and (**) $P < .01$ compared to control. (From Banks RD: *Am J Physiol* 1990; 258:775–780. Used by permission.)

tion in the inner medullary collecting duct through stimulation of prostaglandins which, in turn, inhibit sodium reabsorption.[48] ET-1 may also regulate water excretion as it is synthesized in the collecting duct, inhibits vasopressin-stimulated cAMP in the collecting tubule, and decreases vasopressin-stimulated water reabsorption in this segment of the nephron.[49]

The cardiovascular responses of endothelin include a transient depressor response followed by a long-lived pressor phase, which persists after cessation of the ET infusion for 1 to 3 hours.[1] The transient depressor response has been attributed to endothelin-stimulated release of endothelial-derived relaxing factor (EDRF) and/or prostaglandins.[50] Indomethacin does not uniformly block or reduce the ET-induced vasodepressor response and, hence, it seems likely that EDRF (and possibly atrial natriuretic factor [ANF]) is the more potent mediator of this action. The increased blood pressure is due to large increases in systemic vascular resistance. Although ET-1 has a positive inotropic and chronotropic effect on isolated myocardial preparations, the in vivo effect is generally to reduce cardiac output, probably because of impressive increases in systemic vascular resistance (afterload) and concomitant coronary vasoconstriction.[29, 47]

The endocrine actions of endothelin are to increase the secretion of ANF, increase plasma renin and catecholamines, and increase aldosterone secretion.[29, 51, 52] ET has a direct action on atrial preparations and cultured monocytes to stimulate ANF synthesis and release. ANF is a potent antagonist of the actions of endothelin and concomitant infusion of ANF and ET-1 into the kidney significantly reduces renal vasoconstriction.[46] It is uncertain whether ET increases plasma renin indirectly by virtue of renal ischemic but this is a more likely explanation than a direct stimulatory effect since it probably acts like angiotensin II to directly reduce renin production by the juxtaglomerular apparatus. Increased plasma aldosterone levels have been documented in vivo, and ET-1 directly stimulates aldosterone synthesis in zona glomerulosa cell preparations.[53]

Pathophysiologic Roles of Endothelin

At present, it is difficult to define a pathophysiologic role for endothelin because pharmacologic tools to block endothelin synthesis or endothelin receptors are not available. Hence, as will be discussed, the potential pathophysiologic roles of ET must be inferred from studies of the plasma levels of circulating ET or the use of infusions of anti-ET antisera in the regional circulation of the kidney. Table 5 shows published studies reporting increased plasma levels of ET-1 in diverse abnormalities and diseases. In addition to the difficulties in measuring extremely low levels of plasma ET (0.5 to 2 pg/mL), an additional confounding factor derives from endothelin's role as a paracrine substance rather than a hormone. Most investigators believe that ET release occurs contiguous to the cellular site of action and the ET is not primarily secreted into the plasma as a circulating hormone to act at more distant sites. Plasma levels may represent an overflow

TABLE 5.
Increased Plasma Endothelin-1

Hypertension
Uremia
Cyclosporine toxicity
Congestive heart failure
Myocardial infarction
Shock: cardiogenic or septic (endotoxin)

of ET from endothelial and epithelial cells and may correlate with the synthetic rate of the cell of origin. Increased plasma levels have been reported in patients with hypertension and normal renal function as well as with renal failure regardless of dialysis therapy.[54–56] In one study, the plasma endothelin level was directly correlated with the height of the elevated blood pressure.[57]

Despite these human studies pointing to a role of ET-1 in hypertension, studies of genetic hypertension in experimental animals (spontaneously hypertensive rat or SHR) have not shown enhanced cardiovascular responsiveness to ET-1 in the SHR. Infusions of ET-1 produce comparable increases of blood pressure and decrements of glomerular filtration rate and renal blood flow in SHR and the normotensive control, WKY.[58, 59] ANF completely blocks the effects of ET to increase blood pressure or decrease glomerular filtration rate (GFR) and renal blood flow.[58] The tension developed in isolated mesenteric vessels from 6- and 12-week SHR and WKY was also about the same over a dose range of ET from 10^{-11} to 10^{-8} M.[59] Experimental congestive heart failure in dogs raised plasma endothelin from 0.7 to 3.1 pg/mL, but endothelin infusion into the dogs with heart failure induced smaller changes of blood pressure, systemic vascular resistance, and renal vascular resistance than in the control animals.[60] Acute infusion of cyclosporine A in large quantities induces nephrotoxicity accompanied by an acute transient elevation of plasma ET-1. Infusion of antisera against endothelin into the regional microvasculature of the kidney attenuated or blocked the cyclosporine-induced changes of single nephron GFR, renal plasma flow, and arteriolar resistances.[61] Kon and coworkers have reported a similar protective effect of endothelial antisera against the hypoperfusion and hypofiltration that persists after transient renal ischemia.[62] Endotoxin, in vivo or in vitro, stimulated endothelial secretion of ET and increased plasma levels of ET-1.[63]

All studies heretofore have emphasized the acute effects of endothelin mediated by vasoconstriction. It is important to keep in mind the possible chronic effects of endothelin such as vascular remodeling and regulation of cellular proliferation. ET-1 is a mitogen for cultured vascular smooth muscle cells, fibroblasts, and glomerular mesangial cells.[10, 64] After serum deprivation of cells, ET-1 can be a mitogen without the addition of other growth factors, but most studies show significant potentiation of the proliferative actions of ET-1 by classical growth factors. ET is extremely potent as a mitogen and in our studies of cultured glomerular mesangial cells, ET-1 can increase cellular proliferation at concentrations as low as 0.1nM.[34] It is reasonable to speculate that enhanced local production of ET-1 by vascular endothelium, both macrovasculature and microvasculature, would chronically alter vascular smooth muscle hyperplasia and hypertrophy and lead to vascular remodeling, medial growth, and accentuation of atherogenesis, progressing ultimately to luminal narrowing of the vessel. We have also recently speculated that ET-1 synthesis by glomerular endothelial cells and glomerular mesangial cells may regulate mesangial size and mesangial number, particularly in pathophysiologic conditions in which immune injury, platelet activation, and neutrophil activation result in mesangial proliferation, glomerular remodeling, and glomerulosclerosis, and ultimately glomerular obliteration.[64]

Acknowledgments

We are grateful to Norma Minear for typing the manuscript. Portions of this work were supported by grants from the National Institutes of Health, HL-22563, DK-41684, and HL-37117.

References

1. Yanagisawa M, Kurihara H, Kimura S, et al: A novel potent vasoconstrictor peptide produced by vascular endothelial cells. *Nature* 1988; 332:411–415.
2. Gillespie MN, Owasoyo JO, McMurtry IF, et al: Sustained coronary vasoconstriction provoked by a peptidergic substance release from endothelial cells in culture. *J Pharmacol Exp Ther* 1986; 236:339–343.
3. Hickey KA, Rubanyi G, Paul RG, et al: Characterization of a coronary vasoconstrictor produced by endothelial cells in culture. *Am J Physiol* 1985; 248:550–556.
4. Rubanyi G, Vanhoutte PM: Hypoxia releases a vasoconstrictor substance from the canine vascular endothelium. *J Physiol (London)* 1985; 364:45–56.
5. Inoue A, Yanagisawa M, Kimura S, et al: The human endothelin family: Three structurally and pharmacologically distinct isopeptides predicted by three separate genes. *Proc Natl Acad Sci USA* 1989; 86:2863–2867.
6. Itoh Y, Yanagisawa M, Ohkubo S, et al: Cloning and sequence analysis of cDNA encoding the precursor of a human endothelium-derived vasoconstrictor peptide, endothelin: identity of human and porcine endothelin. *FEBS Lett* 1988; 231:440–444.
7. Saida K, Mitsui Y, Ishida N: A novel peptide, vasoactive intestinal constrictor, of a new (endothelin) peptide family. *J Biol Chem* 1989; 264:14613–14616.
8. Yanagisawa M, Akihiro I, Ishikawa T, et al: Primary structure, synthesis and

biological activity of rat endothelin, and endothelium-derived vasoconstrictor peptide. *Proc Natl Acad Sci USA* 1988; 85:6964–6967.
9. Kloog Y, Sokolovsky M: Similarities in mode and sites of action of sarafotoxins and endothelins. *Trends Pharmacol Sci* 1989; 10:212–214.
10. Simonson MS, Dunn MJ: Cellular signaling by peptides of the endothelin gene family. *FASEB J* 1990; 4:2989–3000.
11. Bloch KD, Eddy RL, Shows TB, et al: cDNA cloning and chromosomal assignment of the gene encoding endothelin 3. *J Biol Chem* 1989; 264:18156–18161.
12. Inoue A, Yanagisawa M, Takuwa Y, et al: The human preproendothelin-1 gene. *J Biol Chem* 1989; 264:14954–14959.
13. MacCumber MW, Ross CA, Glaser BM, et al: Endothelin: visualization of mRNAs by in situ hybridization provides evidence for local action. *Proc Natl Acad Sci USA* 1989; 86:7285–7289.
14. Kosaka T, Suzuki N, Matsumoto H, et al: Synthesis of the vasoconstrictor peptide endothelin in kidney cells. *FEBS Lett* 1989; 249:42–46.
15. Ohta K, Hirata Y, Imai T, et al: Cytokine-induced release of endothelin-1 from porcine renal epithelial cell line. *Biochem Biophys Res Commun* 1990; 169:578–584.
16. Sakamoto H, Sasaki S, Hirata Y, et al: Production of endothelin-1 by rat cultured mesangial cells. *Biochem Biophys Res Commun* 1990; 169:462–468.
17. Shichiri M, Hirata Y, Emori T, et al: Secretion of endothelin and related peptides from renal epithelial cell lines. *FEBS Lett* 1989; 253:203–206.
18. Zoja C, Benigni A, Renzi D, et al: Endothelin and eicosanoid synthesis in cultured mesangial cells. *Kidney Int* 1990; 37:927–933.
19. Yanagisawa M, Masaki T: Endothelin, a novel endothelium-derived peptide. Pharmacological activities, regulation and possible roles in cardiovascular control. *Biochem Pharmacol* 1989; 38:1877–1883.
20. Davenport AP, Nunez DJ, Hall JA, et al: Autoradiographical localization of binding sites for porcine [^{125}I]endothelin-1 in humans, pigs, and rats: Functional relevance in humans. *J Cardiovasc Pharmacol* 1989; 13:166–170.
21. Hoyer D, Waeber C, Palacios JM: [^{125}I]Endothelin-1 binding sites: Autoradiographic studies in the brain and periphery of various species including humans. *J Cardiovasc Pharmacol* 1989; 13:162–165.
22. Kohzuki M, Johnston CI, Chai SY, et al: Localization of endothelin receptors in rat kidney. *Eur J Pharmacol* 1989; 160:193–194.
23. MacCumber MW, Ross CA, Snyder SH: Endothelin in brain: Receptors, mitogenesis, and biosynthesis in glial cells. *Proc Natl Acad Sci USA* 1990; 87:2359–2363.
24. Baldi E, Dunn MJ: Saturable high affinity endothelin binding sites in cultured rat mesangial cells (abstract). *Kidney Int* 1990; 37:363.
25. Clozel M, Fischli W, Guilly C: Specific binding of endothelin on human vascular smooth muscle cells in culture. *J Clin Invest* 1989; 83:1758–1761.
26. Hirata Y, Yoshimi H, Takaichi S, et al: Binding and receptor downregulation of a novel vasoconstrictor endothelin in cultured rat vascular smooth muscle cells. *FEBS Lett* 1988; 239:13–17.
27. Kloog Y, Bousso-Mittler D, Bdolah A, et al: Three apparent receptor subtypes for the endothelin/sarafotoxin family. *FEBS Lett* 1989; 253:199–202.
28. Martin ER, Marsden PA, brenner BM, et al: Identification and characterization of endothelin binding sites in rat renal papillary and glomerular membranes. *Biochem Biophys Res Commun* 1989; 162:130–137.

29. Vane JR, Botting R, Masaki T: Endothelin. *J Cardiovasc Pharmacol* 1989; 13:1–231.
30. Watanabe H, Miyazaki H, Kondoh M, et al: Two distinct types of endothelin receptors are present on chick cardiac membranes. *Biochem Biophys Res Commun* 1989; 161:1252–1259.
31. Badr KF, Munger KA, Sugiura M, et al: High and low affinity binding sites for endothelin on cultured rat mesangial cells. *Biochem Biophys Res Commun* 1989; 161:776–781.
32. Baldi E, Dunn MJ: Endothelin binding and receptor down regulation in rat glomerular mesangial cells. *J Pharmacol Exp Ther* 1991; 256:581–586.
33. Simonson MS, Dunn MJ: Endothelin: Pathways of transmembrane signaling. *Hypertension* 1990; 15:I5–I12.
34. Simonson MS, Wann S, Mene' P, et al: Endothelin stimulates phospholipase C, Na^+/H^+ exchange, c-fos expression, and mitogenesis in rat mesangial cells. *J Clin Invest* 1989; 83:708–712.
35. Thomas CP, Kester M, Dunn MJ: A pertussis toxin sensitive GTP-binding protein couples endothelin to phospholipase C in rat mesangial cells. *Am J Physiol* 1991; 260:F347–F352.
36. Simonson MS, Dunn MJ: Calcium signaling by distinct endothelin peptides in glomerular mesangial cells. *Exp Cell Res* 1991; 192:148–156.
37. Simonson MS, Osanai T, Dunn MJ: Endothelin isopeptides evoke calcium signaling and oscillations of cytosolic free calcium in human mesangial cells. *Biochim Biophys Acta* 1990; 1055:63–68.
38. Simonson MS, Dunn MJ: Endothelin-I stimulates contraction of rat glomerular mesangial cells and potentiates β adrenergic-mediated cAMP accumulation. *J Clin Invest* 1990; 85:790–797.
39. Billah MM, Pai JK, Mullmann TJ, et al: Regulation of phospholipase D in HL-60 granulocytes. *J Biol Chem* 1988; 264:9069–9076.
40. Bocckino SB, Wilson PB, Exton JH: Ca^{2+}-mobilizing hormones elicit PEt accumulation via phospholipase D activation. *FEBS Lett* 1987; 225:201–204.
41. Moolenar WH, Kruiger W, Tilly BC, et al: Growth factor-like action of PA. *Nature* 1986; 323:171–173.
42. Kester M, Simonson MS, McDermott RG, et al: Endothelin stimulates phospholipase D in cultured rat mesangial cells. *J Am Soc Nephrol* 1990; 1:473.
43. Badr KF, Murray JJ, Breyer MD, et al: Mesangial cell, glomerular and renal vascular responses to endothelin in the rat kidney. *J Clin Invest* 1989; 83:336–342.
44. Banks RO: Effects of endothelin on renal function in dogs and rats. *Am J Physiol* 1990; 258:775–780.
45. Cao L, Banks RO: Cardiovascular and renal actions of endothelin: Effects of calcium-channel blockers. *Am J Physiol* 1990; 258:254–258.
46. Katoh T, Chang H, Uchida S, et al: Direct effects of endothelin in the rat kidney. *Am J Physiol* 1990; 258:397–402.
47. Miller WL, Redfield MM, Brunett Jr JC: Integrated cardiac, renal, and endocrine actions of endothelin. *J Clin Invest* 1989; 83:317–320.
48. Zeidel ML, Brady HR, Kone BC, et al: Endothelin, a peptide inhibitor of Na^+-K^+-ATPase in intact renal tubular epithelial cells. *Am J Physiol* 1989; 257:1101–1107.
49. Tomita K, Nonoguchi H, Marumo F: Effects of endothelin on peptide-dependent cyclic adenosine monophosphate accumulation along the nephron segments of the rat. *J Clin Invest* 1990; 85:2014–2018.

50. De Nucci G, Thomas R, D'Orleans-Juste P, et al: Pressor effects of circulating endothelin are limited by its removal in the pulmonary circulation and by the release of prostacyclin and endothelium-derived relaxing factor. *Proc Natl Acad Sci USA* 1988; 85:9797–9800.
51. Brenner BM, Troy JL, Ballermann BJ: Endothelium-dependent vascular responses. Mediators and mechanisms. *J Clin Invest* 1989; 84:1373–1378.
52. Le Monnier de Gouville A-C, Lippton HL, Cevero I, et al: Endothelin—a new family of endothelium-derived peptides with widespread biological properties. *Life Sci* 1989; 45:1499–1513.
53. Cozza EN, Gomez-Sanchez CE, Foecking MF, et al: Endothelin binding to cultured calf adrenal zona glomerulosa cells and stimulation of aldosterone secretion. *J Clin Invest* 1989; 84:1032–1035.
54. Koyama H, Tabata T, Nishizawa Y, et al: Plasma endothelin levels in patients with uraemia. *Lancet* 1989; 1:991–992.
55. Shichiri M, Hirata Y, Ando K, et al: Plasma endothelin levels in hypertension and chronic renal failure. *Hypertension* 1990; 15:493–496.
56. Totsune K, Mouri T, Takahashi K, et al: Detection of immunoreactive endothelin in plasma of hemodialysis patients. *FEBS Lett* 1989; 249:239–242.
57. Kohno M, Yasunari K, Murakawa K-I, et al: Plasma immunoreactive endothelin in essential hypertension. *Am J Med* 1990; 88:614–617.
58. Hirata Y, Matsuoka H, Kimura K, et al: Renal vasoconstriction by the endothelial cell-derived peptide endothelin in spontaneously hypertensive rats. *Circ Research* 1989; 65:1370–1379.
59. Miyauchi T, Ishikawa T, Tomobe Y, et al: Characteristics of pressor response to endothelin in spontaneously hypertensive and Wistar-Kyoto rats. *Hypertension* 1989; 14:427–434.
60. Cavero PG, Miller WL, Heublein DM, et al: Endothelin in experimental congestive heart failure in the anesthetized dog. *Am J Physiol* 1990; 259:312–317.
61. Kon V, Sugiura M, Inagami T, et al: Role of endothelin in cyclosporine-induced glomerular dysfunction. *Kidney Int* 1990; 37:1487–1491.
62. Kon V, Yoshioka T, Fogo A, et al: Glomerular actions of endothelin in vivo. *J Clin Invest* 1989; 83:1762–1767.
63. Sugiura M, Inagami T, Kon V: Endotoxin stimulates endothelin-release in vivo and in vitro as determined by radioimmunoassay. *Biochem Biophys Res Commun* 1989; 161:1220–1227.
64. Simonson MS, Dunn MJ: Endothelin peptides: A possible role in glomerular inflammation. *Lab Invest* 1991; 64:1–4.

Agonists and Antagonists of ATP-Sensitive Potassium Channels

Michel Lazdunski, Ph.D.

Institut de Pharmacologie Moléculaire et Cellulaire du Centre National de la Recherche Scientifique, Sophia Antipolis, Valbonne, France

Henri Bernardi

Institut de Pharmacologie Moléculaire et Cellulaire du Centre National de la Recherche Scientifique, Sophia Antipolis, Valbonne, France

Jan R. de Weille, Ph.D.

Institut de Pharmacologie Moléculaire et Cellulaire de Centre National de la Recherche Scientifique, Sophia Antipolis, Valbonne, France

Christiane Mourre, Ph.D.

Institut de Pharmacologie Moléculaire et Cellulaire du Centre National de la Recherche Scientifique, Sophia Antipolis, Valbonne, France

Michel Fosset, Ph.D

Institut de Pharmacologie Moléculaire et Cellulaire de Centre National de la Recherche Scientifique, Sophia Antipolis, Valbonne, France

The presence of K^+ channels, the activity of which is inhibited by an increase of intracellular adenosine triphosphate (ATP) concentrations, was first described in cardiac cells.[1] These channels have since been identified in pancreatic β cells, in skeletal muscle, in nerve cells, and in smooth muscle.[2] The $[ATP]_{in}$-sensitive K^+ channel (K_{ATP} channel) ensures an essential connection between the bioenergetic level of the cell (ATP) and the electrical properties of excitability of the plasma membrane.

Insulin controls the blood level of glucose and, inversely, the level of blood glucose controls insulin secretion by the β cell. In the absence of exposure to glucose perfusion, the β cell is well polarized (approximately −70 to −60 mV), it behaves as a nonexcitable cell (it does not generate repetitive action potentials), and it does not secrete insulin. This situation (a good polarization, no spontaneous electrical activity) is due to the fact that a number of K^+ channels are then in the open conformation among which are K_{ATP} channels. As soon as the β cell is exposed to a glucose perfusion, it depolarizes, which leads to a spontaneous electrical activity with repetitive action potentials. The β cell has become excitable. The length of the burst of action potential depends on the glucose concentration. After a time, which can be minutes, the β cell will be electrically silent again before starting a new period of spontaneous activity if glucose perfusion persists. It is the spontaneous electrical activity provoked by the glucose perfusion that is largely responsible for insulin secretion.

The molecular mechanism of this electrogenic process is now well understood. Glucose perfusion will activate intracellular mechanisms for ATP production, and this increase of $[ATP]_{in}$ (in fact of the $[ATP]_{in}/[ADP]_{in}$ ratio) will close K^+ channels. This is the key step of the whole process, since this K^+ channel closure will lead to a depolarization that will trigger all the other steps associated with insulin secretion. The depolarization will lead the membrane potential to the threshold of activation of voltage-dependent Ca^{2+} channels. Activation of these Ca^{2+} channels provokes the generation of repetitive action potentials. These Ca^{2+} action potentials will allow Ca^{2+} entry and lead to an increase of the intracellular Ca^{2+} concentration up to the level necessary for insulin secretion. The increase in $[Ca^{2+}]_{in}$ will later produce an activation of Ca^{2+}-dependent K^+ channels. The opening of these later channels will be associated with a repolarization of the β cell membrane, which again will put a distance between the membrane potential and the threshold potential for activation of Ca^{2+} channels and will transiently eliminate repetitive electrical activity.

Sulfonylureas, like glucose, trigger insulin secretion. It was therefore tempting to postulate that this therapeutic class of drugs has a mechanism of action that involves the blockade of K_{ATP} channels. This is indeed how sulfonylureas act.[3] There are two great types of sulfonylureas. Tolbutamide is the prototype of first-generation compounds and glibenclamide the prototype of second-generation compounds. Glibenclamide and other second-generation compounds are potent blockers of K_{ATP} channels. The most potent sulfonylureas, such as glibenclamide, act at concentrations of 0.1 to 1 nM. The less potent sulfonylureas act at concentrations that are 10^3 to 10^5 higher.[3] The most potent inhibitors of K_{ATP} channels are also the most potent antidiabetics (they act at particularly low doses).[3] By blocking K_{ATP} channels, sulfonylureas produce the same effects as glucose itself (which indirectly inhibits the channel by changing the ATP_{in}/ADP_{in} ratio).

Most of what we know today about ionic channels would not have been discovered without strong pharmacologic research. The most potent sulfonylureas have been tritiated, and their receptor has been identified [3] and therefore better understood at the molecular level.[4, 5] The sulfonylurea receptor has been affinity labelled[4, 5] and purified.[5] It is situated on a protein of 150 kDa.

K_{ATP} channels can open without changing $[ATP]_{in}$. If insulin secretion by the β cell is dependent on the level of extracellular concentration of glucose, it is also modulated by a series of hormones. The best known of all of them is somatostatin. Somatostatin inhibits insulin secretion by the β cell. This inhibition is associated with an action of the hormone on K_{ATP}

channel expression.[6] Somatostatin binds to its receptor site, and this binding triggers the activation of a G protein, which triggers the activation of K $_{ATP}$ channels. Somatostatin-activated K_{ATP} channels remain sensitive to blockade by sulfonylureas. Activation of K_{ATP} channels by somatostatin will lead to a hyperpolarization, which will reduce the opening probability of Ca^{2+} channels, the major Ca^{2+} entry system for insulin secretion.

Another hormone, galanin, which was recently discovered, also inhibits insulin secretion and has hyperglycemic effect. It has the same mechanism of action as that which has been previously described for somatostatin.[7, 8]

Thus, the K_{ATP} channel is the target of: (1) antidiabetic sulfonylureas; (2) hormones that inhibit insulin secretion; and (3) glucose, which normally stimulates insulin secretion. It would not be surprising that a defect of structure or regulation of this channel would be the origin of the diabetic state.

The K_{ATP} channel openers, a new class of drugs, has recently attracted considerable interest. These molecules—cromakalim, pinacidil, nicorandil, RP49356, and minoxidil sulfate—relax smooth muscles.[9, 10] Another molecule, diazoxide, which has a structure similar to that of thiazides with a diuretic action, as hyperglycemic effects that are associated with the capacity of the drug to open K_{ATP} channels in the β cell. Diazoxide is also a vasorelaxant and antihypertensive. The opening of K_{ATP} channels polarizes the smooth muscle cell, then decreases the probability of opening of Ca^{2+} channels via L-type Ca^{2+} channels, and therefore inhibits contraction.

K_{ATP} channels that are opened by cromakalim, pinacidil, RP49356, and other K_{ATP} channel openers, are blocked by antidiabetic sulfonylureas. K_{ATP} channel openers are vasorelaxants, and sulfonylureas eliminate this vasorelaxation. Target channels for the K_{ATP} channel openers are K_{ATP} channels.[9, 10] However, it should be kept in mind that channel openers exert their action without changing $[ATP]_{in}$. The sensitivity of K_{ATP} channels in the smooth muscle to sulfonylureas is much lower than that observed in the β cell (approximately 1,000 times). It is then probable that K_{ATP} channels in the smooth muscle are the products of gene(s) that are different from the gene which is expressed in the β cell. Conversely, K_{ATP} channels in the pancreatic β cell are much less sensitive to K_{ATP} channel openers than are those in the smooth muscle cell.

K_{ATP} channel openers in smooth muscle, which are contraction inhibitors, will probably find an application in hypertension (they could be used in combination with other available drugs: Ca^{2+} channel blockers, diuretics, β blockers, inhibitors of the converting enzyme) and also in other pathologic conditions of the smooth muscle such as asthma.

The K_{ATP} channel was identified for the first time in the cardiac cell. Its functional effect in this cell in normal physiologic conditions is still a mystery. In normal conditions, the $[ATP]_{in}$ concentration is such that K_{ATP} channels in the cardiac cell are closed. However these channels may be the target of hormones or neurotransmitters which would act as somatostatin or galanin on the pancreatic β cell. The problem that will be dealt with here is the implication of these channels in cardiac ischemia. Two important events happen when a cardiac cell is ischemic: (1) cytoplasmic acidification; and (2) a decrease of the ATP_{in}/ADP_{in}. The decrease of the ATP_{in}/ADP_{in} opens K_{ATP} channels and shortens the duration of the action potential.[11, 12] It is well known that this shortening is highly involved in the abnormal electrogenicity observed during ischemia.[13] The shortening of the action potential in ischemic cells due to the opening of K_{ATP} channels is suppressed by antidiabetic sulfonylureas.[11, 14]

The problem now is to know what class of drug will be useful in ischemia. Will it be sulfonylureas, which block the K_{ATP} channel or the openers such as cromakalim? If the shortening of the cardiac action potential has a beneficial physiologic effect—linked for example to a decreased Ca^{2+} entry due to the short action potential—then the K_{ATP} channel openers could have a beneficial physiologic effect in ischemia.[15, 16] Patients with diabetes mellitus treated with sulfonylureas may be subject to silent ischemia. This silent ischemia could be associated with a diabetic neuropathy which would decrease or suppress pain perception,[17] or sulfonylureas by inhibiting a K^+ efflux (extracellular K^+ variations should normally lead to a depolarization and then to an activation of the sensory system).

K_{ATP} channels are present in neurons. They have been identified in neurons of the ventromedian hypothalamus where they probably sense variations of glucose concentrations, which play an important role in the control of satiety for sugars. The effect of K_{ATP} channel openers on these channels is unknown.

It is the presence of high-affinity sulfonylurea receptors that has led to the identification of K_{ATP} channels in the central nervous system.[5] Quantitative autoradiography has allowed a precise localization of these channels.[18–20] The highest densities are present in substantia nigra and globus pallidus, but K_{ATP} channels are also located in other brain areas. They are situated in the hippocampus, which is both associated with memory acquisition and deleterious cellular effects linked to anoxia or cerebral ischemia.[21]

What is the physiologic role of K_{ATP} channels in the brain? Are they associated with neurotransmitter secretion as insulin secretion in the β cell? Most of the synapses situated in substantia nigra and globus pallidus contain γ-aminobutyric acid (GABA), the most classic of inhibitory neurotransmitters. GABA inhibits electrical activity of dopaminergic neurons in substantial nigra.[22]

The increase of extracellular glucose concentration stimulates synaptic GABA secretion in substantia nigra[23] as it stimulated insulin secretion in pancreatic islets.

Application of sulfonylureas that stimulate insulin secretion in β cells triggers GABA secretion in substantia nigra.[23] Mechanisms that have been described in endocrine pancreas are then present in the brain. K_{ATP} channels are situated in synapses, and their closing by glucose (indirect) or by sulfonylureas (direct) leads to synaptic depolarization, Ca^{2+} entry via synaptic Ca^{2+} channels, and neurotransmitter secretion. Brain K_{ATP} channels have a pharmacology that is slightly different from that of pancreatic K_{ATP} channels and could well be encoded by one or several distinct genes. What are the physiologic and physiopathologic consequences of these observations?

GABAergic innervation of subsantia nigra has an essential anti-epileptic function.[24] Inhibition of dopaminergic neurones by GABA is key to prevent the propagation of epileptic crises. Hypoglycemia observed in a patient with diabetes mellitus can generate convulsions and coma. Conversely, a hyperglycemic state will lead to a strong inhibition of dopaminergic neurons, which explains (or which can explain) modifications of the locomotor activity observed in the diabetic animal that has been made hyperglycemic and probably also in the patient with diabetes mellitus.

One of the important molecular events of cerebral ischemia, as for cardiac ischemia, is a decrease of the ATP_{in}/ADP_{in}. This decrease occurs during anoxia.[23] In all cases, this alteration of the intracellular ATP_{in}/ADP_{in} will lead to the opening of K_{ATP} channels and to K^+ efflux. We could have here the interpretation of a well-known phenomenon, but which has remained unexplained until now, which is extracellular K^+ accumulation as soon as the animal has had a cardiac arrest.[25] This K^+ efflux with K^+ accumulation in the extracellular space will have dramatic effects on neuron viability, particularly in the hippocampus. Extracellular K^+ accumulation leads to: (1) depolarization of excitatory synapses, which liberates glutamate; (2) activation by glutamate (an excito-toxic transmitter) of specific receptors including the N-methyl-D-aspartate (NMDA) receptor, which is coupled to a Ca^{2+} permeable channel; (3) a massive cellular invasion of Ca^{2+}, which will be unable to go out of the cell which is the target of glutamate, and which won't be able to be stored in endoplasmic reticulum for lack of ATP, prevents the normal functioning of Ca^{2+}-ATPases necessary for extrusion or storage in intracellular stores; and (4) an activation via $[Ca^{2+}]_{in}$ increase of a series of Ca^{2+}-activated enzymes (phospholipases, proteases), which destroy cellular structures as well as a Ca^{2+}-dependent alteration of cytoskeletal structures, all processes leading to cell death.

Anoxia as ischemia liberates glutamate from the hippocampus, and this liberation is inhibited by galanin,[26] which has already been described for its activating action in K_{ATP} channels in the pancreas.

The physiologic role of K_{ATP} channels in skeletal muscle is not well understood.[27] However, intense muscular exercise provokes a K^+ loss and an increase in plasma K^+ concentration, which might be locally beneficial and leads to stimulation of carotid bodies, thus increasing ventilation. Muscle K_{ATP} channels are also regulated by variations of internal pH. A decrease of intracellular pH will occur with ischemia and will decrease the inhibitory effect of ATP and favor opening of the K_{ATP} channel.[28] The K_{ATP} channel in muscle is activated by some of the K_{ATP} channel openers such as pinacidil. The sensitivity of the K_{ATP} channel to openers is observed at concentrations that are much higher than those necessary to activate smooth muscle.[29] However, therapeutic indications could be very interesting in a variety of muscular diseases that are associated with a membrane depolarization, such as periodic paralysis and paramyotonia.

K_{ATP} channels probably play an important role in the regulation of smooth muscle contraction and in the local regulation of blood flow. It is possible or even probable that these channels, the targets of K_{ATP} channel openers, have an important role in the mechanism of action of endogeneous vasorelaxants[30] such as the hyperpolarizing factor derived from endothelium-derived hyperpolarization factor (EDHF), vasoactive intestinal peptide (VIP), or calcitonin gene-related peptide (CGRP).

The analysis of the properties of this class of channels that are sensitive to both antidiabetic sulfonylureas and K^+ channel openers is still in its infancy. The years to come will probably see a series of progresses in the following areas: (1) discovery of new cellular types having K_{ATP} channels and observation of possible application in the pharmacologic and physiopathologic field; (2) discovery of new natural effectors of K_{ATP} channels; and (3) cloning and identification of the different genes in charge of coding for the different subtypes of K_{ATP} channels.

Acknowledgments

This work has benefited from the financial support of the Centre National de la Recherche Scientifique, the Institut National de la Santé et de la Recherchle Médicale (CRE 88.2007), and the Ministère de la Recherche et de la Technologie (grant no. 89.C.0883). Authors are grateful to Drs. H. Schmid-Antomarchi, and S. Amoroso, and to C. Roulinat-Bettelheim.

References

1. Noma A: ATP-regulated K^+ channels in cardiac muscle. *Nature* 1983; 305:147–148.
2. Dunne MJ, Petersen OH: Potassium selective ion channels in insulin-secreting cells: Physiology, pharmacology and their role in stimulus-secretion coupling. *Biochim Biophys Acta Rev Biomembr* 1991; 1071:67–82.
3. Schmid-Antomarchi H, De Weille J, Fosset M, et al: The receptor for antidiabetic sulfonylureas controls the activity of the ATP-modulated K^+ channel in insulin-secreting cells. *J Biol Chem* 1987; 262:15840–15844.
4. Aguilar-Bryan L, Nelson DA, Vu QA, et al: Photoaffinity labeling and partial purification of the β cell sulfonylurea receptor using a novel, biologically active glyburide analog. *J Biol Chem* 1990; 265:8218–8224.
5. Bernardi H, Fosset M, Lazdunski M: Characterization, purification and affinity labelling of the brain [^{3}H]glibenclamide binding protein, a putative neuronal ATP-regulated K^+ channel. *Proc Natl Acad Sci USA* 1988; 85:9816–9820.
6. De Weille JR, Schmid-Antomarchi H, Fosset M, et al: Regulation of ATP-sensitive K^+ channels in insulinoma cells. Activation by somatostatin and kinase C and the role of cAMP. *Proc Natl Acad Sci USA* 1989; 86:2971–2975.
7. Dunne MJ, Bullet MJ, Li G, et al: Galanin activates nucleotide-dependent K^+ channels in insulin-secreting cells via a pertussis toxin-sensitive G-protein, *EMBO J* 1989; 8:413–420.
8. Tatemoto K, Rökaeus AA, Jörnvall H, et al: Galanin-a novel biologically active peptide from porcine intestine. *FEBS Lett* 1983; 164:124–128.
9. Edwards G, Weston AH: Structure-activity relationships of K^+ channel openers. *Trends Pharmacol Sci* 1990; 11:417–422.

10. Quast U, Cook NS: Moving together: K^+ channel openers and ATP-sensitive K^+ channels. *Trends Pharmacol Sci* 1989; 10:431–435.
11. Fosset M, De Weille JR, Green RD, et al: Antidiabetic sulfonylureas control action potential properties in heart cells via high affinity receptors that are linked to ATP-dependent K^+ channels. *J Biol Chem* 1988; 263:7933–7936.
12. Trube G, Hescheler J: Inward-rectifying channels in isolated patches of the heart cell membranes: ATP-dependence and comparison with cell-attached patches. *Pflugers Arch* 1984; 401:178–184.
13. Vleugels A, Vereecke J, Carmeliet E: Ionic currents during hypoxia in voltage-clamped cat ventricular muscle. *Circ Res* 1980; 47:501–508.
14. Gasser RNA, Vaughan-Jones RD: Mechanism of potassium efflux and action potential shortening during ischaemia in isolated mamalian cardiac muscle. *J Physiol* 1990; 431:713–741.
15. Grover GJ, Dzwonczyk S, Sleph PG: Reduction of ischematic damage in isolated rat hearts by the potassium channel opener, RP 52891. *Eur J Pharmacol* 1990; 191:11–198.
16. Grover GJ, McCullough JR, Henry DE, et al: Anti-ischemic effects of the potassium channel activators pinacidil and cromakalim and the reversal of these effects with the potassium channel blocker glyburide. *J Pharm Exp Ther* 1989; 251:98–104.
17. Ashcroft SJH, Ashcroft FM: Properties and functions of ATP-sensitive K-channels. *Cell Signalling* 1990; 2:197–214.
18. Mourre C, Ben Ari Y, Bernardi H, et al: Antidiabetic sulfonylureas: Localization of binding sites in the brain and effects on the hyperpolarization induced by anoxia in hippocampal slices. *Brain Res* 1989; 486:159–164.
19. Mourre C, Widmann C, Lazdunski M: Specific hippocampal lesions indicate the presence of sulfonylurea binding sites associated to ATP-sensitive K^+ channels both post-synaptically and on mossy fibers. *Brain Res* 1990; 540:340–344.
20. Mourre C, Widmann C, Lazdunski M: Sulfonylurea binding sites associated with ATP-regulated K^+ channels in the central nervous system: Autoradiographic analysis of their distribution and ontogenesis, and of their localization in mutant mice cerebellum. *Brain Res* 1990; 519:29–43.
21. Mourre C, Smith ML, Siesjö BK, et al: Brain ischemia alters the density of binding sites for glibenclamide, a specific blocker of ATP-sensitive K^+ channels. *Brain Res* 1990; 526:147–152.
22. Roeper J, Hainsworth AH, Ashcroft FM: Tolbutamide reverses membrane hyperpolarisation induced by activation of D_2 receptors and $GABA_B$ receptors in isolated substantia nigra neurones. *Pflugers Arch* 1990; 416:473–475.
23. Amoroso S, Schmid-Antomarchi H, Fosset M, et al: Glucose, antidiabetic sulfonylureas and neurotransmitter release. Role of ATP-sensitive K^+ channels. *Science* 1990; 247:852–854.
24. Gale K: Role of the substantia nigra in GABA-mediated anticonvulsant action. *Adv Neurol* 1986; 44:343–364.
25. Hansen AJ: Effect of anoxia on ion distribution in the brain. *Physiol Rev* 1985; 65:101–148.
26. Ben Ari Y, Lazdunski M: Galanin protects hippocampal neurons from the functional effects of anoxia. *Eur J Pharm* 1989; 165:331–332.
27. Spruce AE, Standen NB, Stanfield PR: Studies of the unitary properties of adenosine 5′-triphosphate-regulated potassium channels of frog skeletal muscle. *J Physiol* 1987; 382:213–236.

28. Davies NW: Modulation of ATP-sensitive K^+ channels in skeletal muscle by intracellular protons. *Nature* 1990; 343:375–377.
29. Spuler A, Lehmann-Horn F, Grafe P: Cromakalim (BRL 34915) restores in vitro the membrane potential of depolarized human skeletal muscle fibres. *Naunyn-Schmiedeberg's Arch Pharmacol* 1989; 339:327–331.
30. Nelson MT, Patlack JB, Worley JF, et al: Calcium channels, potassium channels, and voltage dependence of arterial smooth muscle tone. *Am J Physiol* 1990; 259:3–18.

The Biological Role, Site, and Regulation of Erythropoietin Production

Kai-Uwe Eckardt, M.D.

Assistant, Physiologisches Institut der Universität Regensburg, Germany

Armin Kurtz, M.D.

Professor, Physiologisches Institut der Universität Regensburg, Germany

With the exception of the growth period, the circulating red blood cell mass and hence the oxygen carrying capacity of blood is normally rather constant. Since the erythron is a continuously regenerating organ, a daily production of 20 mL of red blood cells is required in human adults to compensate for the physiologic demise of 120-day-old erythrocytes. In addition, when increased blood loss occurs or the oxygen saturation of hemoglobin falls, the bone marrow is capable of increasing this normal production rate of red blood cells up to three to fivefold within a few days, and even up to sevenfold under chronic conditions.

Generally, the rate at which blood cells can be released into the circulation depends on the time required by a pluripotent stem cell in the bone marrow to differentiate into red blood cells, white blood cells, or platelets. For each cell line this differentiation comprises multiple steps of cell division and maturation, and an increasing number of hematopoietic growth factors is being recognized as controling these individual steps. While many of these growth factors are produced by bone marrow cells in the direct vicinity of their target cells, the predominant and essential regulator of red blood cell formation, erythropoietin (EPO), is a true hormone in that it is produced outside the bone marrow, mainly in the kidney and to some extent in the liver.

Through the control of EPO production, the kidney becomes the central regulatory organ of red blood cell formation and thereby beyond its role for waste excretion and water and electrolyte homeostasis, carries essential responsibility for tissue oxygenation. As a consequence, chronic renal failure is frequently accompanied by hypoproliferative anemia, resulting mainly from insufficient EPO production. Following the cloning of the EPO gene in 1985,[1, 2] EPO has been produced in abundant quantities with re-

Advances in Nephrology,® vol 21

combinant DNA technology, and the application of this recombinant human EPO (rhEPO) to patients with renal failure has been shown to effectively correct their anemia.[3, 4] First promising results of the application of rhEPO in other hematologic disorders have also been reported.[5–7] The success of EPO in the clinical situation stands in contrast to the state of knowledge of the physiology of this hormone. Not only have the precise mechanisms of action of EPO in the bone marrow not been clearly defined, but neither have the cellular sites of EPO formation and the mechanisms by which circulating EPO levels are adapted to changes in the oxygen supply of the organism. The recent availability of cloned DNA reagents and large quantities of EPO, however, have provided effective tools to address these questions and have turned EPO research into a rapidly developing and expanding field. In the following we will try to outline recent progress in this area and summarize the current state of knowlege on the structure of EPO and its gene, the function of the hormone, its production sites, and the mechanisms of its regulation.

Molecular Structure of EPO and Its Gene

EPO Gene

Cloning of the EPO gene was made possible through the partial purification of a few milligrams of EPO from large amounts of urine from patients with aplastic anemia.[8] Based on limited amino acid sequence information derived from this material, two laboratories succeeded independently in cloning the human EPO gene by screening genomic libraries with synthetic oligonucleotides.[1, 2] With the human EPO gene as a probe, EPO genes subsequently were isolated from the mouse[9, 10] and monkey.[11] A comparison between these genes reveals that EPO is well conserved during evolution, with approximately 80% homology of both the coding region of DNA and the amino acid sequence between man and mouse. The EPO gene appears to be present in the genome as a single copy and there is no evidence for other EPO-related genes or pseudogenes.[1, 2]

The human EPO gene encompasses about 3,000 base pair (bp) and is located on the long arm of chromosome 7.[12, 13] It contains five exons and four introns (Fig 1). EPO is synthesized as a pro-form, containing a 27 amino acid leader peptide, which is processed during secretion, plus a 166 amino acid backbone. Exon I of the EPO gene encodes for part of the leader peptide and contains a relatively long 5′untranslated region, whereas the genetic information of the mature EPO is within exons II to IV. By comparison with the murine EPO gene, it was assumed that the transcriptional start site in the human gene is located at approximately 240 bp 5′ of the translational start site.[10] Recent evidence suggests, however, that multiple transcriptional start sites may exist.[14]

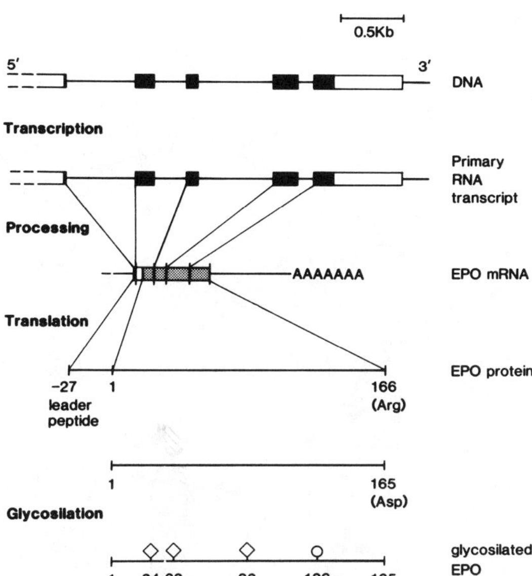

FIG 1.

Schematic presentation of transcription and translation of the human EPO gene and posttranslational modifications of the EPO protein. (Map of EPO gene and EPO mRNA adapted from Jacobs K, Shoemaker C, Rudersdorf R, et al: *Nature* 1985; 313:806–810 and McDonald J, Lin F-K, Goldwasser E: *Mol Cell Biol* 1986; 6:842–848.) Protein encoding portions of the 5 exons of the gene are in black. The EPO gene codes for a 27-amino-acid leader peptide that is considered to be important for secretion of the hormone, plus a 166-amino-acid protein chain. The terminal arginine molecule of the peptide chain is cleaved off at a yet unknown stage of EPO production. This processing appears not to require exposure to serum since it was also found to occur when recombinant EPO was produced under serum-free culture conditions.[15] Approximately 40% of the total molecular weight of mature EPO is due to complex-type carbohydrate additions at three N-linked *(diamond)* and one O-linked *(circle)* glycosylation site (see text for details).

EPO Molecule

The mature EPO molecule is a glycoprotein consisting of an amino acid backbone and complex sugar side chains. The translation of the EPO protein terminates after arginine at position 166 (see Fig 1). However, both recombinant EPO and urinary EPO are missing the carboxy-terminal arginine and contain only 165 amino acids,[15] indicating that the terminal arginine is cleaved off. The physiologic significance of this special processing and the stage of EPO production at which it occurs are unknown.

There are four cysteines in the molecule, forming two disulfide pairs (Fig 2). Disulfide pairing between residues 7 and 161 links both ends of the protein chain, and pairing between residues 29 and 33 forms a small loop.

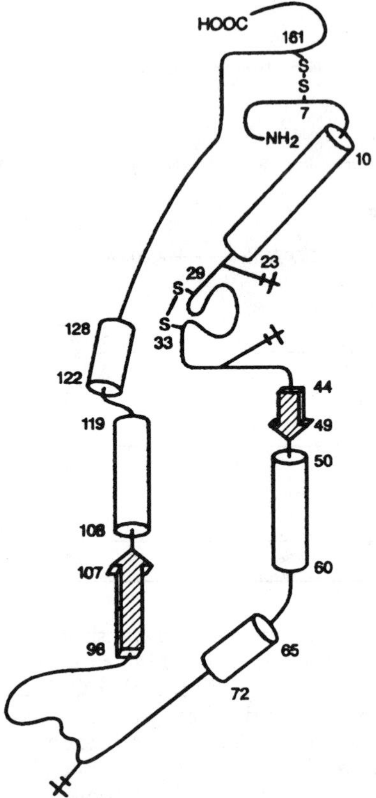

FIG 2.
Model of the secondary structure of human EPO as predicted by the method of Chou and Fasman on the basis of the primary amino acid sequence. Potential α helices are indicated by a cylinder, potential β strands by an arrow, and predicted β turns by a turn in the amino acid backbone. Antennas indicate N-linked glycosylation sites. (From McDonald J, Lin F-K, Goldwasser E: *Mol Cell Biol* 1986; 6:842–848. Used by permission.)

Disulfide pairing is of functional significance, since the biologic activity of EPO is reversibly sensitive to reducing agents.[16, 17] In the mouse, however, cysteine at position 33 is absent, suggesting that the small loop in human EPO may not be absolutely required for activity or that other compensating structural alterations have occurred in the mouse EPO protein.

Approximately 40% of the total molecular weight of EPO (30,400 dalton, as determined by equilibrium sedimentation), is due to carbohydrate additions to the EPO protein. These sugars are linked to the polypeptide chain at three N-linked (Asn 24, 38, 83) and one O-linked (Ser 126) glycosylation sites (see Figs 1, 2). The major component of the O-linked sugar is a disialosyl chain.[18, 19] The N-linked side chains mainly consist of tetraantennary saccharides (about 80%), some of them containing polylactosaminyl repeats. A smaller proportion of triantennary (about 15%) and biantennary (1% to 6%) chains is also present.[18, 20, 21] All of these saccharides are sialylated, although to a different extent. The distribution of these sugar chains varies at each glycosylation site. Chains at position Asn-38 are more heavily sialylated and less frequently of biantennary structure than those at Asn-24. Oligosaccharides at position Asn-83 are relatively homogenous tetra-antennary chains without polylactosaminyl repeats.[19]

The carbohydrate moiety of EPO is not required for action of the hormone on its target cells,[22, 23] and the biologic activity of partially deglycosylated EPO in vitro may even be enhanced.[24, 25] However, the carbohydrate moiety is of considerable importance for the clearance rate of circulating EPO and thus determines its biologic activity in vivo. When recombinant EPO is produced in an unusual cell line that adds only biantennary side chains to the protein, the biologic activity in vivo was found to be decreased sevenfold.[26] Removal of terminal sialic acids of otherwise normal sugar side chains enhances EPO clearance to an extent that its biologic activity is almost totally abolished.[22, 24, 27, 28] This results from rapid uptake via the so-called hepatic asialo receptor, which recognizes the free galactose residues that are exposed by desialylation.[24, 27, 28] Enhanced uptake by the same receptor is also thought to be responsible for increased clearance of those molecules containing polylactosaminyl repeats.[27] Finally, the biologic activity of EPO in vivo is also missing when all sugar residues are removed, but it is unknown where the rapid clearance of deglycosylated EPO occurs.[23]

Because of this important role of the carbohydrate moiety of EPO for its in vivo activity, it was of major clinical importance that the glycosylation pattern of recombinant EPO produced in animal cell lines is almost identical to that of endogenous human urinary EPO.[18, 20, 21] In general, however, the glycosylation of EPO results in some heterogeneity of EPO molecules. Interestingly, clear differences were found in the distribution of oligosaccharide components of urinary EPO among different individuals.[21] It is also possible, though not yet investigated, that within an individual glycosylation may vary with the cellular site and the rate of EPO production, which may affect the biologic efficacy of the hormone.

Site and Mechanism of Action

Target Cells for EPO

Unlike several other hematopoietic growth factors, EPO is largely lineage-specific, influencing almost exclusively the growth of erythroid precursor cells. Those cells within the erythroid lineage that are stimulated by EPO have been defined operationally as erythropoietin-responsive cells (ERC).[29, 30] The current view is that this population of ERC represents erythroid precursors at different developmental stages between a pluripotent stem cell on one side and erythroblasts on the other side, which themselves are both not affected by EPO. Although there appears to be a continuum between these progenitor cells, two major subpopulations have been recognized: the burst forming unit-erythroid (BFU-E), which is closely related to the pluripotent stem cell, and the colony forming unit-erythroid (CFU-E), which is close to the first recognizable erythroblast (Fig 3). In human marrow, BFU-E and CFU-E are present at a frequency of about 20 and 50 per 100,000 nucleated cells, respectively.[31] The maturation from BFU-E to CFU-E progresses with an increasing sensitivity to EPO. Although EPO is considered the main and essential regulator of red blood cell formation, it requires interaction with other growth factors. Thus insulin or insulin-like growth factor I have to be added to purified human CFU-E to induce differentiation into erythroblast colonies in vitro.[32] Purified BFU-E, on the other hand, require interleukin 3, granulocyte-macrophage- and granulocyte-colony-stimulating factor in addition to EPO for maximum development in culture.[33] Furthermore, it is not clear whether under physiologic conditions EPO is actually essential for these

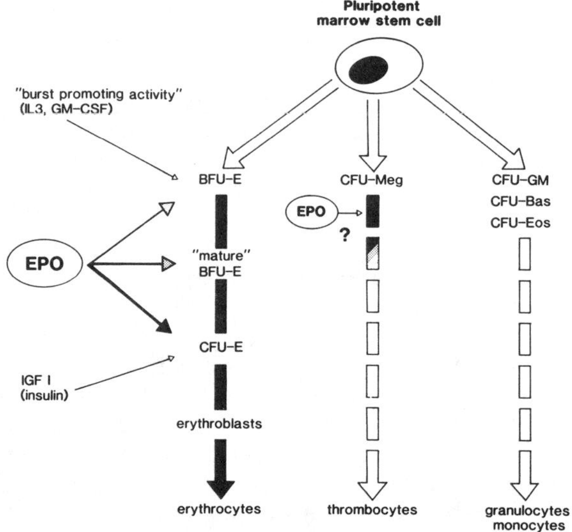

FIG 3.
Simplified scheme of erythropiesis. The various progenitor cells identified in in vitro culture systems are BFU-E (burst-forming unit erythroid), CFU-E (colony-forming unit erythroid), CFU-Meg (colony-forming unit megakaryocyte), CFU-GM (colony-forming unit granulocyte/monocyte), CFU-Bas (colony-forming unit basophil), and CFU-Eos (colony-forming unit eosinophil). EPO is essential for development of erythroid progenitors. The sensitivity of these progenitors toward EPO increases with maturation. In addition to EPO, CFU-E appear to require insulin-like growth factor I or insulin for maturation to erythroblasts. BFU-E are largely dependent on an operationally defined burst promoting activity and this has been assigned to growth factors acting on multiple classes of progenitor cells, such as granulocyte-macrophage colony-stimulating factor (GM-CSF) and interleukin 3 (IL 3). EPO can furthermore promote the differentiation of megacaryocyte progenitors in vitro, but its physiologic role for thrombopoiesis in vivo is not clear.

early precursor cells, because in cultures of unpurified progenitors, BFU-E can proliferate in the absence of any added EPO.[34] The experiments defining the subgroups of erythroid progenitors, their characteristics, and details of their interaction with EPO have recently been comprehensively reviewed.[35]

The EPO Receptor

EPO acts on its target cells via specific surface receptors. Two main approaches have been used to characterize these receptors.

The first approach is based on binding studies of EPO to erythroid cells with the use of iodinated rhEPO that retains full biologic activity and has the same affinity for the EPO receptor as unlabeled EPO.[36] Due to the difficulties in purifying primary BFU-E and CFU-E, most of these experiments have been performed on murine erythroid cell lines,[37, 38] partially purified progenitors derived from mouse and rat fetal livers,[36, 39] and from the spleens of mice treated with phenylhydrazine[25] or infected with the anemia strain of Friend virus (FVA cells).[40, 41] Only recently have binding studies also been carried out on highly purified human CFU-E.[42] Despite these different cells that were studied, many of the results rather conclusively revealed several characteristics of EPO receptors.

First, the number of EPO receptors on the cell surface is comparatively small, in most studies in the order of 800 to 1,200 per cell. Second, two classes of EPO receptors seem to exist with either a low or a high affinity for EPO, with dissociation constants on FVA cells and human CFU-E of 90 to 100 pM and 570 pM, respectively. Different cells either contain both receptor classes or generally the low affinity receptor only. The high affinity receptor seems to be mainly important for erythroid differentiation, since cells lacking this receptor do not differentiate in response to EPO. Furthermore, at concentrations of EPO necessary to maximally stimulate human CFU-E in vitro, about half of the high affinity but none of the low affinity binding sites are occupied,[40, 42] and, finally, given its physiologic concentrations in serum, in vivo EPO probably binds mainly to the high affinity receptor. The third feature of EPO receptors that was revealed by binding of EPO to the cell surface and subsequent chemical cross-linking is the presence of two structural entities with molecular masses of approximately 80 and 100 kilodaltons. When both of these putative receptor proteins are subjected to protease digestion, similar proteolytic fragments are generated, indicating that they may have a common origin.[43] These two proteins do not correspond to the two different binding affinities, since both can be demonstrated with cross-linking when EPO binds to low or high affinity receptors only.[41, 44] This is in accordance with recent evidence indicating that the different affinity of EPO receptors is based on topographic rather than on gross structural differences.[45]

The second, more recent and direct approach to characterizing the EPO receptor was the cloning of its gene in the mouse[46, 47] and in humans.[48, 49] The cDNA and amino acid sequence of both receptors are 82% homologous, which is not surprising in view of the structural similarities of EPO molecules in both species and the long known biologic activity of human EPO in the mouse. Both receptor genes code for a 507 and a 508 amino acid protein in mouse and humans, respectively, which appear to contain single membrane-spanning domains.

Interestingly, although the mouse EPO receptor was cloned from a cell line that possesses only low affinity receptors for EPO, both high and low affinity binding sites appeared when the receptor cDNA obtained from these cells was expressed in COS cells (a transformed monkey kidney cell line), and, furthermore, cross-linking experiments revealed that on both the original and the transfected cells, two receptor proteins of different size, similar to those previously mentioned, are present.[46] While this suggests that the different affinities of EPO receptors and the different molecular size of binding sites have to be explained on the basis of a single receptor gene, and may be due, e.g., to different glycosylation, covalent modification or dimerization, the possibility remains that other yet unidentified proteins are involved in binding of EPO to its target cells.

Although it is generally assumed that the main if not the only physiologically important action of EPO is on erythroid tissue, the presence of EPO receptors has also been reported on some other cells. The demonstration of EPO receptors on megakaryoctes[50] has complemented evidence for a stimulation of thrombopoiesis by high concentrations of EPO in vitro[51–53] and could explain some increase in platelet counts following the intravenous injection of rhEPO in rats,[54] mice,[55] and some patients with renal failure.[4] However, the overall significance of EPO for platelet production may be minor, since deficiency of endogenous EPO in renal disease does not result in thrombocytopenia.

Another organ that was found to contain EPO receptors is murine and rat placenta.[41] This might provide the basis for a maternofetal transport of EPO as was found in mice.[56] However, since the placenta receptors are of the low affinity type, their role would probably be restricted to conditions of highly elevated EPO levels in the mother. Whether the human placenta is able to transport EPO is questionable. Up to tenfold concentration differences of the hormone in either direction have been reported between the maternal and fetal circulation, suggesting that fetal EPO levels are regulated independently.[57]

Finally, very recently EPO receptors with properties different than those previously discussed have been discovered on endothelial cells grown in culture and were found to be associated with proliferation and chemotaxis.[58] Again the physiologic importance of this finding is still unknown, but it will certainly encourage further attempts to search for actions of EPO outside the bone marrow.

Cellular Events

On binding to its receptors, EPO initiates a sequence of events in erythroid cells that results in cell division and at a later stage in the onset of hemoglobin synthesis. The underlying mechanisms appear to comprise an early initiation of RNA synthesis,[59–61] which is followed by protein and DNA synthesis.[62, 63] Internalization of EPO, which occurs rapidly following its binding to the receptor,[25, 40] appears to be unnecessary for its action,[64] but the signal transduction mediating the effects of EPO remains to be determined. Neither cyclic adenosine monophosphate (cAMP)[65] nor cyclic guanosine monophosphate (cGMP)[66] appears to be a direct mediator and the role of an early rise in cytosolic calcium[67, 68] remains questionable,[69] as does the importance of membrane protein phosphorylation.[70]

Irrespective of the precise signal transduction, the final effect of EPO on erythroid percursors could be due to a mitogenic effect of the hormone, an induction of programmed differentiation, or to an action as survival factor that allows an endogenously programmed differentiation to occur. The third possibility, which was proposed several years ago,[71] has been strongly supported by the recent finding that EPO retards DNA breakdown in its target cells.[72]

Production Sites of EPO

Organs Producing EPO

An important role of the kidneys in the formation of EPO was recognized more than 30 years ago. At that time it was found that nephrectomy almost totally blunts an increase in serum EPO levels in response to known stimuli of EPO formation.[73] However, until a few years ago the way by which the kidneys contribute to EPO formation remained controversial. One theory proposed that the kidney produces an enzyme that cleaves EPO from a precursor molecule generated extrarenally. A second hypothesis suggested that the kidneys produce a precursor of EPO, which is then activated by a plasma enzyme. A third theory, which subsequently turned out to be right, namely that no precursor for EPO exists and that EPO is produced as such by the kidneys, was primarily considered less likely. Increasing support for a direct renal synthesis of EPO arose, however, when biologically active EPO was detected in serum-free perfusate of isolated kidneys[74] and, furthermore, could be demonstrated in the homogenate of hypoxic rat kidneys.[75, 76]

Later the cloning of the EPO gene provided a definite answer, since the comparison between the DNA sequence and the amino acid sequence of urinary EPO revealed no evidence for the existence of a proerythropoietin. Moreover, with genomic and cDNA probes for EPO, it was possible to demonstrate EPO mRNA in the kidney.[77, 78] Less, but significant amounts of EPO mRNA were also detected in the liver.[77, 78] This confirmed earlier experiments, in which the remaining EPO production in nephrectomized animals was further reduced by subtotal hepatectomy.[79] Additional experiments on the age dependency of the effect of nephrectomy and/or hepatectomy on EPO formation suggested that the liver is the predominant production site during fetal life, whereas its contribution in adults does not seem to exceed 15% of total EPO formation.[73, 79–81] The time at which a proposed shift in EPO production from liver to kidney occurs seems to be variable among different species. In sheep and rat, a predominance of hepatic EPO formation was found to last beyond birth,[82–85] whereas in a recent quantitative analysis of renal and hepatic EPO mRNA in mice, the majority of EPO mRNA was found in the kidney from mid-gestation on.[56]

EPO mRNA has not been detected in any organ other than the kidney or liver with Northern blot analysis. The possibilty remains that the EPO gene may be expressed elsewhere at levels that are too low to be detected with this method. It is tempting to speculate, for example, that EPO, like other hematopoietic growth factors, may also be produced by bone marrow cells. From the results of in situ hybridization, it was suggested that macrophages in the bone marrow express the EPO gene,[86] a finding, however, that awaits confirmation with other techniques.

In conclusion, there appears to be firm evidence that the physiologically important EPO-producing organs are the kidney and the liver. Since, at least in the adult, the kidney is the predominant organ and very little is yet known about hepatic EPO production, we shall focus on the cellular site and the regulation of renal EPO formation.

Cellular Location of Renal EPO Production

Despite much effort, the question of the renal cell type producing EPO has not yet been definitely answered. While in the past the demonstration of putative EPO immunoreactivity in glomeruli[87] and the finding that cultured mesangial cells produce an in vitro erythropoietic activity[88] favored a glomerular origin of EPO production, this concept had to be revised following the application of hybridization techniques. With RNA blot analysis it was found that after partial disaggregation of hypoxic rat kidneys, EPO mRNA is not present in the glomerular fraction but in the tubular fraction.[78] In accordance with these results, a surprising breakthrough was subsequently made when EPO mRNA was demonstrated on histologic kidney sections by in situ hybridization. Although some investigators using this technique concluded that EPO mRNA is localized in tubular cells,[89, 90] others have quite convincingly shown that after incubation of kidney tissue with either DNA or RNA probes for EPO, hybridization signals arise neither from glomerular nor from tubular cells, but rather originate in cells located between tubuli in the interstitium of the renal cortex and the outer medulla.[91, 92] A peritubular location of EPO-producing cells is also in accordance with our own results (Fig 4).[93] Since a major part of this peritubular space consists of peritubular capillaries, it was suggested that endothelial cells may be the production site of EPO. Nevertheless, other interstitial cells such as fibroblasts or macrophages are possible candidates as well. Beyond in situ hybridization, further evidence for the location of EPO production in the renal interstitium comes from histologic studies in rats that were autoimmunized against EPO.[93] In these animals, immunodeposits surrounded inter-

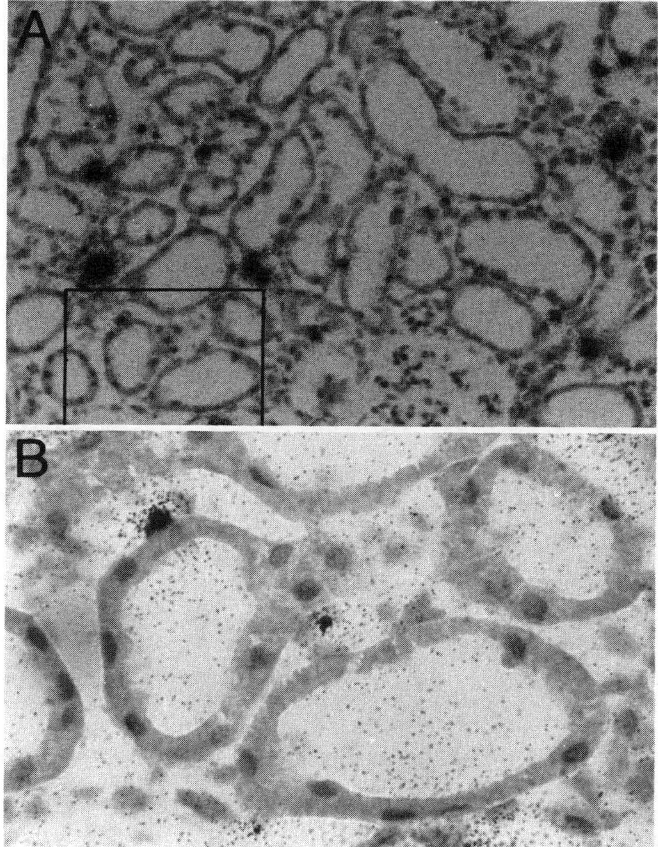

FIG 4.
A, B, in situ hybridization with a ^{35}S-labeled EPO DNA probe on the renal cortex of an adult rat exposed to 0.1% carbon monoxide for 3 hours to induce functional anemia. Silver grains indicate presence of EPO mRNA. **B,** higher magnification shows extratubular location of the labeled cells.

stitial cells in the renal cortex, whereas no deposits were found in association with glomerular or tubular cells.

The difficulty of precisely defining the EPO-producing cells is based on the methodical requirements of in situ hybridization, which tend to reduce the histologic quality of the specimen. So far, it has not been possible to perform on the same specimen both in situ hybridization for EPO and immunohistochemistry against certain cell surface markers, which might be a strategy for definitive identification of the EPO producers. The recent availability of specific antibodies raised against pure rhEPO has also reinitiated attempts to identify EPO-producing cells by direct immunohistochemistry against the hormone. However, apart from the problem that the presence of EPO in a certain cell does not necessarily mean that EPO was actually synthesized by that cell, the results of these studies are conflicting. Whereas one group found discrete signals in cells that they considered to be endothelial,[94] others recently reported signals in glomerular cells[95] and even an intense staining of cortical tubules was found.[90] The majority of investigators, however, failed to detect EPO by means of immunohistochemistry and it is assumed that the reason for this is a constitutive secretion of the hormone, which means that EPO molecules are released immediately after synthesis and that no significant intracellular accumulation of EPO occurs.

Summing up, the available evidence, although not totally conclusive, favors the concept that interstitial cells in proximity to renal tubules in the cortex and the adjacent outer medulla produce the hormone.

Regulation of EPO Production

Plasma EPO Levels

Although little is yet known about the dose-response relationship of EPO, it can be generally stated that (provided an intact bone marrow) the activity of erythropoiesis is proportional to the concentration of EPO in plasma. Over the years, numerous experimental and clinical studies have yielded the concept that circulating EPO levels in turn are related to a ratio of tissue oxygen supply and oxygen need. As a consequence, EPO appears to carefully adapt red blood cell formation to meet the oxygen requirements of the organism. Comparing the role of both oxygen supply and demand for EPO concentrations, the influence of oxygen supply, however, appears to be of major importance and far better defined. The main determinants of oxygen supply are the arterial oxygen content and the oxygen affinity of hemoglobin, and both parameters were found to affect EPO concentrations: EPO levels are positively related to oxygen affinity[96] and inversely related to arterial oxygen content. The latter in turn is determined by oxygen transport capacity and oxygen saturation, and elevations in EPO are regularly found when either of both is reduced.

Thus in chronic anemias, an exponential inverse relationship generally exists between EPO levels and the hemoglobin concentration (Fig 5).[97–99] While normal EPO concentrations in humans are in the order of 10 to 30 mU/mL (corresponding to about 3 to 9pM),[97, 99, 100] up to one-thousand-fold increases occur in severe anemias. The sensitivity of EPO levels toward changes in hemoglobin greatly decreases with increasing hemoglobin, but a significant rise can still be demonstrated when hemoglobin concentrations are only slightly reduced; e.g., following the donation of one unit of red blood cells.[101, 102] Furthermore, also at normal hemoglobin concentrations, EPO levels appear to result from an oxygen-dependent regulation, since they are found to be suppressed on average when oxygen transport capacity is elevated as in polycythemia rubra vera[99, 100, 103, 104] or after hypertransfusion. A clear exception to this inverse relationship of EPO toward hemoglobin can be found in renal disease, where a chronic reduction in hemo-

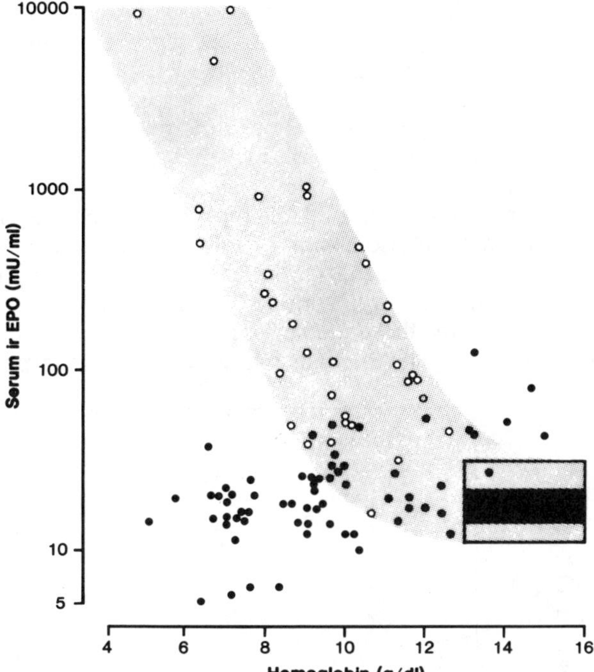

FIG 5.
Relationship between hemoglobin concentrations and serum immunoreactive EPO levels in patients with various types of hyporegenerative and hyperregenerative nonrenal anemias (open symbols) and in patients with chronic renal disease (excluding patients with polycystic kidneys; closed symbols). The rectangle depicts interquartile (dark stippled) and 95% range of EPO values in nonanemic healthy adults. Note in the nonrenal anemias the considerable interindividual variation in EPO levels with more than tenfold differences in patients with the same hemoglobin concentration, which indicates the importance of factors other than oxygen-carrying capacity in modulating EPO concentrations. In chronic renal disease, reductions in hemoglobin are not accompanied by an increase in EPO, but EPO levels remain below, within, or slightly above the normal range and altogether appear to be positively related to hemoglobin. This suggests that in renal disease hemoglobin concentrations are determined by a given amount of EPO produced, which in turn appears to be unresponsive to changes in hemoglobin. (From Kurtz A, Eckardt K-U: *Contrib Nephrol* 1990; 87:15–25. Used by permission.)

globin does not lead to a rise in EPO, and this relative EPO deficiency is considered to be the predominant cause of renal anemias.

Given a constant red blood cell mass, the main determinant of EPO levels is the arterial oxygen tension and hence oxygen saturation of hemoglobin. Following a sudden decrease in oxygen saturation (hypoxic hypoxia), EPO levels start to rise after about 90 minutes and then increase approximately linearly, the slope of this increase being inversely related to arterial oxygen tensions (Fig 6).[105, 106] The arterial oxygen tension, however, does not appear to directly influence EPO levels, since the magnitude of increase in EPO at a given reduction of arterial oxygen tension was found to be suppressed in polycythemic animals.[107] Thus, in conclusion, it appears to be neither arterial oxygen tension nor hemoglobin concentration per se that determines EPO concentrations, but rather the amount of oxygen available to tissues.

As for any other hormone, the effective plasma concentration of EPO is the result of both secretion and clearance rate. The site and mechanisms of EPO clearance are still unknown. Not only do considerable species differences exist, with half-life times of some 2 hours in rats[27, 28, 106, 109] up to 9 hours in dogs,[110] but also the variability of EPO survival in human circulation is remarkably high, with median half-life times of one preparation of

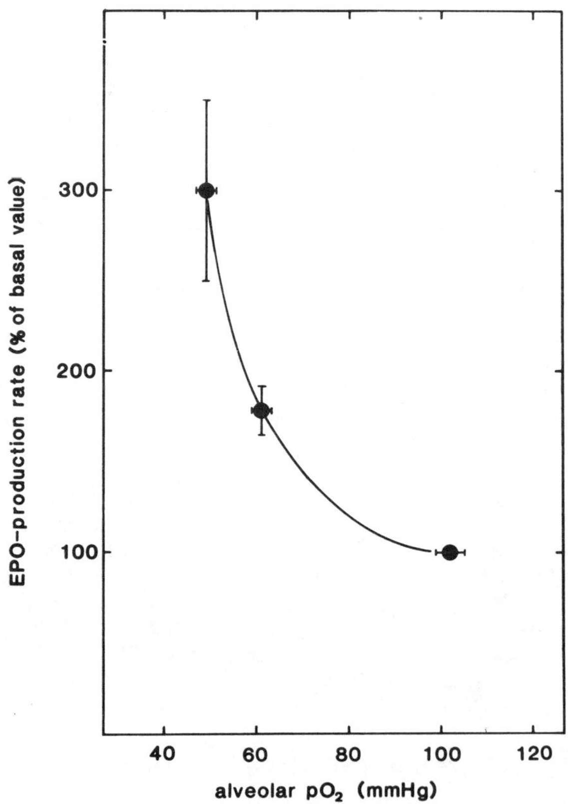

FIG 6.
Relationship between alveolar oxygen tensions and EPO production rates in six male volunteers exposed to simulated altitudes of 3,000 and 4,000 m in a decompression chamber (mean ± SE). Production rates were calculated from the increase in peripheral serum immunoreactive EPO levels. (From Eckardt K-U, Boutellier U, Kurtz A, et al: *J Appl Physiol* 1989; 66:1785–1888. Used by permission.)

rhEPO reported between 2 and 7 hours.[3] However, no evidence so far exists for physiologic regulation of EPO clearance, and in particular hypoxia does not prolong EPO survival in plasma.[106, 111] It can be inferred therefore that the oxygen-dependent alterations in EPO concentrations are due to modulation of renal EPO secretion. Furthermore, since the kidneys contain no storage sites for EPO,[112, 113] the magnitude of EPO secretion appears to directly reflect alterations in its production rate.

EPO Production

EPO production appears to be predominantly regulated at the level of RNA. Under normoxic conditions, renal EPO mRNA content is low and generally below the sensitivity limit of Northern blotting, although with more sensitive methods, such as RNAse protection, it can be demonstrated clearly.[56, 114] Following the onset of hypoxia, an increase in EPO mRNA can be seen within about 60 minutes[78]; it precedes and parallels the rise in EPO serum levels.[78, 107] This rise in EPO mRNA appears to involve an increased rate of EPO gene transcription because EPO production can be blocked by actinomycin D, an inhibitor of RNA polymerase[113, 115] and, furthermore, an enhanced transcription rate of the EPO gene was directly demonstrated in nuclear run-off experiments.[116] It is possible that, in addition, the stability of EPO mRNA may be increased during hypoxia, a concept that was recently suggested on the basis of experiments in an EPO-producing hepatoma cell line.[117] Interestingly, the accumulation of EPO mRNA in the kidney does not appear to result from an increase of EPO mRNA in individual EPO-producing cells, but rather appears to be due mainly to an increasing number of cells expressing the gene.[118] This was demonstrated by in situ hybridization on kidneys from mice with various degrees of anemia, in which an inverse exponential relationship was observed between the number of EPO-producing cells and the hematocrit (Fig 7).

Renal Oxygen Sensor

The regulation of EPO production and hence EPO gene transcription, as previously outlined, requires the ability to perceive alterations in tissue oxygen supply and to transform these alterations into specific signals, which finally result in an interaction with regulatory elements of the EPO gene. This ability, one of the key issues of EPO physiology, can be operationally defined as an oxygen sensor. However, neither the precise location nor the components of this sensor have yet been determined.

The first question that arises when considering this oxygen sensor is whether it is located in the kidney itself or, alternatively, comprises signals generated extrarenally at hypoxia that are then transferred to the kidney via the blood stream or nerve inputs. In this respect, rather convincing evidence has been accumulated indicating that the kidney itself can adjust EPO production to variations in its oxygen supply. The observation re-

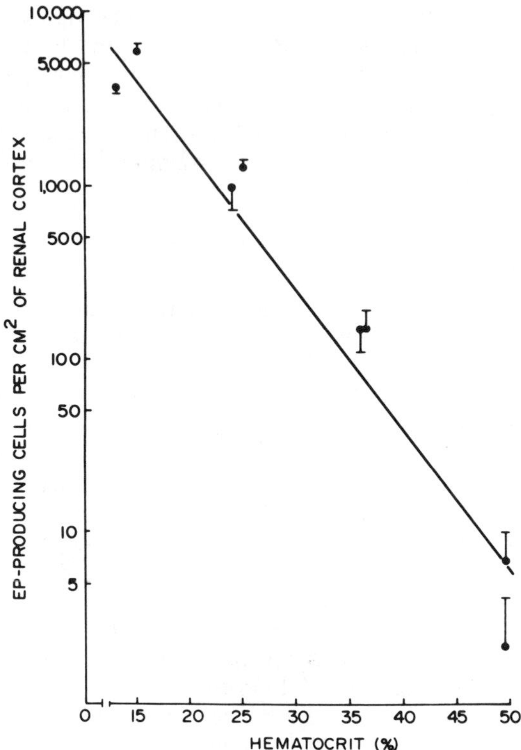

FIG 7.
Relationship between the hematocrit and the number of EPO-producing cells in the renal cortex of mice as determined with in situ hybridization. (From Koury ST, Koury MJ, Bondurant MC, et al: Blood 1989; 74:645–651. Used by permission.)

ported years ago, that an increased amount of erythropoietic bioactivity is released from isolated perfused kidneys upon lowering the oxygen tension of the perfusate,[74, 119, 120] has recently been confirmed by demonstrating oxygen dependent formation of immunoreactive EPO[121, 122] (Fig 8) and modulation of EPO mRNA levels[114] in isolated perfused rat kidneys obtained from normoxic animals. Moreover, in quantitative terms, EPO formation in isolated kidneys perfused at low oxygen tensions is comparable to the in vivo situation.[122] Thus it appears that the kidney is not only the production site of EPO, but in fact the central regulatory organ in the feedback loop that adjusts oxygen supply of the whole organism (Fig 9). Nevertheless, the possibility remains that in certain situations, in particular during anemic hypoxia, when arterial oxygen tension is normal, additional extrarenal signals may contribute to the stimulation of renal EPO formation. The existence of such factors has been postulated from the findings that selective reduction of renal oxygen supply brought about by constriction of renal arteries is only a minor stimulus for EPO formation.[123] and that EPO

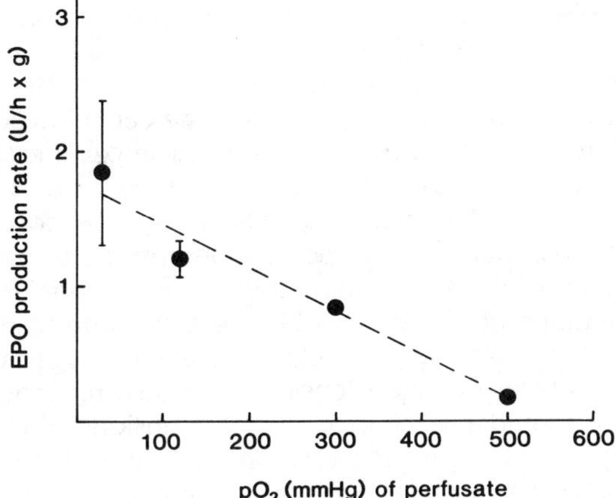

FIG 8.
Relationship between EPO production rate in isolated perfused rat kidneys taken from normoxic animals and oxygen tensions in the perfusate (mean ± SE). (From Scholz H, Schurek HJ, Eckardt K-U, et al: *Pfleugers Arch* 1991; 418:228–233. Used by permission.)

formation in isolated perfused kidneys appeared to be independent of the hemoglobin concentration in the perfusate.[121] Direct evidence for the existence of extrarenal oxygen-dependent signals, however, is lacking.

Proceeding thus from the evidence that the essentials of oxygen sensing are installed in the kidney itself, the question arises whether the EPO-producing cells themselves are oxygen sensitive. Since isolation and in vitro study of these cells has not yet been achieved, this can not be answered at present. In view of the inaccessibility of the native EPO-producing cells, two human hepatoma cell lines, HepG2 cells and Hep3B cells, that, a few

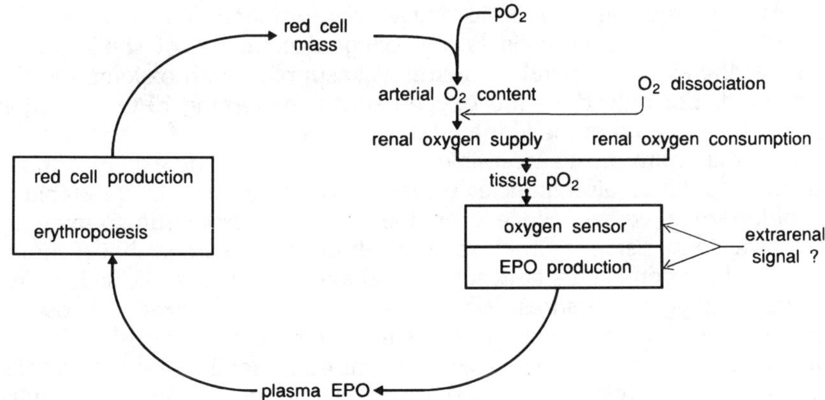

FIG 9.
Feedback regulation of EPO production.

years ago, were discovered to produce EPO in an oxygen-dependent fashion[124] have been used extensively to investigate cellular mechanisms of EPO regulation.[14, 124–126] From these results, it appears that oxygen sensing and EPO production may reside in the same cell. However, it remains unknown to what extent the observations in these cell lines can be transferred to native EPO-producing cells in liver, kidney, or even both organs.

In any case, even if EPO-producing cells in the renal cortex themselves perceive renal oxygen delivery, this perception appears not to be independent of the function of the surrounding tubules. From what was said previously about situations of elevated EPO levels, it can already be inferred that the oxygen dependent signal is related to tissue oxygen tensions, or in other words postcapillary oxygen tensions, because reductions in oxygen carrying capacity would not change oxygen tensions along precapillary vessels. Postcapillary oxygen tensions in turn are dependent on the amount of oxygen removed from blood, which means the local oxygen consumption. Since the major determinant of renal oxygen consumption is tubular sodium reabsorption,[127] site-specific diuretics were used to reduce oxygen demand at different segments along the nephron in an attempt to define those tubular structures involved in oxygen-dependent EPO regulation.[128] It was found that the inhibition of proximal tubular sodium reabsorption was accompanied by a decrease in EPO formation, whereas effective inhibition of sodium reabsorption in the loop of Henle, distal tubule, or collecting duct did not attenuate EPO production, indicating that the proximal tubule plays a role in the oxygen sensing mechanisms. This influence may either be indirect and reside in a reduction of oxygen tensions in the peritubular space where EPO is produced, or in case the EPO-producing cells are not or are only partially oxygen sensitive, the proximal tubule might generate specific signals at hypoxia that are then transferred to EPO-producing cells in its proximity.

At first glance, the location of an oxygen sensor in the kidney appears somewhat surprising, since the volume of oxygen transported to the kidney is rather large compared to its oxygen consumption. In fact, it might be concluded from a comparatively low oxygen extraction of some 8% to 10% that the kidney generally is luxuriously supplied with oxygen. On the other hand, not only does the oxygen sensor governing EPO formation appear to be located in the kidney, but clinical experience teaches that the kidney is the organ most susceptible to hypoxic injury. The explanation for both these putative discrepancies probably resides in the unique architecture of intrarenal vessels. Since arterial and venous vessels run countercurrently over long distances in close association, it is assumed that a shunt-diffusion of oxygen occurs between arterial and venous vessels, which lowers arterial oxygen pressures. While shunt diffusion of oxygen in postglomerular vessels in the vascular bundles is thought to be responsible for the high vulnerability of the thick ascending limb to ischemia,[129, 130] shunt diffusion in preglomerular vessels might well explain the oxygen sensitivity of cortical structures that appears relevant to EPO formation. Support for this concept comes from the observation of oxygen tensions in the renal cortex well below the venous Po_2 of the kidney[131, 132] and from experiments indicating that preglomerular oxygen tensions at the kidney surface are much lower than those in the systemic circulation, this difference increasing greatly with increasing systemic oxygen tensions.[133]

Although these data clearly indicate that the renal oxygen supply is far from being abundant, a direct association between local renal oxygen tensions and EPO production has not been determined. It should be noted that assuming a major oxygen shunting along interlobular vessels predicts an oxygen gradient from the corticomedullary junction to the subcapsular cortex.[133] On the other hand, in situ hybridization for EPO revealed rather the opposite frequency distribution of EPO-producing cells, with the majority of them being located in the inner part of the cortex,[118] indicating that these considerations need refinement. One additional factor that probably has to be taken into account is that shunt diffusion is not limited to oxygen, but also (in the opposite direction) affects carbon dioxide, thereby trapping carbon dioxide to highest values in the outermost subcapsular zone.[134, 135] Since the oxygen dependent control of EPO production is sensitive to increases in Pco_2, as will be discussed, this might partially counterbalance low oxygen tensions in the outer cortex.

Finally, high oxygen sensitivity of the renal cortex is further substantiated by an observation indicating that increased EPO production is not its only response to hypoxia. Within 1 week following the onset of anemia, a marked hypertrophy of peritubular fibroblasts in the cortical labyrinth of rat kidneys was found, with an increased activity of 5′ nucleotidase on the surface of these cells.[136] This enzyme catalyzes the hydrolysis of 5′ adenosine monophosphate (AMP), and its increased activity might thus result in an elevation of local adenosine concentrations. Whether the hypoxia-induced stimulation of these peritubular fibroblasts is of any relevance for EPO formation remains, however, to be clarified.

In conclusion, a rather limited oxygen delivery to the renal cortex on one hand and the high energy consumption of the proximal tubule on the other hand appear to provide the basis for oxygen-dependent regulation of EPO production. Since the tubular oxygen demand depends on the filtered sodium load, which in turn is governed by renal blood flow, a decrease in oxygen supply due to a reduction in blood flow will be counterbalanced by decreased oxygen consumption. This probably, at least partially, explains a relative insensitivity of EPO production toward changes in renal blood flow[123, 137] and, from a teleologic point of view, may be the major advantage of a renal location of the oxygen sensor.[138]

Factors Modulating EPO Production

Indirect evidence obtained in vivo suggests that the sensitivity of the oxygen sensor that governs EPO production is subject to physiologic modulation. Systemic acidosis for instance, whether it is of respiratory or metabolic origin, attenuates the triggering of EPO formation in response to hypoxia and carbon monoxide (-anemia),[108] and in turn the respiratory alkalosis normally occurring in hypoxic hypoxia appears to facilitate the rise in EPO.[139–143] The mechanisms of this pH sensitivity of oxygen sensing still have to be identified. Possible explanations could be changes in tissue oxygenation due to shifts of the oxygen binding curve of hemoglobin,[139–142] alterations of tubular function, or direct effects on energy consumption of EPO-producing cells.[144, 145]

Another factor that influences EPO formation is the duration of hypoxia. Following the onset of hypoxic hypoxia, EPO levels start to rise after about 90 minutes, reaching maximal values after 12 to 24 hours in rodents[106, 112, 141, 146–148] and within 48 hours in man[146, 149] and thereafter decline again despite continued hypoxia to approach steady state levels still above baseline but severalfold lower than peak concentrations (Fig 10). This early decrease in EPO levels occurs before red blood cell mass and therefore oxygen carrying capacity has increased significantly. It appears due to a reduction in EPO mRNA and thus EPO production rather than an increased clearance or consumption of the hormone.[106] Furthermore, this resetting of EPO production appears not to be mediated through a direct or indirect effect of EPO itself, since the application of high amounts of EPO to rats did not blunt the EPO production in response to a subsequent exposure to hypoxia.[106] Although starvation is known to reduce EPO formation[150] and reduced food intake can be observed during continuous hypoxia, this appears

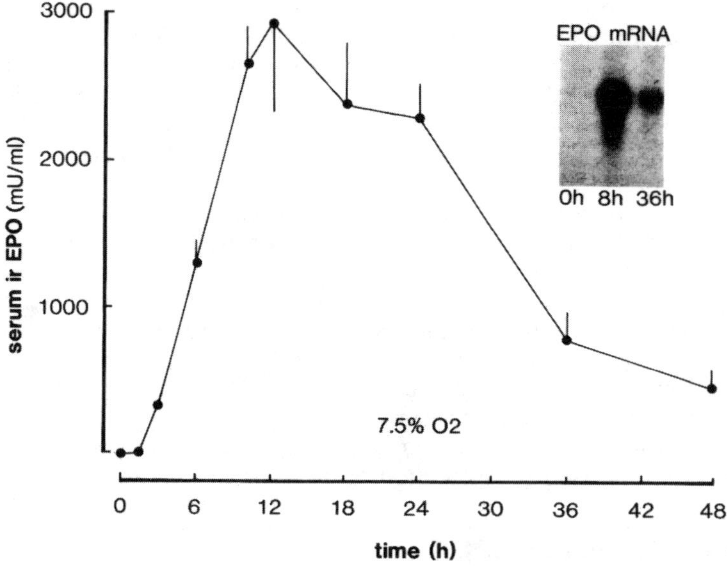

FIG 10.
Temporal pattern of EPO levels in rats continuously exposed to 7.5% O_2 for up to 48 hours. Insert shows the underlying kinetics of renal EPO mRNA. (Northern blot analysis of poly A^+ RNA, hybridized with a genomic mouse EPO probe.) (Adapted from Eckardt K-U, Dittmer J, Neumann R, et al: *Am J Physiol* 1990; 258:1432–1437.)

also not to be responsible for the decline in EPO production, because EPO titers in fed and food-deprived rats were found to increase similarily on repeated hypoxic exposure.[151]

It appears thus that somehow an adaptation of the oxygen sensor occurs during continuous hypoxic hypoxia, but it remains to be clarified whether this is due to systemic, renal, or cellular mechanisms. The kinetics of EPO production in anemic hypoxia have so far not been thoroughly investigated. Although following an acute blood loss some overshoot in EPO levels can be observed, similar to the temporal pattern in hypoxic hypoxia,[101, 152] EPO levels in chronic anemias nevertheless are continuously elevated, suggesting that a putative adaptation is not as effective as it is when oxygen saturation is reduced.

Finally, EPO formation appears not only sensitive to changes in oxygen supply of the organism but also was found to reflect general alterations in oxygen consumption. This concept was first formulated following the observation that hypophysectomized animals that have a low metabolic rate and hence oxygen consumption have a decreased rate of erythropoiesis.[150, 153] More recent evidence confirms that this suppression of erythropoiesis is in part due to diminished EPO levels.[154] and upon hypoxic exposure, EPO production in hypophysectomized rats may be even as low as that in nephrectomized animals.[155, 156] The role of the hypophysis in EPO formation appears to reside in a permissive effect of several hypophysis-dependent hormones, and EPO formation can be restored in hypophysectomized rats through combined replacement therapy with insulin-like growth factor I, thyroxine, and testosterone (our unpublished observations). Again it will require isolation of EPO-producing cells to see if they contain receptors for these hormones, or if the stimulation of EPO production results, e.g., from increased tubular oxygen consumption.

Possible Signal Transduction

In vivo evidence indicates that less than 15 minutes of hypoxia is sufficient to trigger an increase in EPO formation.[108] Protein synthesis appears to be necessary for the cellular events that link changes in oxygen tensions to the production rate of EPO.[116] Furthermore, a number of substances, including prostaglandins,[157, 158] cyclic AMP,[159–161] adenosine,[162, 163] and reactive oxygen metabolites[164] have been suggested to play a role in this signal transduction. However, the physiologic significance of most of the experimental in vitro systems used so far to elaborate possible second messengers in EPO regulation is unknown, and any effect that follows the pharmacologic interaction with certain signal pathways in vivo must raise the question of whether it is specific and direct. Nevertheless, it is of interest that in isolated perfused rat kidneys neither stimulation of cyclic AMP and cyclic guanosine monophosphate formation nor adenosine are able to induce the rise in immunoreactive EPO in the perfusate that can be observed at lowering of the oxygen tension,[122] indicating that these substances probably do not directly mediate an increase in EPO formation in the kidney.

An alternative to classical second messenger pathways has recently been suggested from experiments with EPO-producing Hep3B cells.[125] Based on circumstantial evidence, it was concluded that the oxygen sensor in these cells is a heme protein that undergoes conformational change at reaction with molecular oxygen. It is proposed that the oxy conformation of this heme protein is inactive with regard to EPO production, whereas the deoxy conformation acts to increase EPO expression. This concept is particularly attractive because it may explain the long-known observation that the administration of cobalt stimulates EPO production in vivo.[165] Since cobalt chloride can be converted to cobalt protoporphyrin in vivo,[166] it is possible that cobalt substitutes for ferrous iron in the heme protein, locking it in a deoxy confirmation.[125]

Regulation of the EPO Gene

Finally, the oxygen-dependent signal transduction in EPO-producing cells will have to affect regulatory elements of the EPO gene. These have so far not been defined, but are the subject of intense current investigation. From structural analysis of the EPO gene, a possible regulatory role was suggested for highly conserved sequences in the first intron and in a region encompassing 140 base pairs upstream from the putative transcriptional start site, including the sequence GATAACA that is related to the canonical TATA box often seen in eukaryotic promotors.[9, 10] More recent studies performed in transfected Hep3B cells and in transgenic mice[14, 23] revealed, however, that additional inducing and suppressing elements must be present, probably at both sides of the gene and at a distance extending more than 6 kb 5′ and/or 0.7 kb 3′ to the gene. Interestingly, the experiments in transgenic mice have also indicated that regulation of the EPO gene in kidney and liver are quite different.[14, 167]

Conclusions

Although several important questions on the physiology of EPO remain to be resolved, the cloning of its gene and the subsequent expression of EPO complementary DNA in mammalian cell lines has definitely terminated the elusiveness of this renal hormone. The availability of sufficient quantities of EPO and of its gene probes has greatly facilitated precise and reproducible assays and a number of experimental approaches to elucidate the action and production of EPO.

Cloning of the EPO receptor has initiated studies that will lead to a better understanding of how EPO acts to induce differentiation and maturation of erythroid precursor cells. The regulation of EPO production, on the other hand, has been shown to occur at the level of RNA, and the major production site of EPO has been confined to the peritubular space of the renal cortex and the outer medulla. A functional entity of proximal tubular cells and peritubular EPO-producing cells has been conceptualized as the site of oxygen-dependent regulation of EPO. Demonstration of EPO mRNA might eventually allow unequivocal definition and even isolation of native EPO-producing cells from kidney and liver and to test the physiologic significance of attractive concepts on the cellular regulation of EPO that have recently been elaborated in permanent cell lines.

Acknowledgment

We thank Christian Gasser for doing the artwork.

References

1. Jacobs K, Shoemaker C, Rudersdorf R, et al: Isolation and characterization of genomic and cDNA clones of human erythropoietin. *Nature* 1985; 313:806–810.
2. Lin F-K, Suggs S, Lin C-H, et al: Cloning and expression of the human erythropoietin gene. *Proc Natl Acad Sci USA* 1985; 82:7580–7584.
3. Cotes PM, Pippard MJ, Reid CDL, et al: Characterization of the anaemia of chronic renal failure and the mode of its correction by a preparation of human erythropoietin (r-HuEPO). An investigation of the pharmacokinetics of intravenous erythropoietin and its effects on erythrokinetics. *Q J Med* 1989; 262:113–137.
4. Eschbach JW, Abdulhadi MH, Browne JK, et al: Recombinant human erythropoietin in anemic patients with end-stage renal disease. *Ann Intern Med* 1989; 111;992–1000.
5. Halpérin DS, Wacker P, Lacourt G, et al: Effects of recombinant human erythropoietin in infants with the anemia of prematurity: A pilot study. *J Pediatr* 1990; 116:779–786.
6. Ludwig H, Fritz E, Kotzmann H, et al: Erythropoietin treatment of anemia associated with multiple myeloma. *N Engl J Med* 1990; 322:1693–1699.
7. Oster W, Herrmann F, Gamm H, et al: Erythropoietin for the treatment of anemia of malignancy associated with neoplastic bone marrow infiltration. *J Clin Oncol* 1990; 8:956–962.
8. Miyake T, Kung CK-H, Goldwasser E: Purification of human erythropoietin. *J Biol Chem* 1977; 252:5558–5564.
9. McDonald J, Lin F-K, Goldwasser E: Cloning, sequencing, and evolutionary analysis of the mouse erythropoietin gene. *Mol Cell Biol* 1986; 6:842–848.
10. Shoemaker CB, Mitsock LD: Murine erythropoietine gene: Cloning, expression, and human gene homology. *Mol Cell Biol* 1986; 6:849–858.
11. Lin F-K, Lin C-H, Lai P-H, et al: Monkey erythropoietin gene: Cloning, expression and comparison with the human erythropoietin gene. *Gene* 1986; 44:201–209.
12. Law ML, Cai G-Y, Lin F-K, et al: Chromosomal assignment of the human erythropoietin gene and its DNA polymorphism. *Proc Natl Acad Sci USA* 1986; 83:6920–6924.
13. Watkins PC, Edy R, Hoffman N, et al: Regional assignment of the erythropoi-

etin gene to human chromosome region 7 q22. *Cytogenet Cell Genet* 1986; 42:214–218.

14. Semenza GL, Dureza RC, Traystman MD, et al: Human erythropoietin gene expression in transgenic mice: Multiple transcription initiation sites and cis-acting regulatory elements. *Mol Cell Biol* 1990; 10:930–938.
15. Recny M, Scoble HA, Kim Y: Structural characterization of natural human urinary and recombinant DNA-derived erythropoietin. *J Biol Chem* 1987; 262:17156–17163.
16. Sytkowski AJ: Denaturation and renaturation of human erythropoietin. *Biochem Biophys Res Commun* 1980; 96:143–149.
17. Wang FF, Kung CK-H, Goldwasser E: Some chemical properties of human erythropoietin. *Endocrinology* 1985; 116:2286–2292.
18. Sasaki H, Bothner B, Dell A, et al: Carbohydrate structure of erythropoietin expressed in chinese hamster ovary cells by a human erythropoietin cDNA. *J Biol Chem* 1987; 262:12059–12076.
19. Sasaki H, Ochi N, Del A, et al: Site-specific glycosilation of human recombinant erythropoietin: Analysis of glycopeptides or peptides at each glycosilation site by fast atom bombardment mass spectrometry. *Biochemistry* 1988; 27:8618–8626.
20. Takeuchi M, Takasaki S, Miyazaki H, et al: Comparative study of the asparagine-linked sugar chains of human erythropoietins purified from urine and the culture medium of recombinant chinese hamster ovary cells. *J Biol Chem* 1988; 263:3657–3663.
21. Tsuda E, Goto M, Murakami A, et al: Comparative study of N-linked oligosaccharides of urinary and recombinant erythropoietins. *Biochemistry* 1988; 27:5646–5654.
22. Lukowsky WA, Painter RA: Studies on the role of sialic acid in the physical and biological properties of erythropoietin. *Can J Biochem Cell Biol* 1972; 50:909–917.
23. Smith Dordal M, Wang FF, Goldwasser E: The role of carbohydrate in erythropoietin action. *Endocrinology* 1985; 116:2293–2299.
24. Goldwasser E, Kung CK-H, Eliason J: On the mechanism of erythropoietin-induced differentiation XIII. The role of sialic acid in erythropoietin action. *J Biol Chem* 1974; 249:4202–4206.
25. Mufson RA, Gesner TG: Binding and internalization of recombinant human erythropoietin in murine erythroid precursor cells. *Blood* 1987; 69:1485–1490.
26. Takeuchi M, Inoue N, Strickland TW, et al: Relationship between sugar chain structure and biological activity of recombinant human erythropoietin produced in Chinese hamster ovary cells. *Proc Natl Acad Sci USA* 1989; 86:7819–7822.
27. Fukuda MN, Sasaki H, Lopex L, et al: Survival of recombinant erythropoietin in the circulation: The role of carbohydrates. *Blood* 1989; 73:84–89.
28. Spivak JL, Hogans BB: The in vivo metabolism of recombinant human erythropoietin in the rat. *Blood* 1989; 73:90–99.
29. Porteous DD, Lajtha LG: Restoration of stem cell function after irradiation. *Ann NY Acad Sci* 1968; 149:151–155.
30. Stephenson JR, Axelrad AA: Separation of erythropoietin-sensitive cells from hemopoietic spleen colony-forming stem cells of mouse fetal liver by unit gravity sedimentation. *Blood* 1971; 34:417–427.
31. Eaves CJ, Eaves AC: Erythropoiesis, in Golde DW, Takaku F (eds): *Hematopoietic Stem Cells.* New York, Marcel Dekker, 1985, p 19.

32. Sawada K, Krantz SB, Dessypris EN, et al: Human colony-forming units-erythroid do not require accessory cells, but do require direct interaction with insulin-like growth factor I and/or insulin for erythroid development. *J Clin Invest* 1989; 83:1701–1709.
33. Sonoda Y, Yang YC, Wong GG, et al: Analysis in serum-free culture of the targest of recombinant human hemopoietic growth factors: Interleukin 3 and granulocyte/macrophage-colony-stimulating factor are specific for early developmental stages. *Proc Natl Acad Sci USA* 1988; 85:4360–4364.
34. Iscove NN: Erythropoietin-independent stimulation of early erythropiesis in adult marrow cultures by conditioned medium for lectin-stimulated mouse spleen cells, in ICN-UCLA Symposium on Hematopoietic Cell Differentiation. New York, Academic Press, 1978, pp 37–82.
35. Graber SE, Krantz SB: Erythropoietin: Biology and clinical use. *Hematol Oncol Clin North Am* 1989; 3:369–400.
36. Mayeux P, Billat C, Jacquot R: The erythropoietin receptor of rat erythroid progenitor cells. Characterization and affinity cross-linkage. *J Biol Chem* 1987; 262:13985–13990.
37. Broudy VC, Lin N, Egrie J, et al: Identification of the receptor for erythropoietin on human and murine erythroleukemia cells and modulation by phorbol ester and dimethyl sulfoxide. *Proc Natl Acad Sci USA* 1988; 85:6513–6517.
38. Todokoro K, Kanazawa S, Amanuma H, et al: Specific binding of erythropoietin to its receptor on responsive mouse erythroleukemia cells. *Proc Natl Acad Sci USA* 1987; 84:4126–4130.
39. Fukamachi H, Saito T, Tojo A, et al: Binding of erythropoietin to CFU-E derived from fetal mouse liver cells. *Exp Hematol* 1987; 15:833–837.
40. Sawyer ST, Krantz SB, Goldwasser E: Binding and receptor-mediated endocytosis of erythropoietin in Friend virus-infected erythroid cells. *J Biol Chem* 1987; 262:5554–5562.
41. Sawyer ST, Krantz SB, Sawada K: Receptors for erythropoietin in mouse and human erythroid cells and placenta. *Blood* 1989; 74:103–109.
42. Sawada K, Krantz SB, Sawyer ST, et al: Quantitation of specific binding of erythropoietin to human erythroid colony-forming cells. *J Cell Physiol* 1988; 137:337–345.
43. Sawyer ST. The two proteins of the erythropoietin receptor are structurally similar. *J Biol Chem* 1990; 264:13343–13347.
44. Sawyer ST: Receptors for erythropoietin: Distribution, structure, and role in receptor mediated endocytosis in eryxthroid cells. *Subcell Biochem* in press.
45. Sawyer ST, Sawada K, Krantz SB, et al: Conversion of the low affinity binding sites for erythropoietin into higher affinity binding sites by chymopain digestion of the cell surface in mouse and human erythroid cells (abstract). *Blood* 1989; 74:152.
46. D'Andrea AD, Lodish HF, Wong GG: Expression cloning of the murine erythropoietin receptor. *Cell* 1989; 57:277–285.
47. Youssoufian H, Zon LI, Orkin SH, et al: Structure and transcription of the mouse erythropoietin receptor gene. *Mol Cell Biol* 1990; 10:3675–3682.
48. Jones SS, D'Andrea AD, Haines LL, et al: Human erythropoietin receptor: Cloning, expression, and biologic characterization. *Blood* 1990; 76:31–35.
49. Winkelmann JC, Penny LA, Deaven LL, et al: The gene for the human erythropoietin receptor: Analysis of the coding sequence and assignment to chromosome 19p. *Blood* 1990; 76:24–30.
50. Fraser JK, Tan AS, Lin F-K, et al: Expression of specific high-affinity binding

sites for erythropoietin on rat and mouse megakaryocytes. *Exp Hematol* 1989; 17:10–16.
51. Burstein SA, Ishibashi T: Erythropoietin and megakaryocytopoiesis. *Blood Cells* 1989; 15:193–201.
52. Dessypris EN, Gleaton JH, Armstrong OL: Effect of human recombinant erythropoietin on human marrow megakaryocyte colony formation in vitro. *Br J Haematol* 1987; 65:265–269.
53. Ishibashi T, Koziol JA, Burstein SA: Human recombinant erythropoietin promotes differentiation of murine megakaryocytes in vitro. *J Clin Invest* 1987; 79:286–289.
54. Berridge MV, Fraser JK, Carter JM, et al: Effects of recombinant human erythropoietin on megakaryocytes and on platelet production in the rat. *Blood* 1988; 72:970–977.
55. McDonald TP, Cottrell MB, Clift RE, et al: High doses of recombinant erythropoietin stimulate platelet production in mice. *Exp Hematol* 1987; 15:719–721.
56. Koury MJ, Bondurant MC, Graber SE, et al: Erythropoietin messenger RNA levels in developing mice and transfer of ^{125}I-erythropoietin by the placenta. *J Clin Invest* 1988; 82:154–159.
57. Thomas RM, Canning CE, Cotes PM, et al: Erythropoietin and cord blood haemoglobin in the regulation of human fetal erythropoiesis. *Br J Obstet Gynaecol* 1983; 90:795–800.
58. Anagnostou A, Lee ES, Kessimian N, et al: Erythropoietin has a mitogenic and positive chemotactic effect on endothelial cells. *Proc Natl Acad Sci USA* 1990; 87:5978–5982.
59. Koury MJ, Bondurant MC: Maintenance by erythropoietin of viability and maturation of murine erythroid precursor cells. *J Cell Physiol* 1988; 137:65.
60. Krantz SB, Goldwasser E: On the mechanism of erythropoietin-induced differentiation II. The effect on RNA synthesis. *Biochim Biophys Acta* 1965; 103:325–332.
61. Piantadosi CA, Dickerman HW, Spivak JL: Sequential activation of splenic nuclear RNA polymerases by erythropoietin. *J Clin Invest* 1976; 57:20–26.
62. Dukes PP: In vitro studies on DNA synthesis of bone marrow cells stimulated by erythropoietin. *Ann NY Acad Sci* 1968; 149:437–444.
63. Gross M, Goldwasser E: On the mechanism of erythropoietin-induced differentiation. VII. The relationship between stimulated deoxyribonucleic acid synthesis and ribonucleic acid synthesis. *J Biol Chem* 1970; 245:1632–1636.
64. Roodman GD, Spivak JL, Zanjani ED: Stimulation of erythroid colony formation in vitro by erythropoietin immobilized on agarose-bound lectins. *J Lab Clin Med* 1981; 98:684–690.
65. Graber SE, Carillo M, Drantz SB: Lack of effect of erythropoietin on cyclic adenosine 3′, 5′-monophosphate levels in rat fetal liver cells. *J Lab Clin Med* 1974; 83:288–295.
66. Graber SE, Bomboy JD, Salmon WD, et al: Evidence that endotoxin is the cyclic 3′, 5′-GMP-promoting factor in erythropoietin preparations. *J Lab Clin Med* 1979; 93:25–31.
67. Miller BA, Scaduto RC, Tillotson DL, et al: Erythropoietin stimulates a rise in intracellular free calcium concentration in single early human erythroid precursors. *J Clin Invest* 1988; 82:309–315.
68. Mladenovic J, Kay NE: Erythropoietin induces rapid increases in intracellular

free calcium in human bone marrow cells. *J Lab Clin Med* 1988; 112:23–27.
69. Imagawa S, Smith BR, Palmer-Crocker R, et al: The effect of recombinant erythropoietin on intracellular free calcium in erythropoietin-responsive cells. *Blood* 1989; 73:1452–1457.
70. Choi H-S, Wojchowski DM, Sytkowski AJ: Erythropoietin rapidly alters phosphorylation of pp43, an erythroid membrane protein. *J Biol Chem* 1987; 262:2933–2936.
71. Eaves CJ, Humphries RK, Krystal G, et al: Hemoglobins in development and differentiation, in Stamatoyannopoulos G, Nienhius AW (eds). New York, 1981, p 63.
72. Koury MJ, Bondurant MC: Erythropoietin retards DNA breakdown and prevents programmed death in erythroid progenitor cells. *Science* 1990; 248:378–381.
73. Jacobson LO, Goldwasser E, Fried W, et al: Role of the kidney in erythropoiesis. *Nature* 1957; 179:633–634.
74. Erslev AJ: In vitro production of erythropoietin by kidneys perfused with a serum-free solution. *Blood* 1974; 44:77–85.
75. Fried W, Barone-Varelas J, Berman M: Detection of high erythropoietin titers in renal extracts of hypoxic rats. *J Lab Clin Med* 1981; 97:82–86.
76. Jelkmann W, Bauer C: Demonstration of high levels of erythropoietin in rat kidneys following hypoxic hypoxia. *Pfluegers Arch* 1981; 392:34–39.
77. Bondurant MC, Koury MJ: Anemia induces accumulation of erythropoietin mRNA in the kidney and liver. *Mol Cell Biol* 1986; 6:2731–2733.
78. Schuster SJ, Wilson JH, Erslev AJ, et al: Physiologic regulation and tissue localization of renal erythropoietin messenger RNA. *Blood* 1987; 70:316–318.
79. Fried W: The liver as a source of extrarenal erythropoietin production. *Blood* 1972; 40:671–677.
80. Lucarelli G, Howard D, Stohlman F: Regulation of erythropoiesis. XV. Neonatal erythropoiesis and the effect of nephrectomy. *J Clin Invest* 1964; 43:2195–2203.
81. Zanjani ED, Poster J, Burlington H, et al: Liver as the primary site of erythropoietin formation in the fetus. *J Lab Clin Med* 1977; 89:640–644.
82. Carmena AO, Howard D, Stohlman F: Regulation of erythropoiesis XXII. Erythropoietin production in the newborn animal. *Blood* 1968; 32:376–382.
83. Peschle C, Marone G, Genovese A, et al: Erythropoietin production by the liver in fetal-neonatal life. *Life Sci* 1975; 17:1325–1330.
84. Schooley JC, Mahlmann LJ: Extrarenal erythropoietin production by the liver in the weanling rat. *Proc Soc Exp Biol Med* 1974; 145:1081–1083.
85. Zanjani ED, Ascensai JL, McGlave PB, et al: Studies on the liver to kidney switch of erythropoietin production. *J Clin Invest* 1981; 76:1183–1188.
86. Vogt C, Pentz S, Rich IN: A role for the macrophage in normal hemopoiesis: III. In vitro and in vivo erythropoietin gene expression in macrophages detected by in situ hybridization. *Exp Hematol* 1989; 17:391–397.
87. Fisher JW, Taylor G, Porteous DD: Localization of erythropoietin in glomeruli of sheep kidney by fluorescent antibody technique. *Nature* 1965; 205:611–612.
88. Kurtz A, Jelkmann W, Sinowatz F, et al: Renal mesangial cell cultures as a model for study of erythropoietin production. *Proc Natl Acad Sci USA* 1983; 80:4008–4011.
89. Maples PB, Smith DH, Beru N, et al: Identification of erythropoietin-produc-

ing cells in mammalian tissues by in situ hybridization (abstract). *Blood* 1986; 68:170.
90. Maxwell AP, Lappin TRJ, Johnston CF, et al: Erythropoietin production in kidney tubular cells. *Br J Haematol* 1990; 74:535–539.
91. Koury ST, Bondurant MC, Koury MJ: Localization of erythropoietin synthesizing cells in murine kidneys by in situ hybridization. *Blood* 1988; 71:524–527.
92. Lacombe C, Da Silva J-L, Bruneval P, et al: Peritubular cells are the site of erythropoietin synthesis in the murine hypoxic kidney. *J Clin Invest* 1988; 81:620–623.
93. Kurtz A, Eckardt K-U, Neumann R, et al: Site of erythropoietin formation. *Contrib Nephrol* 1989; 76:14–23.
94. Suzuki T, Sasaki R: Immunocytochemical demonstration of erythropoietin immunoreactivity in peritubular endothelial cells of the anemic mouse kidney. *Arch Histol Cytol* 1990; 53:121–124.
95. Fukushima Y, Yanagisawa M, Nakamoto Y, et al: Localization of renal erythropoietin and the role of Ia antigen expression in hypoxic rat glomeruli. *Tohoku J Exp Med* 1990; 160:129–140.
96. Lechermann B, Jelkmann W: Erythropoietin production in normoxic and hypoxic rats with increased blood O_2 affinity. *Respir Physiol* 1985; 60:1–8.
97. Cotes PM: Immunoreactive erythropoietin in serum I. Evidence for the validity of the assay method and the physiological relevance of estimates. *Br J Haematol* 1982; 50:427–438.
98. Erslev AJ, Wilson J, Caro J: Erythropoietin titers in anemic, nonuremic patients. *J Lab Clin Med* 1987; 109:429–433.
99. Garcia JF, Ebbe SN, Hollander L, et al: Radioimmunoassay of erythropoietin: Circulating levels in normal and polycythemic human beings. *J Lab Clin Med* 1982; 99:624–635.
100. Rege AB, Brookins J, Fisher JW: A radioimmunoassay for erythropoietin: Serum levels in normal human subjects and patients with hemopoietic disorders. *J Lab Clin Med* 1982; 100:829–834.
101. Lorentz A, Jendrissek A, Eckardt K-U, et al: Serial immunoreactive erythropoietin levels in patients predonating autologous blood for erythropoietic hip surgery. *Transfusion,* in press.
102. Miller ME, Cronkite EP, Garcia JF: Plasma levels of immunoreactive erythropoietin after acute blood loss in man. *Br J Haematol* 1982; 52:545–549.
103. Cotes PM, Coré CJ, Liu Yin JA, et al: Determination of serum immunoreactive erythropoietin in the investigation of erythrocytosis. *N Engl J Med* 1986; 315:283–287.
104. Erslev AJ, Caro J: Pure erythrocytosis classified according to erythropoietin titers. *Am J Med* 1984; 76:57–61.
105. Eckardt K-U, Boutellier U, Kurtz A, et al: Rate of erythropoietin formation in humans in response to acute hypobaric hypoxia. *J Appl Physiol* 1989; 66:1785–1788.
106. Eckardt K-U, Dittmer J, Neumann R, et al: Decline of erythropoietin formation at continuous hypoxia is not due to feedback inhibition. *Am J Physiol* 1990; 258:1432–1437.
107. Kurtz A, Eckardt K-U, Tannahill l, et al: Regulation of erythropoietin production. *Contrib Nephrol* 1988; 66:1–16.
108. Eckardt K-U, Kurtz A, Bauer C: Triggering of erythropoietin formation by hypoxia is inhibited by respiratory and metabolic acidosis. *Am J Physiol* 1990; 258:678–683.

109. Steinberg SE, Garcia JF, Matzke GR, et al: Erythropoietin kinetics in rats: Generation and clearance. *Blood* 1986; 67:646–649.
110. Fu J-S, Lertora JJL, Brookins J, et al: Pharmacokinetics of erythropoietin in intact and anephric dogs. *J Lab Clin Med* 1988; 111:669–676.
111. Piroso E, Flaharty K, Caro J, et al: Erythropoietin half-life in rats with hypoplastic and hyperplastic bone marrows (abstract). *Blood* 1989; 74:270.
112. Jelkmann W: Temporal pattern of erythropoietin titers in kidney tissue during hypoxic hypoxia. *Pfluegers Arch* 1982; 393:88–91.
113. Schooley JC, Mahlmann LJ: Evidence for the de novo synthesis of erythropoietin in hypoxic rats. *Blood* 1972; 40:662–671.
114. Ratcliffe PJ, Jones RW, Phillips RE, et al: Oxygen-dependent modulation of erythropoietin mRNA levels. *J Exp Med* 1990; 172:657–660.
115. Giger K: Wirkung von Actinomycin D auf die Erythropoietinbildung während der Hypoxie bei der Ratte. *Klin Wochenschr* 1968; 46:42–44.
116. Schuster SJ, Badiavas EV, Costa-Giomi P, et al: Stimulation of erythropoietin gene transcription during hypoxia and cobalt exposure. *Blood* 1989; 73:13–16.
117. Goldberg MA, Gaut CC, Bunn HF: Erythropoietin mRNA levels are regulated by both transcriptional events and by changes in RNA stability (abstract). *Blood* 1989; 74:191.
118. Koury ST, Koury MJ, Bondurant MC, et al: Quantitation of erythropoietin-producing cells in kidneys of mice by in situ hybridization: Correlation with hematocrit, renal erythropoietin mRNA, and serum erythropoietin concentration. *Blood* 1989; 74:645–651.
119. Fisher JW, Langston JW: The influence of hypoxemia and cobalt on erythropoietin production in the isolated perfused dog kidney. *Blood* 1967; 29:114–125.
120. Kuratowska Z, Lewartowski B, Michalak E: Studies on the production of erythropoietin by isolated perfused organs. *Blood* 1961; 18:527–534.
121. Pagel H, Jelkmann W, Weiss C: Renal production of erythropoietin - studies in the isolated perfused rat kidney (abstract). *Pfluegers Arch* 1990; 415:41.
122. Scholz H, Schurek HJ, Eckardt K-U, et al: Oxygen dependent erythropoietin production by the isolated perfused rat kidney. *Pfluegers Arch* 1991; 418:228–233.
123. Pagel H, Jelkmann W, Weiss C: A comparison of the effects of renal artery constriction and anemia on the production of erythropoietin. *Pfluegers Arch* 1988; 413:62–66.
124. Goldberg MA, Glass GA, Cunningham JM, et al: The regulated expression of erythropoietin by two human hepatoma cell lines. *Proc Natl Acad Sci USA* 1987; 84:7972–7976.
125. Goldberg MA, Dunning SP, Bunn HF: Regulation of the erythropoietin gene: Evidence that the oxygen sensor is a heme protein. *Science* 1988; 242:1412–1415.
126. Nielsen OJ, Schuster SJ, Kaufman R, et al: Regulation of erythropoietin production in a human hepatoblastoma cell line. *Blood* 1987; 70:1904–1909.
127. Kramer K, Deetjen P. Beziehung des O_2 Verbrauchs der Niere zu Durchblutung und Glomerulusfiltrat bei Änderung des arteriellen Druckes. *Pfluegers Arch* 1960; 271:782–796.
128. Eckardt K-U, Kurtz A, Bauer C: Regulation of erythropoietin formation is related to proximal tubular function. *Am J Physiol* 1990; 256:942–947.
129. Brezis M, Rosen S, Silvio P, et al: Selective vulnerability of the medullary

thick ascending limb to anoxia in the isolated perfused rat kidney. *J Clin Invest* 1984; 73:182–190.
130. Schurek HJ, Kriz W. Morphological and functional evidence for oxygen deficiency in the isolated perfused rat kidney. *Lab Invest* 1985; 53:145–155.
131. Aukland K, Krog J: Renal oxygen tension. *Nature* 1960; 188:671.
132. Baumgärtl H, Leichtweiss HP, Lübbers DW, et al: The oxygen supply of the dog kidney: Measurements of intrarenal pO_2. *Mirovasc Res* 1972; 4:247–257.
133. Schurek HJ, Jost U, Bertram H, et al: Preglomerular cortical oxygen diffusion shunt: A prerequisite for effective erythropoietin regulation? *Contrib Nephrol* 1989; 76:57–66.
134. DuBose TD, Bidani A: Kietics of CO_2 exchange in the kidney. *Ann Rev Physiol* 1988; 50:653–667.
135. Sohtell M: CO_2 along the proximal tubules in the rat kidney. *Acta Physiol Scand* 1979; 105:146–155.
136. Le Hir M, Eckardt K-U, Kaissling B: Anemia induces 5′-nucleotidase in fibroblasts of cortical labyrinth of rat kidney. *Renal Physiol Biochem* 1989; 12:313–319.
137. Fisher JW, Samuels AI: Relationship between renal blood flow and erythropoietin production in dogs. *Proc Soc Exp Biol Med* 1967; 125:482–485.
138. Erslev AJ, Caro J, Besarab A: Why the kidney? *Nephron* 1985; 41:213–216.
139. Cohen RA, Miller ME, Garcia JF, et al: Regulatory mechanism of erythropoietin production: Effects of hypoxemia and hypercarbia. *Exp Hematol* 1981; 9:513–521.
140. Miller ME, Howard D: Modulation of erythropoietin concentrations by manipulation of hypercarbia. *Blood Cells* 1979; 5:389–403.
141. Schooley JC, Mahlmann LJ: Hypoxia and the initiation of erythropoietin production. *Blood Cells* 1975; 1:429–448.
142. Wolf-Priessnitz J, Schooley JC, Mahlmann LJ: Inhibition of erythropoietin production in unanaesthetized rabbits exposed to an acute hypoxic-hypercapnic environment. *Blood* 1978; 52:153–162.
143. Zucali JR, Lee M, Mirand EA: Carbon dioxide effects on erythropoietin and erythropoiesis. *J Lab Clin Med* 1978; 92:648–655.
144. Gores GJ, Nieminen A-L, Wray BA, et al: Intracellular pH during chemical hypoxia in cultured rat hepatocytes. Protection by intracellular acidosis against the onset of cell death. *J Clin Invest* 1989; 83:386–396.
145. Penttila A, Trump BJ: Extracellular acidosis protects Ehrlich ascites tumor cells and rat renal cortex against anoxic injury. *Science* 1974; 185:277–278.
146. Abbrecht PH, Littell JK: Plasma erythropoietin in men and mice during acclimatization to different altitudes. *J Appl Physiol* 1972; 32:54–58.
147. Caro J, Erslev AJ: Biologic and immunolgic eythropoietin in extracts from hypoxic whole rat kidneys and in their glomerular and tubular fractions. *J Lab Clin Med* 1984; 103:922–931.
148. Fried W, Johnson C, Heller P: Observations on the regulation of erythropoiesis during prolonged periods of hypoxia. *Blood* 1970; 36:607–616.
149. Reynafarje C, Ramos J, Faura J, et al: Humoral control of erythropoietic activity in man during and after altitude exposure.*Proc Soc Exp Biol Med* 1964; 116:649–650.
150. Fried W, Plzak L, Jacobson LO, et al: Erythropoiesis. II. Assay of erythropoietin in hypophysectomized rats. *Proc Soc Exp Biol Med* 1956; 92:203–207.

151. Jelkmann W, Kurtz A, Bauer C: Effects of fasting on the hypoxia-induced erythropoietin production in rats. *Pfluegers Arch* 1983; 396:174–175.
152. Miller ME, Rørth M, Stohlman F, et al: Effects of acute bleeding on acid-base balance, erythropoietin (Ep) production and in vivo P50 in the rat. *Br J Haematol* 1976; 33:379–385.
153. Crafts RC, Meineke A: The anemia of hypophysectomized animals. *Ann NY Acad Sci* 1990; 77:501–517.
154. Kurtz A, Zapf J, Eckardt K-U, et al: Insulin-like growth factor I stimulates erythropoiesis in hypophysectomized rats. *Proc Natl Acad Sci USA* 1988; 85:7825–7829.
155. Halvorsen S, Roh BL, Fisher JW: Erythropoietin production in nephrectomized and hypophysectomized animals. *Am J Physiol* 1968; 215:349–352.
156. Peschle C, Rappaport IA, Magli MC, et al: Role of the hypophysis in erythropoietin production during hypoxia. *Blood* 1978; 51:1117–1124.
157. Fisher JW. Prostaglandins and kidney erythropoietin production. *Nephron* 1980; 25:53–56.
158. Kurtz A, Jelkmann W, Pfeilschifter J, et al: Role of prostaglandins in hypoxia-stimulated erythropoietin production. *Am J Physiol* 1985; 249:3–8.
159. Kurtz A, Jelkmann W, Pfuhl A, et al: Erythropoietin production by fetal mouse liver cells in response to hypoxia and adenylate cyclase. *Endocrinology* 1986; 118:567–572.
160. Schooley JC, Mahlmann LJ: Stimulation of erythropoiesis in the plethoric mouse by cyclic-AMP and its inhibition by antierythropoietin. *Proc Soc Exp Biol Med* 1971; 137:1298–1292.
161. Sherwood JB, Burns ER, Shouval D: Stimulation by cAMP of erythropoietin secretion by an established human renal carcinoma cell line. *Blood* 1987; 69:1053–1057.
162. Paul P, Rothmann SA, Meagher C: Modulation of erythropoietin production by adenosine. *J Lab Clin Med* 1988; 112:168–173.
163. Ueno M, Brookins J, Beckman B, et al: A1 and A2 adenosine receptor regulation of erythropoietin production. *Life Sci* 1988; 43:229–237.
164. Ueno M, Brookins J, Beckman B, et al: Effects of reactive oxygen metabolites on erythropoietin production in renal carcinoma cells. *Biochem Biophys Res Commun* 1988; 154:773–780.
165. Goldwasser E, Jacobson LO, Fried W, et al: Studies on erythropoiesis. V. The effect of cobalt on the production of erythropoietin. *Blood* 1958; 13:55–60.
166. Sinclair P, Gibbs AH, Sinclair JF, et al: Formation of cobalt protoporphyrin in the liver of rats: A mechanism for the inhibition of liver haem biosynthesis by inorganic cobalt. *Biochem J* 1979; 178:529–538.
167. Semenza GL, Traystman MD, Gearhart JD, et al: Polycythemia in transgenic mice expressing the human erythropoietin gene. *Proc Natl Acad Sci USA* 1989; 86:2301–2305.

Part III

Therapy in Renal Patients

The New Treatments of Hyperparathyroidism Secondary to Renal Insufficiency

Albert Fournier, M.D.

Professor of Medicine, Service de Néphrologie, Centre Hospitalier Régional et Universitaire d'Amiens, France

Tilman Drüeke, M.D.

Director, Associate Professor, INSERM U90, Department of Nephrology, Necker Hospital, Paris, France

Philippe Morinière, M.D.

Service de Néphrologie du Centre Hospitalier Régional et Universitaire d'Amiens, France

Johanna Zingraff, M.D.

Department of Nephrology, Necker Hospital, Paris, France

Bernard Boudailliez

Practicien Hospitalier, Service de Pédiatrie I du Centre Hospitalier Regional et Universitaire, d'Amiens, France

Jean Michel Achard

Chef de Clinique, Service de Néphrologie du Centre Hospitalier Régional et Universitaire d'Amiens, France

For the 1981 Necker Seminars in Nephrology, we reviewed the pathophysiology and treatment of hyperparathyroidism secondary to renal insufficiency. In this update, we will discuss the advances in this field over the past 10 years.

Pathophysiology of Hyperparathyroidism Secondary to Renal Insufficiency

Figure 1A shows the conceptualization in 1981 of the pathophysiologic mechanisms contributing to the stimulation of parathyroid hormone (PTH)

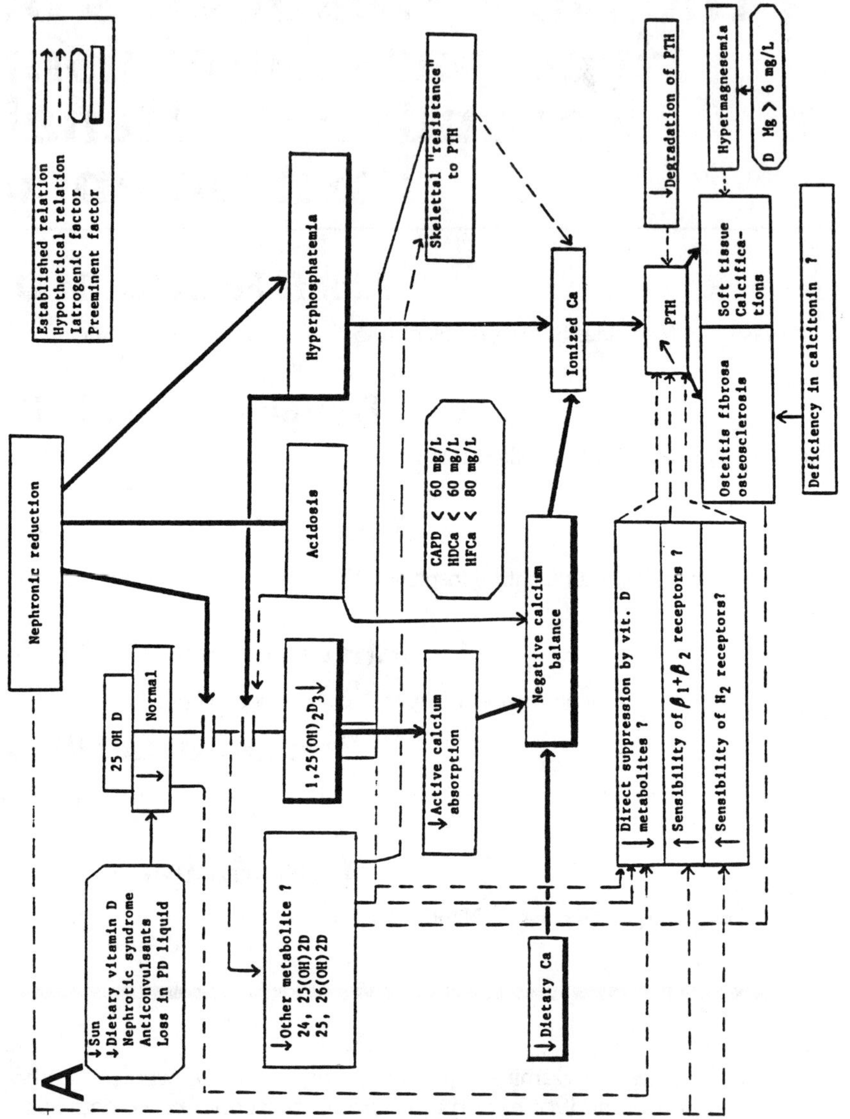

FIG 1.
A, 1981 diagram of pathophysiology of hyperparathyroidism secondary to renal insufficiency. **B,** 1991 diagram of pathophysiology of hyperparathyroidism secondary to renal insufficiency. Effect of $CaCO_3$: It corrects the negative Ca balance, prevents hyperphosphatemia and intraepithelial retention of PO_4, and partially corrects acidosis, In consequence it partially restores calcitriol synthesis and the upward shift of the calcium set point of the calcium regulated PTH secretion. *Solid arrows* = established role; *broken arrows* = hypothetical role; *dotted arrows* = suppressive effect; *hatched boxes* = iatrogenic factor.

B
Intraepithelial PO4 retention
Acidosis
CaCO3
Plasma calcitriol (production)
Nephronic reduction
Uremic toxins
Active intestinal Ca absorption
Negative Ca balance
Hypocalcemia
Bone resistance to PTH
Parathyroid hyperplasia
SYNTHESIS / SECRETION OF PTH
Osteitis fibrosa
Deficiency in 24,25 (OH)2 D3
Deficiency in calcitonin ?
Anti convulsant
Plasma PO4 in advanced renal failure
Sun exposure
Milk intake
Anticonvulsants
D binding protein loss
CAPD
nephrotic syndrom
Deficiency in 25 OH vit. D3
Dietary Ca due to protein restriction
Dialyse- hemofiltration fluid
CAPD : Ca < 6.5 mg/L
HD : Ca < 6.5 mg/l
HF : Ca < 7.0 mg/l
CaCO3
Diabete hypothyroïdisme
Intoxication with Àlu - Fe Calcitriol

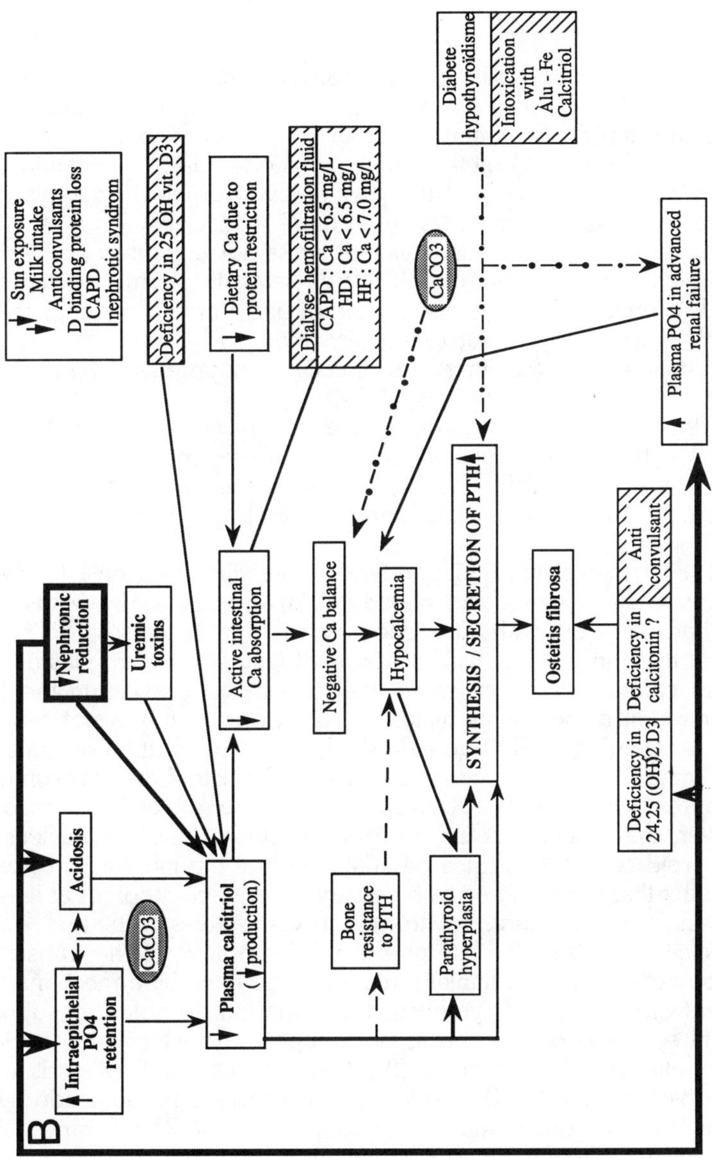

FIG 1 (cont.).

secretion in renal insufficiency.[1] Figure 1B shows our present understanding of these mechanisms.

Figure 1, **B** is not very different from that presented 10 years ago, except for four points:

a. The direct suppressive effect of calcitriol and inversely the stimulating role of its deficiency on PTH synthesis is now well established and its molecular mechanism has been determined. This effect appears to override that of other vitamin D metabolites, namely 24,25-$(OH)_2$ vitamin D3 and 25,26-$(OH)_2$ vitamin D3,[2–4] the plasma levels of which may also be decreased (although not consistently) in renal insufficiency.[5, 6]

b. hyperphosphatemia also has a direct stimulating effect on PTH secretion[7] and indirect effects through the decrease in plasma ionized calcium related to physicochemical disequilibrium and through the suppression of 25-OH vitamin D - 1α-hydroxylase activity;

c. uremic toxins also intervene directly by suppressing 1α-hydroxylase activity;

d. other factors, on the contrary, may abnormally suppress PTH secretion through associated disease such as diabetes mellitus[8] or intoxication such as by aluminum[8] or possibly iron overload,[9] or more simply because of overtreatment by oral calcium and calcitriol.[10]

In 1981,[1] the calcium-independent suppressive effect on PTH secretion of intravenous calcitriol had already been established by Madsen et al. They had obtained, with intravenous calcitriol, a decrease in PTH plasma concentration in patients with acute renal failure in whom plasma ionized calcium concentration was maintained constant by lowering the calcium concentration of peritoneal dialysis fluid. However, it was not certain that this was unambiguously due to a direct effect of calcitriol on parathyroid cells because in vitro studies on the action of calcitriol on PTH synthesis by parathyroid cells in culture showed contradictory results. It was recognized, however, that calcitriol could be fixed on cytosol and the nucleus of the parathyroid cells. It has since been shown that the inconsistency was due to the fact that the cells had to be incubated with calcitriol for at least 12 to 24 hours.[11] Furthermore, in vitro and in vivo studies in the rat[2–4] showed that calcitriol directly inhibits prepro-PTH synthesis at the transcriptional level by acting on the 5'flanking region of the gene by a mechanism independent of new protein synthesis. It is important to note that suppression of PTH synthesis by calcitriol is dose-dependent, which may explain the greater efficacy of intravenous (IV) than oral calcitriol. At odds with the rapid onset (within 2 to 3 minutes) of PTH secretion modulation by extracellular calcium concentration, the suppression of PTH synthesis by calcitriol occurs only after 12 to 24 hours. It is preceded by a progressive decrease in the steady state levels of the prepro-PTH mRNA. Plasma calcium concentration changes not only influence PTH secretion within a few minutes but, on a longer term basis, also act on transcription, which is stimulated by hypocalcemia and inhibited by hypercalcemia. The mechanism by which hypercalcemia suppresses transcription differs from that of calcitriol since only calcitriol suppression is prevented by dexamethasone.[11] The calcitriol suppressive effect on PTH transcription is stronger than that of hypercalcemia because when hypocalcemia is induced in the rat by hyperphosphatemia or by calcitonin, the induced stimulation of PTH transcription is prevented by simultaneous administration of calcitriol.[2] However, dietary calcium deficiency has a stronger stimulating effect (five times) than vitamin D deficiency (two times) on the expression of the PTH gene.[3]

Calcitriol has not only a plasma calcium-independent suppressive effect on PTH synthesis but may also alter the release of synthesized PTH, so that its deficiency in renal insufficiency explains the increase of the set-point of calcium-regulated PTH secretion; i.e., the plasma concentration able to suppress by 50% the maximal secretion of parathyroid cells. The calcium set-point is 1mM for normal parathyroid cells in culture and 1.26mM for cells from uremic hyperplastic parathyroid glands.[11] This increased set-point of calcium-regulated PTH secretion is also responsible for the increased calcium concentration necessary to inhibit adenylate cyclase activity of membranes prepared with uremic parathyroid glands. Thus, when plasma calcitriol concentration is subnormal, plasma calcium concentration should be above normal to prevent PTH hypersecretion. Inversely, increase of plasma calcitriol concentration to normal or even supranormal levels by oral or intravenous bolus of calcitriol should decrease this calcium set-point.[12, 13]

A decrease in the number of calcitriol receptors on the uremic parathyroid glands has been reported[14, 15] without a change in their affinity for calcitriol. This decrease, together with the low plasma levels of calcitriol, could contribute to stimulation of PTH synthesis and secretion. However, the reliability of these findings has recently been questioned by work of the Ritz group (personal communication), which incriminates artifactual bench protelysis of the receptor as being at the origin of the decrease in the number of receptors.

Finally, it should be stressed that low plasma calcitriol levels contribute to stimulation of PTH synthesis not only by increasing the activity of each cell but also by increasing the number of cells (proliferation); i.e., by promoting hyperplasia of the parathyroid glands, a process which is experimentally better prevented than cured.[16]

Hyperphosphatemia has long been known to favor hyperparathyroidism, and numerous works of Slatopolsky and his team have clearly established the value of its prevention for the control of hyperparathyroidism.[11] The mechanism of this effect is not yet fully established. A decrease in ionized calcium due to physicochemical disequilibrium in the plasma when plasma phosphate increases is insufficient to explain stimulation of PTH secretion, especially at the beginning of renal insufficiency.[17] The trade-off hypothesis Bricker et al. put forth in the 1960s regarding the pathogenesis of hyperparathyroidism in early renal insufficiency should now be abandoned. (It considered that phosphate retention secondary to a decrease in glomerular filtration should transiently lead to hyperphosphatemia and therefore to hypocalcemia, thus stimulating PTH secretion that would correct hyperphosphatemia [and therefore hypocalcemia] by decreasing phosphate tubular reabsorption.) Furthermore, it had been shown that fractional PO_4 reabsorption could decrease in renal insufficiency in the absence of PTH. At the end of the 1970s, it was thus proposed that phosphate retention intervened essentially by decreasing 25-OH vitamin D - 1α-hydroxylase activity. It was considered that in early renal insufficiency, despite normal plasma phosphate concentration, the reduction in nephron mass led to an increase in the filtered load of PO_4 in the individual nephron because of increased glomerular filtration rate (GFR) of the remnant nephrons. This would in turn lead to an increased tubular intraepithelial concentration of PO_4 and depression of 1α-hydroxylase activity. The resulting calcitriol deficiency was even considered a homeostatic adaptation phenomenon for phosphate retention since it leads to a decrease in intestinal absorption of phosphate.[18] Because of the direct suppressive effect of calcitriol on PTH secretion, this calcitriol deficiency leads to hyperparathyroidism. Therefore, the latter should no longer be interpreted as a consequence of an ionic disturbance of the extracellular milieu but rather as a consequence of an endocrine deficiency.[19]

The parathyroid response may be such that the plasma concentrations of calcitriol in early renal insufficiency may remain normal in absolute value. However, the synthesis reserve of calcitriol is decreased according to Ritz et al.,[19] who showed that maximal stimulation of 1α-hydroxylase by exogenous 1-34 PTH was less in early renal insufficiency than in control subjects. Such a decrease in calcitriol synthesis reserve could not be demonstrated by Prince et al.,[20] who only submaximally stimulated 1α-hydroxylase by calcium deficiency. Due to this hyperparathyroidism, plasma phosphate level can remain in the normal range and even at the lower range of normal because of accelerated hyperphosphaturia after an oral load of phosphate since the tubular reabsorption of phosphate is more readily suppressed.[21] In fact, in four patients with mild renal insufficiency, Llach et al.[22] obtained normalization of hyperparathyroidism and postprandial hyperphosphaturia only by several weeks' restriction of dietary phosphate, whereas plasma concentrations of calcitriol normalized. The possibility of increasing plasma concentrations of calcitriol by phosphate restriction was confirmed in normal individuals by Portale et al.[23] but not by Seidel et al.[24] It was also confirmed in early renal insufficiency (between 30 and 60 mL/min GFR), the phosphate restriction being reinforced by $Al(OH)_3$[25] or by calcium carbonate.[26] It disappears, however, in more severe renal insufficiency (GFR <20 mL/min)[27, 28] even when $Al(OH)_3$ is used. In this situation, Takamoto actually found a decrease in plasma calcitriol concentration and incriminated the toxicity of aluminium on 1α-hydroxylase.

To Lopez Hilker et al.[7] goes credit for demonstrating a direct stimulating effect of hyperphosphatemia on PTH secretion. They showed that phosphate restriction could prevent hyperparathyroidism in uremic dogs while plasma calcium levels remained normal and plasma calcitriol concentration low. A direct effect of phosphate on PTH secretion is also supported by the observation of Dabbaugh et al.[29] that phosphate restriction prevents hyperparathyroidism in the vitamin D-deficient rat maintained normocalcemic. The mechanism of this direct effect of phosphate on PTH secretion is not yet elucidated. Modification of phospholipid composition of the parathyroid cell membrane, with changes in calcium channels, and of calcitriol receptors has been incriminated.[7]

That uremic toxins affect the pathogenesis of hyperparathyroidism by decreasing 1α-hydroxylase activity was demonstrated by Hsu and Patel,[30] who perfused rats with their own phosphate free urine and showed that calcitriol synthesis was inhibited proportionally to the oral protein load. Guadinosuccinic acid, a well recognised uremic toxin, may be implicated since it decreases the circulating levels of calcitriol in normal rats.[31]

In recent years, we have learned to recognize the role of factors that could abnormally suppress PTH secretion and therefore induce adynamic bone disease.[8] Some factors are diseases that may cause renal insufficiency, such as diabetes mellitus and hypothyroidism.[8] Others are iatrogenic, essentially aluminum through water used for the dialysate preparation and not appropriately treated with reverse osmosis or deionization or through the aluminum phosphate binders,[32] and possibly iron brought by transfusions and injections.[9] Such factors may suppress PTH secretion to such a point that a relative hypoparathyroid state is induced with either only moderately elevated C-terminal PTH levels[10] or even normal 1-84 PTH levels,[33] leading to adynamic bone. However, such factors may not be detected. This was the case in our studies describing for the first time an idiopathic adynamic bone disease in patients receiving dialysis[34] and in not yet dialyzed patients with uremia.[10] In the latter study, abnormally high levels of plasma calcitriol induced by a 25-OH D_3 supplement were incriminated. This study also suggested a role of uremia per se in this adynamic state, since this histologic pattern was observed in patients in whom C-terminal PTH plasma levels were similar to those of patients with normal bone but more advanced renal failure. It thus seems that hyperparathyroidism protects the patient with uremia from bone adynamism and that if it is too strongly suppressed, an adynamic bone pattern due to uremia is unmasked.

The other pathophysiologic mechanisms involved in hyperparathyroidism are conceptualized in 1991 as they were in 1981. The crucial importance of negative calcium balance is still recognized. It is favored by the conjunction of decreased intake of calcium due to protein and phosphate restriction and of defective adaptative stimulation of active intestinal calcium absorption due to calcitriol deficiency. This deleterious mechanism can, however, easily be bypassed by oral administration of high-dose calcium. When elemental calcium intake is over 1.5 g per day (which can easily be obtained with 3 g of $CaCO_3$ or 1,200 mg of elemental calcium plus 400 mg of calcium in a diet without milk products), calcitriol is no longer necessary to prevent the negative calcium balance since thanks to the calcium concentration gradient between the intestinal lumen and the blood, passive calcium absorption by paracellular pathways occurs.[35, 36] This increase in passive calcium absorption may even become a problem when control of hyperphosphatemia necessitates higher doses of $CaCO_3$. In such cases, hypercalcemia may occur even if oral calcium is taken with food to better complex the phosphate and decrease calcium absorption. Figure 1B indicates the role of oral calcium as phosphate binder: by binding phosphate in the gut, it prevents phosphate retention in the tubular cell and therefore inhibition of 25-OH D-1α-hydroxylase activity[25,26] as well as hyperphosphatemia, thus preventing the direct stimulating effect of the latter on PTH secretion.[7,11]

Hypothetical stimulation of β2 adrenergic receptors and histaminergic H2-receptors is not seen in Fig. 1B. No new data support a pathophysiologic role of these receptors or a therapeutical advantage of their blockade by β-blockers or anti-H2 drugs. Explaining hyperparathyroidism by resistance of uremic bone to PTH always remains hypothetical. The prevention of hyperparathyroidism by phosphate restriction is not consistently associated with disappearance of resistance to the hypercalcemic effect of exogenous PTH.[37, 38] It should be pointed out that this concept was difficult to integrate when it was thought that PTH induces hypercalcemia by stimulating osteoclastic resorption since the latter is actually increased in uremia. In fact, the rapid hypercalcemic effect of PTH seems due to calcium transfer from a rapidly exchangeable calcium pool situated around the osteocyte across the osseous membrane formed by the lining cells that separate bone from extracellular fluid. Increased osteoclastic resorption is only responsible for the delayed occurrence after PTH infusion of prolonged hypercalcemia.[39] The concept of resistance of the uremic bone to PTH effect is in fact erroneous. Recent studies have shown that the uremic bone is actually more sensitive to the resorptive effect of PTH, probably as a result of a deficiency in 24,25-$(OH)_2$D3, as we shall discuss.[40, 41]

Regarding mechanisms other than PTH hypersecretion in the genesis of the histologic lesions of osteitis fibrosa, the role of calcitonin deficiency remains hypothetical. The recent study by Malluche et al.[42] did not confirm the inverse correlations that Kanis et al. had observed between the plasma levels of PTH and those of calcitonin in patients with uremia and frank elevation of alkaline phosphatase levels. On the other hand, the role of 24,25-$(OH)_2$ vitamin D3 deficiency has again been emphasized by new studies. In 1981, we pointed out that Lieberherr had suggested that 24,25-$(OH)_2$ vitamin D3 could decrease the osteoclastic effect of PTH since, in vitro, the stimulation by PTH of bone alkaline and acid phosphatases and the calcium release from a rat calvaria could be inhibited by 24,25-(OH)2 vitamin D3, whereas calcitriol had the reverse effect. Furthermore, our group had shown that patients receiving dialysis who improved bone hyperresorption by treatment with 1α-OH vitamin D3 plus 25-OH vitamin D3 were those whose plasma levels of 24,25-$(OH)_2$ vitamin D3 were increased either before or during treatment and finally normalized; patients whose bone did not improve were those whose plasma 24,25-$(OH)_2$ vitamin D levels remained low.[5] The deficiency in 24,25-$(OH)_2$ vitamin D3 in patients with uremia is thus not constant, which may be explained by the fact that 24-hydroxylase is present not only in the kidney but also in the gut and the bone and that it may be stimulated by calcium and phosphate repletion secondary to calcitriol administration.[37]

Thus as early as 1981, a potential therapeutic effect of 24,25-$(OH)_2$ vitamin D3 had been suggested mainly related to its local protective effect against the osteoclastic action of PTH. Its suppressive effect on PTH secretion has always been controversial, having been found in the uremic dog by Canterbury et al.,[43, 44] but not by Olgaard et al.[45] This was probably due to different calcium intake since suppression of PTH was observed by Canterbury et al.[44] only when the dogs had a high calcium diet.

Since 1981, numerous experimental and clinical works have supported this protective effect of 24,25-$(OH)_2$ vitamin D3. In the uremic rat, Main et al.[46] showed it to be as effective as calcitriol in preventing decreased calcified bone mass induced by a phosphate-rich diet. A Norwegian group has also shown that in normal rats, 24,25-$(OH)_2$ D3 has a physiologic role, decreasing PTH stimulation of osteoblast membrane adenyate cyclase activity and potentiating its stimulation by calcitonin, whereas calcitriol has only trivial effects on these phenomena.[40] The same group has further shown (using 2 bone biopsy specimens, one for histomorphometric study, the other for studying in vitro stimulation by exogenous 1-84 PTH of bone cell membrane adenylate cyclase activity) that in normal humans and in patients with uremia or primary hyperparathyroidism, the increase in adenylate cyclase activity induced by PTH is inversely correlated to circulating plasma concentrations of 24,25-$(OH)_2$ vitamin D. In addition, the ratio of adenylate cyclase activity to plasma 24,25-$(OH)_2$ vitamin D was linearly correlated to bone resorption.[41] These data suggest a protective role of 24,25-$(OH)_2$ vitamin D3 against the osteoclastic effect of PTH. To further support their hypothesis, these authors[17] then studied the effect of injection into rats of 26,25-$(OH)_2$ vitamin D3, 25-OH vitamin D_3, and 1,25-$(OH)_2$ vitamin D3 during 12 weeks. They observed that the PTH-induced increase in adenylate cyclase activity of the calvaria membrane was completely abolished in rats treated with 24,25-$(OH)_2$ vitamin D3; this could explain the lack of increase in alkaline phosphatases, hydroxyprolinuria, and in plasma and urinary calcium levels. In animals treated with 25-OH vitamin D3 or calcitriol, the increase in alkaline phosphatases and in hydroxyprolinuria was not prevented, and calciuria increased. Plasma calcium levels did not, however, increase with 25-OH vitamin D3 whereas they did with calcitriol. The same group, further exploring the mechanism of interaction of PTH-sensitive adenylate cyclase activity with 24,25-OH vitamin D3, showed that 24,25-$(OH)_2$ vitamin D3, interrupts the coupling of the PTH receptor to the guanosine triphosphate (GTP)-binding protein G.[47a] Furthermore, recent works[48] have shown that 24,25-$(OH)_2$ vitamin D3 inhibits fusion of precursors for human osteoclastlike cells.

Results of Rubinger et al.[49] in the uremic rat also support a protective role of 24,25-$(OH)_2$ vitamin D3 for bone. They show that calcitriol and not

24,25-$(OH)_2$ vitamin D3 increases intestinal calcium absorption and plasma calcium concentration but that their association decreases hypercalcemia without decreasing fractional absorption of calcium, suggesting decreased calcitriol-induced calcium release by the bone.

Finally acidosis may contribute both to hypersecretion of PTH and to enhancement of its action on bone.[50] Acidosis favors a negative calcium balance, hyperphosphatemia,[50, 51, 52] and deficient calcitriol synthesis.[36, 38] In fact, correction of acidosis in patients receiving dialysis who have osteitis fibrosa, compared to control patients in whom acidosis was not corrected, prevented increased plasma concentrations of PTH and osteocalcine and was associated with improvement in the histologic degree of osteitis fibrosa.[50]

The Iatrogenic Vicious Circle of the Association of 1α-Hydroxyvitamin D Derivatives, Aluminum Phosphate Binders, and Deferoxamine Treatment

For Malluche and Faugere, treatment of renal osteodystrophy is still in 1990 an unmet challenge.[53] We agree with this negative judgment when considering the practical results of therapeutic advice given by most textbooks 5 to 10 years ago.[21, 53–57] This advice consisted of giving 1α-hydroxyvitamin D derivatives in association with aluminum phosphate binders and small doses of oral calcium. Figure 2 illustrates this vicious circle.

The use of 1α-hydroxylated hydroxyvitamin D metabolites (either calcitriol or 1α-OH vitamin D3, transformed into calcitriol by hepatic 25 hydroxylation) is logical since, as pointed out above, there is absolute or relative defective synthesis of this active metabolite, which stimulates PTH hypersecretion by inducing a negative calcium balance and by nonsuppression of PTH gene transcription in parathyroid cells. However, correction of calcitriol deficiency will stimulate intestinal absorption not only of calcium but also of phosphate and aluminum.

Increase in phosphate absorption by calcitriol is well documented by balance studies in patients with uremia. Coburn et al.[58] showed that with a daily dose of 0.68 and 2.7 μg calcitriol, net intestinal absorption of phosphate increased by 2.5 and 6 mmol/day whereas that of calcium increased by 2 and 6.5 mmol/day. This effect is not necessarily followed by increased plasma phosphate because when hyperparathyroidism is severe (with elevated plasma alkaline phosphatases), its suppression by calcitriol will decrease the phosphate release from bone, preventing the increase in plasma phosphate. It is well known that increased plasma concentration of phosphate and calcium after treatment of severe hyperparathyroidism by calcitriol occurs only when plasma alkaline phosphatases normalize. The increase in plasma phosphate leads to an increased dose of $A1(OH)_3$, and the absorption of aluminum will increase. Furthermore, intestinal absorption of aluminum is very likely directly increased by calcitriol as shown by the experimental work of Adler and and Berlyne[59] on everted duodenum

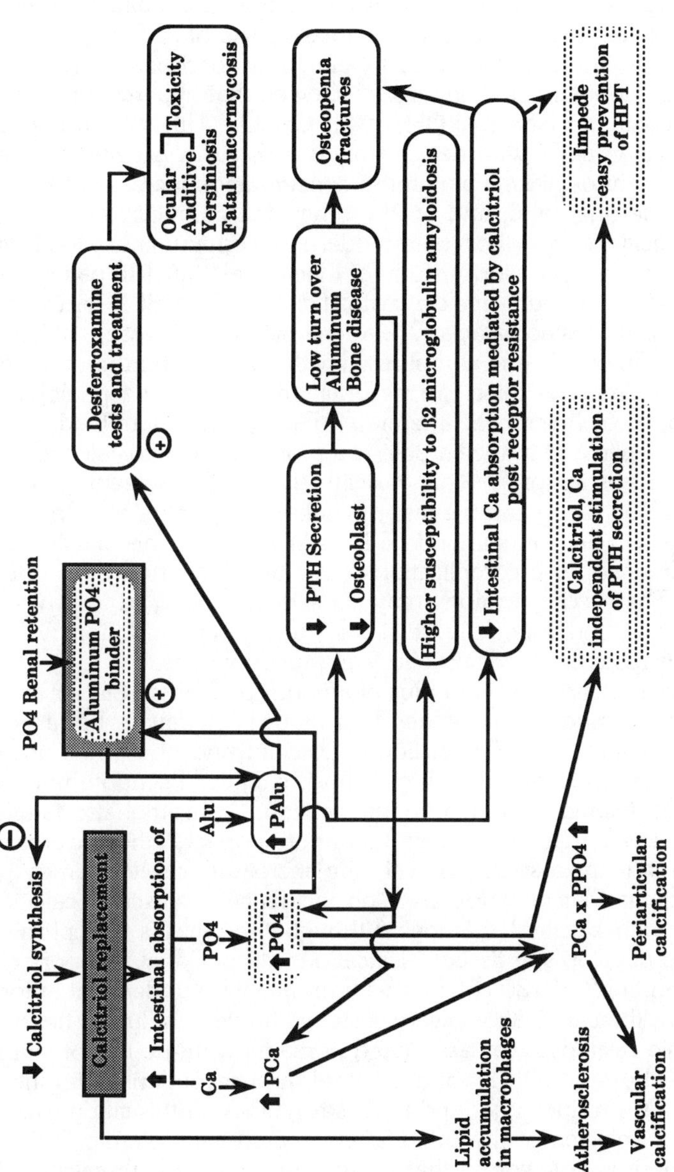

FIG 2.
Association of calcitriol, aluminum phosphate binders, and desferoxamine: the iatrogenic vicious circle.

segment. We brought indirect clinical evidence of this phenomenon, showing that 1α-OH D3 increases plasma aluminum in patients receiving dialysis only when they are absorbing a fixed dose of $Al(OH)_3$.[60, 61]

The aluminum load induced by aluminum phosphate binder is well recognized. Moriniere et al. in 1982[62] showed that hyperaluminemia could be corrected by replacing $Al(OH)_3$ with $CaCO_3$. This was further supported by Sebert et al.,[63] who demonstrated a correlation between bone aluminum content or plasma aluminum concentration increase after deferoxamine on the one hand, and on the other, the cumulative dose of $Al(OH)_3$. The toxicity of this phosphate-binder-induced aluminum load was clearly shown with a bone biopsy study of Llach et al.[57] in 140 patients always dialyzed with aluminum-free dialysate. It disclosed that 30% had aluminic bone disease (23% osteomalacia, 7% adynamic bone disease), which could become symptomatic and complicated with fractures. Furthermore, this aluminum load may be toxic for the brain (myoclonic encephalopathy)[54] and erythropoiesis (microcytic anemia).[56] Finally, aluminum load may favor β2 microglobulin and induce a post-receptor resistance to calcitriol for calcium intestinal absorption.[64] This toxicity justifies the screening of aluminum overload by deferoxamine test (a chelating agent for aluminum and iron) as proposed by Cannata and de Broe.[65] However this practice is not without risk since toxic complications have been reported even after a single test.[56] These complications may be serious: cecity, not always reversible ototoxicity; and especially yersiniosis and fungal infection with rhizopus, which is responsible for usually fatal mucormycosis.

The association calcitriol plus aluminum phosphate binder can also promote soft tissue calcifications. This association favors bone adynamism, which prevents bone deposition of calcium and phosphate and therefore favors hypercalcemia and hyperphosphatemia. Pseudotumoral calcinosis has been related to aluminum intoxication.[66] Calcitriol also favors lipid accumulation in macrophages and therefore possibly atherosclerosis.[67] These phenomena in association with the increased calcium times phosphate product may account for the high incidence of vascular calcification observed with calcitriol therapy. Although the child is less prone than the adult to develop soft tissue calcification, Milliner et al.[68] reported such calcification in 72 of 120 children with uremia who underwent autopsy. In 43 children, the calcifications were systemic (in vessels, lungs, heart, kidneys). Systemic calcinosis was associated primarily with the use of vitamin D, dihydrotachysterol (DHT), and calcitriol, and secondarily with increased Ca times PO_4 product, age, and male sex. Although this study was retrospective and only ten of the 60 children treated with vitamin D had received calcitriol, it is noteworthy that the risk was higher with calcitriol than with native vitamin D. Vitamin D was also associated with more severe calcinosis since eight of the ten children who died before the age of 3 years from lung or heart calcinosis had received vitamin D. This should suggest extreme caution even in children regarding use of the high doses of calcitriol recommended by some authors.[69]

Parathyroid Gland Suppression by Oral Calcium Taken Primarily as Phosphate Binder

Justification of Oral Calcium as Primary Step Therapy

As shown on Figure 1B, oral calcium given with meals to complex dietary phosphate has multiple beneficial effects. It prevents phosphate retention, a mechanism stimulating PTH secretion at all stages of renal insufficiency. In early renal failure, prevention of PO_4 retention by oral calcium allows restoration, to a certain extent of the normal synthesis of calcitriol, as shown by Turner et al.,[26] who with $CaCO_3$ obtained supraphysiologic plasma levels of calcitriol. Normalization of calcitriol synthesis with calcium carbonate involves not only correction of phosphate retention but also of acidosis since acidosis has been proven to decrease 1α-hydroxylase activity.[36] The alkalinizing effect of $CaCO_3$ is more marked in patients not yet receiving dialysis[70] in whom plasma bicarbonate may increase by 6 mmol/L; in patients receiving dialysis, plasma bicarbonate increases only by 1 to 2 mmol/L.[62] Since calcium doses necessary to complex the phosphate are generally above 1.5 g of elemental calcium, they suffice to correct the negative calcium balance of renal insufficiency by promoting passive calcium absorption.

In more severe renal failure, correction of phosphate retention by oral calcium no longer corrects defective calcitriol synthesis[27, 28] but contributes to suppressing PTH secretion by correcting hypocalcemia and hyperphosphatemia, the latter then playing a direct stimulating role on PTH secretion.

Finally, oral calcium prevents osteomalacia, the other major component of renal osteodystrophy.[37, 71, 72] Figure 3 shows its pathophysiology, which is not yet well explained, but uremic osteomalacia appears mainly related to a negative calcium balance and acidosis. However, the most prevalent etiology of osteomalacia in patients with uremia is not uremia per se, but rather vitamin D depletion and intoxication by aluminum from water and/or phosphate binders.[36, 38, 56] When these factors are absent, osteomalacia is unusual even when plasma calcitriol levels are low as in anephric patients receiving dialysis.[73]

Administration Modalities of Oral Calcium

Schiller et al.[74] demonstrated that when the aim of giving calcium is phosphate chelation, oral calcium should be given with the meals rich in phosphate. This modality should always be respected in renal insufficiency even at its early stage because intratubuloepithelial retention of phosphate decreasing calcitriol synthesis may already exist even though plasma phosphate concentrations are still normal or even low. It is only when frank hypophosphatemia occurs because of malnutrition or malabsorption that calcium is primarily given as a calcium supplement either in the fasting state or between meals to increase its absorption.

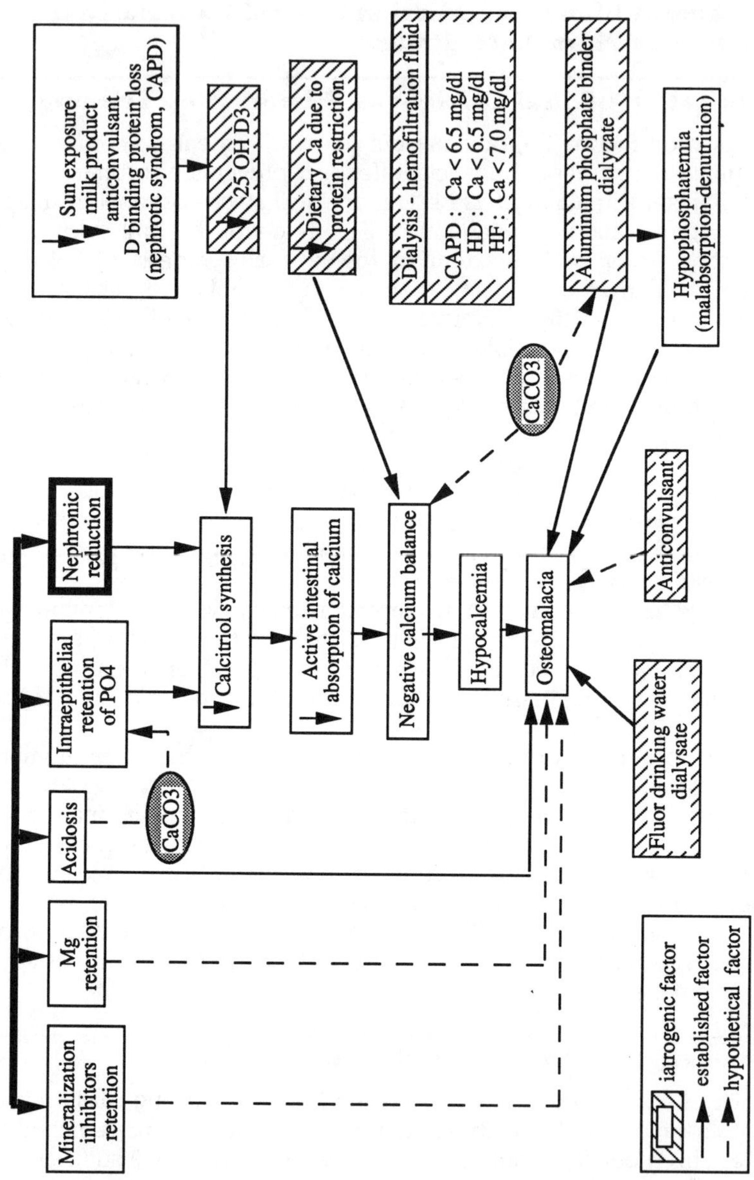

FIG 3.
Pathophysiology of osteomalacia in the uremic patient: effect of $CaCO_3$. It replaces aluminum phosphate binder, corrects the negative Ca balance, partially corrects the acidosis, and promotes calcitriol synthesis by correcting phosphate retention and acidosis.

Which calcium salts should be preferred? Since the initial publication of Moriniere et al.[62] in 1982 showing that oral intake of 9 g of $CaCO_3$ can efficiently control predialytic hyperphosphatemia, most works on the use of oral calcium as phosphate binder have been performed with $CaCO_3$.[51]

Table 1 shows a summary of these studies and that $CaCO_3$ is an effective phosphate binder, failure being observed in 0% to 30% of cases, mainly because of hypercalcemia or hyperphosphatemia related to poor compliance.[61, 76–86] $CaCO_3$ is mainly preferred because it is an alkalinizing salt (Cl_2Ca is contraindicated because it favors acidosis) and has a higher calcium content (40%) than other salts (lactate 12%, gluconate 9%, acetate 23%, alginate 10%, and citrate 21%). Calcium citrate (Citracal) is widely used in the United States but should never be given in association with $Al(OH)_3$, since citrate ion favors aluminum absorption.[85] Regarding the calcic ketoanalogs of Fresenius Laboratory, a Ketosteril tablet contains 50 mg of elemental calcium[86] and a Ketovaline tablet 93 mg[87]; thus the daily dose necessary to control hyperphosphatemia is an unwieldly 12 to 18 tablets. Polystyrene sulfonate of calcium (Calcium Sorbisterit, a resin exchanging calcium for potassium) contains 36 mmol or 1,440 mg of elemental calcium for 20 g of resins.

Thus $CaCO_3$ provides its elemental calcium in smaller volume, and numerous galenic forms have been prepared and are palatable and convenient to take (such as in France, Calcidia [Lefranc Laboratory], Calcium Sandoz Forte, and the orange-flavored suspension of Valpan Laboratory). In our experience, $CaCO_3$ has better gastrointestinal tolerance than calcium acetate, but a double-blind trial is necessary to establish this difference. Based on past experience. $CaCO_3$ would be the form of first choice. However the works of Sheikh et al.[88] in healthy control subjects and Mai et al.[89] in patients receiving dialysis with intestinal lavage have suggested that acetate was a better complexant for phosphate than $CaCO_3$, since for the same dose of 1,000 mg of elemental calcium, more phosphate was complexed. As shown in Table 2, this amount is 174 vs. 112 mg in healthy control subjects and 106 vs. 43 mg in the dialyzed patient receiving dialysis. The reason for this difference would be better solubilization of calcium acetate at the alkaline pH of the intestine. In addition, calcium absorption is slightly lower with acetate so that the amount of complexed phosphate per milligram of absorbed calcium is two to three times that observed with $CaCO_3$.

Since these data suggested that half the dose of elemental calcium given as acetate would complex the same amount of phosphate as $CaCO_3$, we tested whether this dose of calcium acetate would control predialysis plasma phosphate as well as $CaCO_3$. In a cross-over study, eight patients receiving chronic hemodialysis received, for 10 weeks each, acetate, then $CaCO_3$, and finally acetate again. The same control of phosphate (1.7 mmol/L) was obtained with 650 mg of elemental calcium given as acetate as that with 1,300 mg of elemental Ca given as $CaCO_3$ (Table 3).[83, 90–92] Our results agree with those of Schaeffer et al.[91] and of Slatopolsky et al.,[83] who observed the same control of hyperphosphatemia with 1,020

TABLE 1.
Control of Hyperphosphatemia in Adult Hemodialyzed Patients by Moderate-to-High Doses of $CaCO_3$

First Author, yr	References	No. Patients	Duration (mo)	Previous Treatment $CaCO_3$ g/L	Previous Treatment $Al(OH)_3$* g/L	Previous Treatment Vitamin D (No. pts)
Moriniere, 1982	62	16	6	3	4.3 ± 3	—
		7	6	3	5 ± 4	7
Moriniere, 1985	76	15	6	8.5 ± 1	—	—
Addison, 1985	77	38	5 ± 1.5	—	1.42*	16
Monnier, 1986	78	15	36	—	0.5–15	—
Slatopolsky, 1986	79	20	2	—	5.6	—
Hercz, 1987	80	39	3–14	—	6.8 ± 0.6	Yes
Mactier, 1987	81	41	4	—	2.9	—
Sawyer, 1989	82	15	6	—	0.5–1.5*	2
Slatopolsky, 1989	83	21	7	—	5.1	—
Malberti, 1989	84	20	12	2.4	0	17

*Expressed in g/day of elemental aluminum.
†Plasma PTH and alkaline phosphatase increased when the dialysate Ca concentration was lowered from 1.75 to 1.5 mmol.

and 1,400 mg of elemental calcium given as acetate as that with 1,880 and 2,800 mg of elemental calcium given as carbonate, respectively. In the study of Tielemans et al.,[92] the same dose of 1,000 mg of elemental calcium was given as acetate and carbonate and better control of predialysis plasma phosphate was observed with acetate (1.40 mmol/L) than with carbonate (1.56 mmol/L). On the basis of these data, it would seem at first glance logical to recommend the use of acetate rather than carbonate since the amount of absorbed calcium would be expected to be reduced by half, hence less frequent hypercalcemia. However such a lower incidence has not been observed in our experience (nor in those of Schaeffer et al. and Slatopolsky et al., at least when calcitriol was used simultaneously). The reason for this paradox is not clear. If, according to

Treatment Evaluated				
$CaCO_3$ g/d	**Vitamin D (No. pts)**	**Dialysate Calcium mmol/L**	**No. Episodes Ca> 110 mg/L (No. pts)**	**Percent Failures**
9 ± 6	—	1.7 ± 0.05	1–8 (7)	11
14 ± 5		1.7 ± 0.05		
8.7 ± 1	—	1.7 ± 0.05	22 (8)	0
6	15	1.75	2	5
6 (2-12)	Yes	1.75	Not reported	0
8.5 (2.5-17)	—	1.6	7	30
5.8 ± 0.4	—	1.75	34 (14)	30
9.2	—	1.75/105	11	5
6	2	1.75/1.35/1.05	8	0
10.5 ± 7	—	1.25	5	0
2.4	17	1.75/1.5	6.5/6.8 (%)	PTH ↑ †

acute intestinal absorption studies with the lavage technic, it is assumed that the amount of calcium absorbed is half with calcium acetate because the ingested amount is half, it may be suggested that calcium phosphate deposition in the bone and soft tissue would be less with acetate than with $CaCO_3$. Therefore only a long-term study comparing the effect of these two salts on bone mass and soft tissue calcification will show which is preferable in renal insufficiency. However, we will see as follows that results of acute intestinal absorption studies may not be reliable for evaluation of medium-term calcium net absorption, and recent in vitro studies by Gertz (personal communication) have shown that the bioavailablity of calcium to be absorbed was greater after 24 hours of incubation of PO_4 with $CaCO_3$ than with Ca acetate.

TABLE 2.
Effect of the Oral Intake of 1,000 mg of Elemental Calcium as Acetate or Carbonate on the Net Absorption of Ca and on Po_4 Complexation*

	Phosphate (mg)			Calcium (mg)		
Chelators	**Placebo**	**Acetate Ca**	**$CaCO_3$**	**Placebo**	**Acetate Ca**	**$CaCO_3$**
Absorption (mg)						
Healthy controls†	263	89	151	42	190	251
Uremic‡	181	75	138	−28	314	355
	Complexation of PO_4§ (mg)			Complexation of PO_4/mg of absorbed Ca¶		
Healthy controls†		174	112		1.1	0.53
Uremic‡		106	43		0.3	0.11

*After a meal containing 395 mg PO_4 and 214 mg Ca, using intestinal lavage technique.
†From Sheikh: *JCI* 1989; 83:67–73.(n = 10).
‡From Mai: *Kidney Int* 1989; 36:690–695. (n = 6).
§Complexation power: net absorption with Ca − net absorption with placebo.
¶Amount of absorbed calcium coming from the Ca salt: net absorption with the Ca salt − net absorption with placebo.

Side Effects of Oral Calcium and Their Prevention

Besides gastrointestinal intolerance (more often diarrhea than constipation and long-term distaste, which may be prevented by changing the preparation) the major problem is hypercalcemia. It does not seem to be related only to the dose ingested but rather to bone turnover as shown by the recent study of Meric et al.[93] In 39 patients receiving dialysis who developed hypercalcemia when $CaCO_3$ had completely replaced $Al(OH)_3$, plasma calcium was already higher than in those who remained eucalcemic and the biochemical markers of bone turnover (PTH, osteocalcin, and alkaline phosphatases) were lower, whereas $CaCO_3$ dose and dietary calcium were similar, as were age, sex, duration of dialysis, physical activity, and aluminum overload (deferoxamine test). Since aluminum overload may be a factor favoring adynamic bone disease,[8] it should be sought when hypercalcemia occurs. In the absence of aluminum overload, hypercalcemia may suggest idiopathic adynamic bone disease on the basis of low plasma values for alkaline phosphatase, osteocalcin, and 1-84 PTH. It is then logical to decrease dialysate calcium concentration while monitoring these parameters. When these etiologies are excluded, $CaCO_3$ doses can be incriminated. In patients receiving dialysis, two therapeutic approachs are possible: maintain the oral $CaCO_3$ dose and decrease dialysate calcium concentration or decrease $CaCO_3$ and add a moderate dose of magnesium derivatives while decreasing dialysate magnesium concentration in order to prevent the risk of hypermagnesemia. Both approaches are obviously excluded in patients not yet on dialysis.

When 1α-OH vitamin D metabolites are considered not absolutely necessary, magnesium hydroxide or carbonate associated with oral calcium appears up to now forces the best approach. Relatively high doses of $CaCO_3$ can then be used in association with relatively low doses of magnesium derivatives so that the dialysate concentration of magnesium is only mildly decreased from 0.7 to 0.37 mmol/L[94, 95] and not to zero as proposed by O'Donnovan et al.,[96] who used high doses of magnesium carbonate (2.5 to 7.5 g/day) as sole phosphate binder without inducing hypermagnesemia or hyperkalemia. With this latter approach, there is risk of magnesium depletion with its own hazards (cramps, cardiac arrythmia) in case of poor patient compliance for magnesium derivatives. We confirmed that with 0.37 mmol/L magnesium in the dialysate, slight hypermagnesemia (1.5 ± 0.2 mmol/L) was induced with a mean dose of 2 ± 0.5 g of $Mg(OH)_2$. Its only side effect was the need to increase potassium chelators. Calcium polystyrene sulfonate (Calcium Sorbisterit) was then used as chelator rather than sodium polystyrene sulfonate (Kayexalate) to prevent sodium load and alkalosis (due to binding of magnesium on the resin in sodium exchange and liberation of hydroxide ions).[97] This side effect may, on the contrary, lead to use of Kayexalate in case of severe acidosis. Mild hypermagnesemia has no long-term deleterious effect on bone: after 18 months of treatment, no mineralization defect was observed.[97] It is probably preferable to prevent mild hypermagnesemia, however, by fur-

TABLE 3.
Medium-Term Comparative Studies of Ca Acetate and Ca Carbonate as Phosphate Binder (mean ± SD)

	Acetate						
First Author (reference)	No. Patients	Duration (wk)	Ca dose (mg/d)	Other Binder	Plasma Ca (mmol/L)	Plasma PO_4 (mmol/L)	No. Patients with HCa* (episodes)
Morinière (90)	8	10	650	0	2.55 ± 0.14	1.75 ± 0.38	6
Schaeffer (91)	12	7	1,020	0	2.53 ± 0.39	1.51 ± .39	0
Tielemans (92)	12	6	1,000	$Al(OH)_3$: 37 ± 5 mEq	2.5 ± .02	1.4 ± .06†	4 pt (5)‡
Slatopolsky (83)	20	4	1,400	—	2.5	1.7†	3 pt (7)§

*HCA-hypercalcemia.
†Significantly lower or higher than with $CaCO_3$.
‡Patients also had a fixed dose of 1α-OH vitamin D3.
§Eight patients were receiving a fixed dose of IV calcitriol.

ther decreasing the dialysate magnesium concentration to 0.2 mmol/L.

When 1α-OH vitamin D derivatives are considered necessary and when a dialysate calcium concentration below 1.62 mmol/L (or 65 mg/L) is preferred in order to prevent negative intradialytic calcium balance, $CaCO_2$ cannot be given because of the high incidence of hypercalcemia, and $Mg(OH)_2$ as sole phosphate binder with a dialysate magnesium of 0.2 mmol/L has been considered by us as an alternative possibility. We thus compared intravenous 1α-OH vitamin D3, in association with Mg $(OH)_2$ as sole phosphate binder, to $CaCO_3$ associated or not with Mg $(OH)_2$ but not with vitamin D. This approach proved feasible but unsatisfactory since the doses of Mg $(OH)_2$ (>6g per day) needed to control 1α-OH vitamin D3-induced hyperphosphatemia were poorly tolerated (diarrhea and hyperkalemia), so that these doses had to be decreased as well as those of 1α-OH vitamin D3, which resulted in control of hyperparathyroidism not better than that given by the simple association of oral $CaCO_3$ and Mg $(OH)_2$ at lower doses. Therefore we now advise keeping $CaCO_3$ as sole phosphate binder and if necessary decreasing dialysate calcium concentration to 60 to 50 and even 40 mg/L (1.5, 1.25, or 1 mmol/L) as proposed by Mactier et al.,[81] Sawyer et al.,[82] and Slatopolsky et al.[98]

We do not advise, however, to routinely decrease dialysate calcium below 65 mg/L (1.62 mmol/L), which for Malberti et al.[84] is the concentration at which intradialytic calcium balance is null with a body weight loss about 3 kg. In fact, this weight loss causes a loss of about 180 mg ultrafiltrable calcium, which is why the bath calcium concentration should be

			Carbonate			
No. Patients	**Duration (wk)**	**Ca Dose (mg/d)**	**Other Binder**	**Plasma Ca (mmol/L)**	**Plasma PO_4 (mmol/L)**	**No. Patients With HCa* (episodes)**
8	10	1,310	0	2.56 ± 0.13	1.74 ± 0.32	4
12	7	1,880	0	2.53 ± .19	1.34 ± 0.40	0
12	6	1,000	$Al(OH)_3$: 40 ± 5 mEq	2.5 ± .02	1.56 ± .06	4 pt (4)‡
20	4	2,800	—	2.5	1.57	7 pt(8)§

above 6.0 mg/dL (normal concentration of ultrafiltrable calcium) to prevent negative intradialytic calcium balance. Since the intestinal calcium balance of the patient with uremia is spontaneously negative (about -80 mg/day[70]), it is evident that with a dose of $CaCO_3$ below 3 g day (minimal intake to prevent negative intestinal calcium balance), long-term overall calcium balance will be negative if a DCa below 6.5 mg/dL is used. Stimulation of hyperparathyroidism will ensue, reflected only by increased plasma concentration of PTH and alkaline phosphatases, the plasma calcium decrease being inconstant. This sequence occurred in the patients of Malberti et al.,[84] who took only 3 g of $CaCO_3$ in spite of concomitant calcitriol 0.2 μg/day (see Table 1). When the mean daily dose of CaCO3 is 9 to 12 g, dialysate calcium (DCa) can be decreased to 5.0 mg/dL; Slatopolsky et al. verified that in this case plasma PTH concentrations remained stable after 6 months without vitamin D therapy.[98]

In patients receiving continuous ambulatory peritoneal dialysis (CAPD) Hutchinson and Gokal[99] also reported stable control of hyperparathyroidism by 10 ± 5 g $CaCO_3$ without vitamin D, whereas DCa was reduced to 5.0 mg/dL. In hemofiltration, the Ca balance per session with 30 L of exchange and 3 kg of weight loss is: ultrafiltrable calcium × 30 liters = substitution fluid calcium × [30 L −(3 kg body weight loss + 1 L for priming the circuit)]. Thus, for null intrasession calcium balance, calcium concentration in the substitution fluid is about 7.0 mg/dL. This concentration can be further decreased when the amount of $CaCO_3$ taken by the patient is greater than 6 g/day. Kaye et al.[100] propose using zero calcium dialysate when hypercalcemia occurs with $CaCO_3$ and reinfusing less calcium than usually necessary to maintain null calcium balance (about 41 ± 1 mmol per session). Reinfusing only 7 or 20 mmol per dialysis prevented recurrence of hypercalcemia in two patients receiving $CaCO_3$ by inducing a negative intradialytic calcium balance of 30 and 23 mmol while plasma-intact PTH levels remained between one and two times the upper limit of normal for 4 to 12 months.[101] This technique has the further advantage of allowing bicarbonate dialysis with the common dialysis machine with a single dialysate concentrate containing bicarbonate and no calcium. The amount of calcium reinfused is critically dependent on dialyser area and weight loss. When these factors are overlooked, severe postdialytic hypocalcemia may ensue. In our experience, it is necessary to infuse 22 to 30 mL/hour of 10% Cl_2Ca (i.e., about 10 to 13 mmol/hour) when weight loss is 2 to 3 kg, the duration of dialysis 4 hours, dialyser area 1 m^2, blood flow 300 mL/min, and dialysate flow 500 mL/min.

Long-Term Efficacy of Oral Calcium Alone in Control of Hyperparathyroidism: Comparison With 1αOH Vitamin D Derivatives

No long-term study (≥ 6 months) has yet been published on the effect of calcium acetate on plasma PTH levels. However, many studies show that $CaCO_3$ alone without 1α-OH vitamin D derivatives prevents worsening or even improves moderate hyperparathyroidism (without subperiosteal resorption).

In the Patient Receiving Maintenance Dialysis

Moriniere et al.[61] first showed in seven patients that substitution of $Al(OH)_3$ and 1α-OH vitamin D3 by high doses of $CaCO_3$ (14 g/day) maintained plasma concentrations of Ca, PO_4, cPTH, and alkaline phosphatases for 6 months whereas plasma aluminum concentrations decreased. Since it is well proven that aluminum overload suppresses PTH secretion,[102] the stability of PTH levels demonstrates the greater suppressive effect of $CaCO_3$ on PTH secretion. To better compare the suppressive effect of $CaCO_3$ and that of 1α-OH vitamin D3 associated with $Al(OH)_3$, we performed a controlled trial[76] for 6 months in 15 and 12 dialysis patients previously receiving only 9 g of $CaCO_3$. In the control group, treatment was unchanged. In the experimental group, 1α-OH vitamin D3 and $Al(OH)_3$ were introduced after reduction of $CaCO_3$ from 9 to 3 g. Doses of 1α-OH vitamin D3 had to be gradually decreased from 1 to 0.25 μg/day and those of $Al(OH)_3$ increased from 2 to 6 g/day to prevent hyperphosphatemia. Both groups kept constant plasma concentrations of calcium and phosphate, whereas plasma aluminum concentrations decreased in the $CaCO_3$ group from 2 to 0.8 μmol/L and remained stable in the 1α group. Despite decreased plasma aluminum in the $CaCO_3$ group, plasma concentrations of C terminal and midregion PTH remained stable at levels eight and five times the upper limit of normal. Mean plasma alkaline phosphatases remained normal in both groups, but a patient in the $CaCO_3$ group developed vitamin D-deficient osteomalacia (plasma 25-OH vitamin D = 3 ng/mL) with increased alkaline phosphatases, which remitted with 25-OH vitamin D3 at 70 μg/week.

In the third study, we compared $CaCO_3$ with intravenous 1α-OH vitamin D3.[103] Forty-seven patients receiving dialysis with no radiologic subperiosteal resorption while treated with $CaCO_3$ alone and a dialysate concentration of Ca of 1.62 mmol/L and of Mg of 0.2 mmol/L were selected and randomized into a control group maintaining the same treatment, and an experimental group receiving intravenous 1α (at increasing doses of 1 to 4 μg after each of three weekly dialyses during the first 4 weeks) in association with Mg $(OH)_2$ as sole phosphate binder. Since we had previously shown that histologically frank osteitis fibrosa (increased bone formation rate and increased osteoclastic resorption) is present only when plasma concentration of intact PTH is above twice the upper limit of normal, we analyzed the results in relation to initial levels of intact PTH. In 60% of our patients no frank osteitis fibrosa was noted and intact PTH plasma levels remained under twice the upper limit of normal in both the control and 1α groups, with the exception of two patients in each group. For patients with initial frank hyperparathyroidism, plasma levels of intact PTH remained stable in the $CaCO_3$ group but decreased significantly during the first 2 months in the 1α group, thereafter returning to initial value. This escape phenomenon was due to the decrease in 1α-OH vitamin D3 doses to 0.6 μg/dialysis at the sixth month because of increased plasma calcium (2.6 mmol/L) and especially increased plasma phosphate, at 2.3 mmol/L at the second month despite the increase in Mg $(OH)_2$ to 6 g/day; i.e., the maximal tolerable dose not inducing diarrhea or hyperkalemia. It thus appears that long-term intravenous 1α with Mg(OH)2 as sole phosphate binder does not control frank hyperparathyroidism better than $CaCO_3$.

Prevention of frank hyperparathyroidism (high plasma alkaline phoshatases) by $CaCO_3$ associated or not with $Mg(OH)_2$ was further evaluated in our dialysis center by the number of patients in whom it was necessary to add 1α-OH vitamin D3 to stop the increase in alkaline phosphatases or to perform parathyroidectomy. This study was performed in 1988[94] on 57 patients treated for 1 to 5 years with $CaCO_3$, associated for 26 of them with $Mg(OH)_2$, and having plasma aluminum of 0.8 μmol/L. Low doses of oral 1α-OH vitamin D3 had to be added in 9 and parathyroidectomy had had to be performed in the 5 previous years in 7: 1 case of neglected primary hyperparathyroidism; 2 of poor compliance to preventive treatment; 2 of severe hyperparathyroidism at the beginning of treatment with $CaCO_3$; thus, preventive treatment actually failed in only 2 cases, a 56-year-old woman receiving dialysis for 12 years and a 42-year-old man receiving dialysis for 9 years but chronically underdialyzed because of difficult vascular access.

We also compared our present preventive treatment of $CaCO_3 \pm Mg(OH)_2$ without 1α-OH vitamin D3 with our classical treatment given 10 years ago, using only 3 g $CACO_3$, moderate doses of $Al(OH)_3$, and if necessary oral 1α-OH vitamin D3.[95, 104] The two patient groups were matched for age, sex, duration on dialysis, and dialysate calcium. After 2 to 4 years of follow-up, prevention of hyperparathyroidism was confirmed by stable plasma alkaline phosphatases in the normal range. Bone biopsy specimens after 24 months in 13 patients of the Ca ± Mg group and 19 of the aluminum ± 1α group showed similar prevalence and severity of histologic osteitis fibrosa, with aluminic bone disease present in four of the aluminum ± 1α group but absent in the Ca ± Mg group. In the Ca ± Mg group, there were four cases of idiopathic adynamic bone disease associated with relative hypoparathyroidism with only slightly elevated plasma C terminal PTH and normal plasma intact PTH levels.[34]

It should be pointed out that 18 of the 47 patients in our recent study with intravenous 1α had normal plasma levels of intact PTH; according to Cohen Solal's study,[10] half of them should have histologically adynamic bone despite the absence of aluminum overload. These observations demonstrate the efficacy of hyperparathyroidism control with $CaCO_3$ alone or associated with $Mg(OH)_2$. In the absence of 1α-OH vitamin D3, this treatment has even exceeded its target in 9 patients, i.e., in 1/5 cases.

In the Patient With Uremia Not Yet on Dialysis

We studied $CaCO_3$ (3 g/day) associated with non-hypercalcemic doses of 25-OH vitamin D3 (10 to 25 μg/day) to treat hyperparathyroidism in not yet dialyzed adult patients with uremia (Table 4).[52, 71] In 21 patients with initial creatinine clearance of 15 to 29 mL/min, plasma alkaline phosphatases decreased from 148 to 110 and 112 IU (normal <170 IU) after 1 and 2 years of treatment; plasma cPTH concentration remained stable despite plasma creatinine increased from 370 to 440 μmol/L, which should have induced increased plasma levels of cPTH due to decreased catabolism of the C terminal fragments secondary to decreased GFR. Two subsequent bone biopsies performed at 15-month intervals in 12 of these patients showed a significant decrease in osteoid volume and osteoblastic surface and a nonsignificant decrease in osteoclastic hyperresorption. More recently we found that two of 16 patients similarly treated developed a histologic pattern of adynamic bone disease with relative hypoparathyroidism compared to the degree of renal insufficiency. These patients had similar C terminal PTH plasma levels but higher plasma creatinine than those with normal histologic bone. The reason for this hypoparathyroidism was abnormal elevation of plasma levels of calcitriol, explained in one case by a very high level of 25-OH vitamin D probably due to inadvertent 25-OH vitamin D3 overdose.[10]

The efficacy of $CaCO_3$ in the treatment of renal rickets in children was shown by Curtis et al.[105] without vitamin D but with a phosphate supplement for paradoxical hypophosphatemia. As discussed as follows, treatment of renal rickets, however, usually necessitates both $CaCO_3$ and 1α-OH vitamin D3 derivatives.

TABLE 4.
Use of 1α-OH Vitamin D3 Derivatives in Predialytic Renal Insufficiency in Comparison With $CaCO_3$ ± 25-OH D3

	Massry 1985	Coen 1986	Nordal 1988	Baker 1989	Fournier 1988
Experimental conditions					
Creatinine clearance, mL/min (initial range/final mean)	15–55/35	10–30/13	10–40/20	20–59/31	29–15/19
Slope 1/plasma creatinine (dL/mg/mo)	Stable	Smaller	Stable	Stable	Smaller
Vitamin D (μg/day)	1.25:1–0.5	1.25:0.25	1.25:0.25	1.25:0.25	25-OH vitamin D:10–25
Ca intake (mg/day)	?	500	?	800	1,200
Protein intake (g/kg)	?	0.8	?	?	0.8
PO_4 intake (mg/kg)	?	12	?	15	13
Experimental group (*n*)	17	15	14	8	21
Control group (*n*)	16	23	14	8	—
Duration (mo)	12	12	8	12	12–24
Results					
Urinary calcium mg/24 hr (before/after)			36/80	60/100	40/80
Plasma calcium, mg/L (before/after)	↑	91/94*	92/100	98/102	94/94
Reversible hypercalcemia (episodes)	11	0	8	4	0
Plasma PO_4, mg/L (before/after)†	↔	40/46*	58/58	42/41	35/44
Alkaline phosphatase	↓	207/126*	201/155*	74/56*	148/110*
PTH	↓	2/1.9	1.4/1.0	0.87/0.63	138/132
Osteoid volume	?	↔	↓	↓	↓ ↓
Osteoblast	?	↓		↓	↓
Osteoclast	↓	↓	↓	↓	↔

*Significant variation at $P < .05$.
†$Al(OH)_3$ administration was excluded except in the study of Nordal.

Long-Term Use of $CaCO_3$ and the Risk of Soft Tissue Calcifications

Soft tissue calcifications are common in patients with uremia, especially those receiving long-term dialysis. Coburn and Slatopolsky[36] distinguish them into three types with different pathogenesis: (1) conjunctival and periarticular calcification related to the increased Ca × PO_4 product and to PTH hypersecretion because they improve with control of hyperphosphatemia and/or parathyroidectomy; (2) vascular calcification of the media and intima in which hyperphosphatemia and hypomagnesemia are incriminated while the role of hyperparathyroidism is less certain because parathyroidectomy does not consistently lead to improvement; (3) visceral calcification of the lungs, heart, and kidneys for which they propose no pathogenesis or treatment.

Recently Zins et al.[66] stressed that pseudo-tumoral periarticular calcifications could be related to aluminum intoxication, which induces adynamic bone disease preventing Ca and PO_4 deposition in bone and thus increased plasma concentration of calcium and phosphate. A recent work by Milliner et al.[68] on 120 autopsies from children with uremia showed that the main risk factor of systemic calcifications was the use of vitamin D, DHT, and calcitriol.

Does $CaCO_3$ as phosphate binder also favor soft tissue calcification? In theory, certainly. If the data of Mai et al.[89] obtained after a single meal including 1,000 mg of elemental calcium given as $CaCO_3$ (which induces a net absorption of 355 mg calcium) are extrapolated to the day, daily calcium balance is 710 or 1,420 mg when 2 or 4,000 mg of elemental calcium are given as 5 or 10 g $CaCO_3$ (the usual doses). Urinary calcium loss being negligible in patients receiving dialysis, all absorbed calcium should be deposited in the organism unless eliminated later through the feces. This latter possibility is highly probable because of the discrepancy between the net absorption of calcium extrapolated from Mai's data and that obtained by the balance technique over 3 weeks by Clarkson et al.[70] In this princeps study, 20 g $CaCO_3$ was given per day to patients with uremia not yet receiving dialysis; net intestinal absorption was 660 mg and not 2,840 mg/24 hr as expected from the data of Mai. However if Clarkson's data are extrapolated to the long term with a daily dose of 10 g $CaCO_3$, an annual positive calcium balance of 0.330 × 365 days = 120 g can be estimated. Since on the other hand, Clarkson et al. showed that despite increased fecal phosphate, phosphate balance became positive (up to +62 mg/day, because of the greater decrement of phosphaturia), it is wise to consider possible induction of soft tissue calcifications with $CaCO_3$ therapy, since all the retained calcium phosphate may not necessarily go into bone. Therefore before deciding to use exclusively high doses of $CaCO_3$ as phosphate binder in 1980, we reviewed the literature.

We were relatively sure that the retained calcium phosphate was going primarily into bone on the basis of the data of Curtis et al.,[105] who reported cure of renal rickets without soft tissue calcifications and those of Meyrier et al.[108] who observed fewer metastatic calcifications and higher bone remineralization in patients receiving dialysis and $CaCO_3$ (5 to 20 g/day) and $Al(OH)_3$ than in those without oral treatment. We then undertook with Renaud et al.[109] a study of the risk factors for vascular calcifications in patients receiving dialysis and both $Al(OH)_3$ and $CaCO_3$ (3 to 6 g/day). The annual extension of radiologically visible calcifications was not related to the $CaCO_3$ dose but to, in decreasing order, age, male sex, diastolic blood pressure, blood triglycerides, blood glucose, and lastly plasma concentrations of Ca and PO_4. Thus the hypothesis that $CaCO_3$ per se could favor vascular calcifications was unlikely since the two parameters were not correlated. The correlation between vascular calcification and the $Ca \times PO_4$ product in this and Nichols' study[110] suggests that to prevent soft tissue calcifications, the main measure is to prevent hypercalcemia and hyperphosphatemia.

There are few data on the long-term evolution of soft tissue calcifications in treatments with $CaCO_3$ or calcitriol associated with $Al(OH)_3$. For $CaCO_3$, Moriniere et al.[62] noted, in a first study, two cases of occurrence or worsening of vascular calcifications after 6 months of treatment in 23 patients and, in a second study,[76] 3 cases within 6 months in each of the two groups (one treated by $CaCo_3$ alone and the other by 1α-OH vitamin D3 and $Al[OH]_3$). The interest of the study by Monnier et al.[78] should be stressed since they report on $CaCO_3$ treatment over 36 months, with no calcification in 7 patients who were intially without calcification, and worsening in 4 of 8 who already had vascular calcifications, only during the first 12 months of treatment.

To compare $CaCO_3$ to $Al(OH)_3$ associated with 1α-OH vitamin D3 derivatives in preventing hyperparathyroidism and soft tissue calcifications, we evaluated 32 patients treated for over 24 months with $CaCO_3$ (mean daily dose, 8 g) associated with $Mg(OH)_2$ (2.6 g/day) in half of the cases, and 30 patients treated 10 years earlier with low dose $CaCO_3$ (3 g/day), $Al(OH)_3$, and if necessary, 1α-OH vitamin D3.[95] Patients were matched for age, sex, and duration of dialysis. Dialysate calcium was similar (6.5 to 7.0 mg/dL), but dialysate magnesium was lower (0.8 mg/dL vs. 1.7 mg/dL) in the $CaCO_3 \pm Mg$ than in the aluminum $\pm$ 1α group to prevent hypermagnesemia. Plasma concentrations of Ca, PO_4, triglycerides, cholesterol, uric acid, and blood pressure were not significantly different, suggesting that other risk factors of calcification were comparable. The initial extent and subsequent increase in vascular and periarticular calcifications were similar in the two groups after 2 to 4 years (Table 5). Although historical and not parallel, this controlled comparison suggests that moderate doses of $CaCO_3 \pm Mg(OH)_2$ do not expose to a greater risk of vascular calcification than low doses of $CaCO_3 + Al(OH)_3 \pm$ 1α-OH vitamin D3. Although moderate, extension of vascular calcification occurs. This stresses the necessity of caution in monitoring these patients and of initiating further long-term studies to compare $CaCO_3$ with Ca acetate for this risk.

TABLE 5.
Changes of the Vascular and Periarticular Calcifications in Patients Treated With $Al(OH)_3$ ± 1α Vitamin D3 in Comparison With Those Treated With Moderate Doses of $CaCO_3$ ± $Mg(OH)_2$*

	Ca ± Mg				Al ± 1 α			
Time (mo)	**0**	**24**	**36**	**48**	**0**	**24**	**36**	**48**
No. of Patients	**32**	**32**	**17**	**9**	**30**	**30**	**15**	**8**
Mean length of vascular calcifications (cm ± SD)	14 ± 21	21 ± 28§	35 ± 34§	30 ± 26‡	19 ± 12	27 ± 18§	37 ± 27§	35 ± 33‡
Periarticular calcifications†								
Severity + (No. patients)	4	7	4	1	5	6	2	0
Severity + + (No. patients)	1	3	2	2	0	4	2	1
Severity + + + (No. patients)	0	0	0	0	1	1	1	0

*Significance of the difference vs. T0 in the same group: ‡ = P <.05; § = P < .01. At no time was the difference between the two therapeutic groups significantly different.

†Severity + :1 small calcification of less than 5 mm of diameter; severity + + :2 small calcifications or 1 with a diameter >5 mm; severity + + + : 3 small calcifications or 1 with a diameter > 10 mm.

Use of Vitamin D and its Derivatives in Treatment of Hyperparathyroidism Secondary to Renal Insufficiency

Use of Native Vitamin D, Dihydrotachysterol, and 25-OH Vitamin D3

Native vitamin D2 and D3 have long been used in the treatment of renal osteodystrophy, mainly at pharmacological doses (0.5 to 12 mg/day) to force the vitamin D resistance state induced by uremia and explained by deficient calcitriol synthesis. This state explains why physiologic doses (800 IU or 20 μg/day) are ineffective in increasing plasma calcium in uremia patients.[37]

Dihydrotachysterol or AT[10] is a synthetic product that does not necessitate hydroxylation in position 1 because of the one stereochimic place taken by its hydroxyl in position 3 due to the double-link 5-6, which determines a transposition of ring A. This explains why hypercalcemic doses of DHT are less than those of native vitamin D2 or D3 (250 to 370 μg/day).[37]

25-OH vitamin D3 has a hypercalcemic effect in uremic patients when given only at a daily dose equal to or above 50 μg. At such doses, it has the same effect on hyperparathyroidism as 1α- OH vitamin D3 given at 1-2 μg/day. It also normalizes the decreased mineralization front for a lower elevation of the Ca × PO_4 product than does 1α-OH vitamin[111] D3.

The availability of 1α-OH vitamin D3 derivatives with a more rapid hypercalcemic effect (1 to 2 weeks vs. 4 to 8 for 25-OH vitamin D3) and of shorter duration when the drug is discontinued (1 vs. 4 weeks)[111] led to abandoning these older forms of vitamin D. However, they remain useful in treatment of vitamin D depletion, which is not rare in patients with renal insufficiency; plasma concentration of 25-OH vitamin D is decreased despite normal hepatic 25-hydroxylase activity in about one third of patients receiving dialysis in Northern Europe, where sun is scarce. This is seldom observed in the United States, where food is industrially fortified. Even in sunny Arab countries, vitamin D depletion may often occur because of social habits, the infants being kept inside the home, the women protected by tchador and the bread made with a phytate rich flour (chuppaty), which binds not only calcium but also vitamin D metabolites in the gut, disrupting the hepatoenteric vitamin D cycle. Racial pigmentation enhances the risk of vitamin D depletion because the melanine pigment competes with 7-dihydrocholesterol for ultraviolet photons. The depressive effect of uremia on skin synthesis of vitamin D3 is observed in Florida in blacks but not in whites.[112] Furthermore, plasma concentrations of 25-OH vitamin D can be diminished in the patient with uremia because of loss of urinary vitamin D binding protein in nephrotic syndrome[113] or through the peritoneal fluid of patients receiving CAPD[114–116] or because of increased hepatic catabolism of 25-OH vitamin D induced by anticonvulsant agents.[117]

This decrease in 25-OH vitamin D plasma concentration may lead to decreased plasma concentration not only of 24,25-$(OH)_2$ vitamin D3 but also of 1,25-$(OH)_2$ vitamin D3; contrary to those in healthy individuals, in uremia, plasma calcitriol levels are correlated to those of plasma 25-OH vitamin D. This explains why native vitamin D-sensitive osteomalacia is not rare in patients with uremia in France and England and why vitamin D depletion may favor osteitis fibrosa, as we suggested on finding lower plasma 25-OH vitamin D concentration in patients receiving dialysis who developed subperiosteal resorption than in those who did not. For us, these findings justify routine supplementation with native vitamin D2 or D3 or 25-OH vitamin D3 in patients with uremia to bring 25-OH vitamin D plasma concentration to the upper limit of normal (30 ng/mL). The doses required vary from 70 to 140 μg/week in patients receiving hemodialysis to 350 to 700 μg/week in patients receiving CAPD.[114]

Use of 1α-OH Vitamin D3 Derivatives in Patients With Uremia

The first part of this review discussed the rationale for the use of 1α-OH vitamin D3 derivatives and the second stressed the risk of its association with aluminum phosphate binder. The third showed that oral calcium taken with meals could replace this dangerous aluminum phosphate binder. Since 1α-OH vitamin D3 derivatives increase fractional absorption of calcium, their use is compromised by frequent hypercalcemia if oral calcium is taken as phosphate binder. Thus, the use of 1α-OH vitamin D3 derivatives is relatively uncomplicated in only two situations: (1) in early renal failure (GFR >20 mL/min) when hyperphosphatemia is not yet present; and (2) in patients receiving dialysis because, to prevent hypercalcemia, it is possible to decrease either the dialysate concentration of calcium when oral calcium is used as phosphate binder or of magnesium concentration when $Mg(OH)_2$ or Mg carbonate is used.

Use of 1α-OH Vitamin D3 Derivatives in Adult Patients With Uremia Not Yet on Dialysis

In the adult, these derivatives were first used in advanced renal failure (GFR <20 mL/min) in association with $Al(OH)_3$. Results on bone parameters were disappointing while degradation of renal function accelerated because of the increased Ca × PO_4 product.[118] Later, these derivatives were used without phosphate binder ($Al(OH)_2$ or calcium) in moderate or mild renal insufficiency (see Table 5). Although, compared to lower doses, the close of 0.5 to 1 μg/day used by Massry et al.[119] was more effective on hyperparathyroidism, it also induced frequent hypercalcemia. We recommend therefore the 0.25 μg/day used by Coen et al.,[119a] Baker et al.,[120] and Nordal et al.,[121] which much less frequently induced hypercalcemia or hyperphosphatemia (without associated $Al(OH)_3$ except in the study of Nordal). The improved biochemical and histologic parameters of hyperparathyroidism in these studies was similar to those we obtained with 3 g $CaCO_3$ and nonhypercalcemic doses of 25-OH vitamin D3 (10 to 25 μg/day).

It is interesting that in these studies, renal failure decelerated rather than accelerated. However, plasma creatinine concentration and creatinine clearance are not good parameters of vitamin D nephrotoxicity. Bertoli et al.[122] showed that 0.5 μg/day calcitriol for 4 months induced a significant increase in plasma creatinine (from 494 to 602 μmol/L), which disappeared 2 months after discontinuation of the drug. In parallel, creatinine clearance decreased from 22 to 19 mL/min, whereas urinary creatinine increased from 8.4 to 9.3 mmol/24 hour. Blood urea did not increase and inulin clearance remained stable (13 and 12 mL/min). The explanation for the increase in creatinuria would be a greater muscular creatinine production due to improvement in uremic myopathy by calcitriol. The comparatively greater increase of plasma creatinine would be explained by a decrease of creatinine secretion induced by calcitriol.

In summary, in the adult with moderate renal insufficiency (defined as GFR between 15 and 60 mL/min), small doses of calcitriol alone are as effective and safe as 3 g $CaCO_3$ associated with 10 to 25 μg/day 25-OH vitamin D3 in preventing hyperparathyroidism. No data exist regarding the use of these drugs before this degree of renal insufficiency. According to Reichel et al.,[123] such prevention would not yet be justified because plasma concentrations of intact PTH increase over 1.5 of the upper limit of normal only when GFR decreases below 60 mL/min. However earlier prevention may be useful in patients at higher risk of hyperparathyroidism before dialysis because of more severe acidosis and longer duration of uremia, namely in interstitial nephritis and polycystic kidney disease and in patients who receive furosemide, which increases calciuria and plasma PTH.[123]

The preferential choice between $CaCO_3$ associated with 25-OH vitamin D3 and low dose calcitriol will be possible only after a long-term study with comparable dietary intake of protein, phosphate, and calcium and with therapy-induced increases in calciuria in the same range (100 to 120 mg/24 hours since above this range hypercalcemia may occur[120]). $CaCO_3$ and 25-OH vitamin D3 treatment theoretically has the advantage of not favoring PO_4 absorption and therefore being homeostatically more logical,[18] as well as of being easily continued until the patient is receiving dialysis; below a GFR of 15 mL/min the use of 1α hydroxylated vitamin D3 derivatives is hazardous because it worsens hyperphosphatemia and therefore accelerates renal function deterioration.[118] We thus presently recommend in the adult: (1) begin with associating $CaCO_3$ (3 g/day) and 25-OH vitamin D3 (10 to 20 μg/day); (2) monitor urinary and plasma calcium and phosphate, plasma 25-OH vitamin D, and plasma intact PTH levels; and (3) add 1α-OH vitamin D derivatives only if plasma-intact PTH levels increase above twice the upper limit of normal, provided urinary calcium does not exceed 120 mg/24 hour, plasma calcium 10.7 mg/dL, plasma PO_4 4.5 mg/dL, and plasma 25-OH vitamin D concentration 30 ng/mL.

Use of 1α-OH Vitamin D Derivatives in the Patient Receiving Dialysis

The problem varies according to clinical severity of hyperparathyroidism; i.e., whether radiologic subperiosteal resorption and increased plasma alkaline phosphatases are present.

Treatment of Severe Hyperparathyroidism.—When subperiosteal resorption and/or increased plasma alkaline phosphatase activity occur in a patient previously treated with oral calcium as phosphate binder, use of 1α-OH vitamin D3 derivatives is justified when plasma phosphate is below 1.7 mmol (5.5 mg/dL) and plasma calcium below 2.4 mmol/L (9.6 mg/dL). This situation occurs in one of six patients in our center.[94]

The classical mode of administration is 0.25 to 2 μg calcitriol/day orally and 0.5 to 4 μg/day 1α-OH vitamin D3. Efficacy of these derivatives is well documented in open trials for calcitriol[69, 128] and 1α-OH vitamin D3[126] and in controlled trials.[127] However, aluminum-phosphate binders were always used. On beginning treatment, $Al(OH)_3$ doses could obviously be decreased, but had to be increased, usually to levels higher than initially, as plasma alkaline phosphatases normalized. Thus it cannot be concluded that improved hyperparathyroidism was due only to 1α-OH vitamin D3 derivatives; we showed in a previous study that a decrease in plasma phosphate by $Al(OH)_3$ alone could also decrease osteoclastic hyperresorption.[128]

When oral daily administration of 1α-OH vitamin D3 derivatives fails to control hyperparathyroidism because of hypercalcemia, they can be given by intermittent intravenous injection or oral bolus two to three times a week. Slatopolsky et al.[129] showed that short term IV administration of calcitriol decreases plasma PTH levels before plasma ionized calcium concentration increases. Improved sensitivity of the parathyroid glands to plasma calcium after IV calcitriol was further demonstrated by studying the sigmoidal relationship of PTH levels (ordinate) and plasma calcium levels (abcissa) while increasing or decreasing plasma calcium concentrations by changing dialysate calcium concentration. After IV calcitriol, the curve is shifted downward and to the left, the set-point of calcium being significantly decreased in the study of Delmez et al.[12] but not in that of Dunlay et al.,[13] suggesting a direct suppression of PTH secretion. Decrease of calcium and phosphate release from bone can predominate over calcitriol stimulation of intestinal absorption of calcium and phosphate so that a decrease in plasma calcium and phosphate may occur during the first 8 weeks.[130]

Evidence that long-term treatment by IV calcitriol is effective in treating severe hyperparathyroidism not cured by oral daily administration of calcitriol because of hypercalcemia was brought by Andress et al.[130a] In 12 selected patients, IV calcitriol significantly decreased plasma alkaline phosphatases and PTH levels, although the latter remained respectively over two or three times the upper limit of normal. Bone histomorphometric parameters also improved, but in about half of the patients, bone resorption and bone formation rate remained abnormal, the number of osteoclasts even increasing in four cases. These spectacular but partial results were, however, obtained by discontinuing all calcium intake and keeping $Al(OH)_3$ as phosphate binder. Therefore, although Aluminon staining was negative in several cases on second biopsy, it is not sure that the treatment did not increase the aluminum overload, since absence of staining for aluminum can be explained by persistence of severe hyperparathyroidism, protecting the osteoid-calcified bone interface from aluminum deposition. Thus the possibility of late occurrence of aluminic osteomalacia or adynamic bone disease cannot be disregarded, when eventually the hyperparathyroidism is actually cured.[131]

Partial efficacy of intravenous calcitriol has been recently confirmed by the Italian cooperative study[132] on 76 patients with initial plasma intact PTH levels about ten times the upper limit of normal. In 3 of 4 of these patients, PTH levels decreased by 50% after 4 months. However, this was obtained only at the expense of increasing aluminum phosphate binder because of worsening hyperphosphatemia. Thus the study of Laut et al.[133] is of more interest, showing that IV calcitriol controlled severe hyperparathyroidism in 14 patients receiving dialysis while hyperphosphatemia was controlled exclusively with oral calcium while dialysate calcium was decreased from 7.0 to 6.0 or 5.0 mg/dL. After 14 months, plasma alkaline phosphatases were decreased by a factor of 4 and plasma levels of intact PTH by a factor of 7. This success was limited by increased plasma calcium from 9.0 to 11.0 mg/dL and plasma phosphate from 5.5 to 6.7 mg/dL, therefore by increased risk of soft tissue calcification.

1α-OH vitamin D3 can also be given intravenously, since this synthetic derivative is transformed into calcitriol by hepatic 25 hydroxylation, with plasma peaks of 100 pg/mL calcitriol 10 hours after injection of 4 μg (whereas 2 μg of calcitriol give a peak of 450 pg/mL 15 minutes later, and levels of 100 pg/mL 10 hours later). Results reported by Brandi et al.[134] and Lunghall et al.[135] have, however, the same shortcomings as most studies with intravenous calcitriol, namely that decreased PTH plasma levels were obtained at the price of worsening hyperphosphatemia (respectively from 1.9 to 2.4 and 2.1 to 2.4 mmol/L), despite maintaining aluminum-phosphate binders with the consequent double risk of long-term aluminum intoxication and soft tissue calcification. To preclude these risks, we used intravenous 1α-OH vitamin D3 (Etalpha) with $Mg(OH)_2$ as sole phosphate binder,[103] without success, since tolerable doses of IV 1α-OH vitamin D3 and $Mg(OH)_2$ were insufficient for long-term decrease of high intact PTH plasma levels. We then performed a multicentric trial treating 20 patients with severe hyperparathyroidism (since all had increased plasma alkaline phosphatases) with IV 1α-OH vitamin D3 given three times a week at a mean dose of 2 μg/dialysis; hyperphosphatemia was controlled only with $CaCO_3$ and hypercalcemia was prevented by decreasing dialysate calcium concentration to 5.0 mg/dL (1.25 mmol/L)[136]; 6 months later, plasma alkaline phosphatases were normalized, plasma levels of intact PTH decreased from 486 to 125 (normal <55 pg/mL), plasma calcium concentrations increased only from 2.35 to 2.47, and plasma phosphate from 1.56 to 1.64 mmol/L.

Intermittent oral administration of calcitriol or 1α-OH vitamin D3 bolus also appears quite effective, although it has not been compared with IV. administration. Brandi et al.[137] showed that once suppression of hyperparathyroidism was obtained with intravenous 1α-OH vitamin D3, it could be maintained for 1 year by the same dose as oral bolus. Fukagawa et al.[138] even reported ultrasonographic regression within 12 weeks of hyperplastic parathyroid glands. Given the uncertain reproducibility of this technique, such results must await confirmation. In the study of Tsukamoto et al.,[139] two oral boli of 4 μg calcitriol per week significantly decreased PTH and alkaline phosphatase levels while previous daily treatment had been ineffective. Six months later, however, plasma calcium had increased to 10.6 mg/dL and plasma phosphate was maintained at 5.9 mg/dL only with $Al(OH)_3$. With one weekly oral bolus of 8 to 12 μg 1α-OH vitamin D3, $CaCO_3$ as sole phosphate binder and dialysate calcium (DCa) decreased to 1.25 or 1.5 mmol/L. Akizawa et al.[140] observed better control of hyperparathyroidism than in a control group taking 0.4 μg/day 1α-OH vitamin D3 orally. Evidence that intermittent was superior to daily administration is, however, weakened by the fact that the total dose of 1α-OH vitamin D3 per week and plasma concentration of calcium and PO_4 were greater in the experimental group. A recent study[141] further questions the superiority of intermittent oral administration of calcitriol since the decrease in plasma PTH levels and alkaline phosphatases were comparable in nine patients taking 2.6 μg three times a week and in six patients taking 2.0 μg daily. (It should be pointed out that in this study hypercalcemia was prevented by a dialysate Ca of 4.0 mg/dL, and hyperphosphatemia by the use of $Al(OH)_3$ 3 g/day in addition to $CaCO_3$. Therefore we think that the main advantage of intermittent oral bolus of 1α-OH vitamin D3 derivatives (while awaiting an intravenous form) is that it is more reliably given, since administered under nurse supervision during the dialysis session. This point is important because patients with severe hyperparathyroidism are poorly compliant to treatment.

Critical review of the literature on the new means of administering 1α-OH vitamin D3 derivatives yields modest results. In only two studies has intravenous calcitriol[133] or intravenous 1α-OH vitamin D3[136] treated severe hyperparathyroidism with efficacy without aluminum phosphate binders; i.e., with $CaCO_3$ as sole phosphate binder while hypercalcemia was prevented by decreasing DCa to 6.0 or 5.0 mg/dL. Since the follow-up is still relatively short (14 and 6 months), it is not certain whether surgical parathyroidectomy will finally not be necessary. The treatment will be beneficial, however, even if parathyroidectomy is finally necessary, since the preparathyroidectomy skeleton will be somewhat remineralized, decreasing the postparathyroidectomy risk of hypocalcemia and hypophosphoremia due to hungry bone syndrome.

Treatment of Infraradiologic Hyperparathyroidism (or Prevention of Radiologic Hyperparathyroidism).—There are few controlled trials demonstrating an advantage of using 1α-OH vitamin D3 derivatives in the prevention of radiologic renal bone disease. In the three studies we found,[142–144] plasma concentrations of PTH decreased more profoundly in experimental than in control groups but, in all trials, hyperphosphatemia was controlled with $Al(OH)_3$, at often increasing doses. In the only study with bone histologic studies,[144] it was found that the improvement or prevention of osteitis fibrosa was counterbalanced by induction of aluminic osteomalacia, the prognosis of which is worse than that of osteitis fibrosa. In our own open trials with 1α-OH vitamin D3[145] or calcitriol[146] we found that improvement of osteoclastic resorption was primarily related to control of hyperphosphatemia, which was at that time obtained by associating 3 g of $CaCO_3$ and moderate doses of $Al(OH)_3$. This approach prevented aluminic osteomalacia but not aluminic adynamic bone disease.[34] Thus we disagree with Malluche and Faugere who in their 1990 review still advise the use of low dose $Al(OH)_3$ associated with $CaCO_3$ and calcitriol, because according to their own works, aluminic adynamic bone disease leads to osteopenia.

A recent study from Geneva[147] suggests, however, that low doses of oral calcitriol (0.25 μg/day) could be beneficial since compared to a control group otherwise similarly treated over 20 months, calcitriol prevented increased plasma concentrations of PTH and osteocalcin and decreased bone density measured with biphotonic absorption. On the contrary, bone density increased at the lumbar vertebrae and femur shaft. $Al(OH)_3$ was not excluded and it is not absolutely excluded that the increased density of lumbar vertebrae may be explained by increased aortic calcification. Histologic data in these patients would be interesting to prove the actual benefit of this therapy.

We agree with Okada et al.[149] that the role of 1α-OH vitamin D3 derivatives in preventing radiologic hyperparathyroidism is limited to its addition, when possible, to $CaCO_3$ given as phosphate binder while DCa remains at 6.5 mg/dL to prevent intradialytic negative calcium balance. MgOH or Mg carbonate as sole phosphate binder in association with 1α-OH vitamin D3 derivatives (even as intermittent intravenous bolus) did not lead to better long-term control of hyperparathyroidism than with $CaCO_3 \pm Mg(OH)_2$. Furthermore a general strategy associating low DCa (1.25 mmol/L) oral calcium as sole phosphate binder and intravenous 1α-OH vitamin D3 derivatives does not seem reasonable for the moment because of pratical difficulties to use it on a large scale and the higher cost of the drug itself and of its monitoring. A long-term comparative evaluation of the cost-benefit ratio of this approach is therefore necessary before recommending it. It must also be kept in mind that patients without radiologic osteitis fibrosa or increased alkaline phosphatases represent about half of our dialysis population provided they are treated with a DCa of 6.5 mg/dL and the association $CaCO_3 \pm Mg(OH)_2$ as phosphate binder.

Use of Nonhypercalcemic Derivatives of Vitamin D: 24,25-$(OH)_2$ Vitamin D3 and 22 oxa Calcitriol

Clinical Use of 24,25-$(OH)_2$ Vitamin D3

In part I, we saw the pathophysiologic interest of compensating 24,25-$(OH)_2$ vitamin D3 deficiency not for its direct suppressive effect on PTH synthesis but rather for its protective role against osteoclastic resorption favored by PTH and possibly calcitriol. Clinical evidence of the usefulness of giving 24,25-$(OH)_2$ vitamin D3 to treat renal osteodystrophy is, however, still tenuous. Muirhead et al.[150] showed in 1982 that 2 μg/day 24,25-$(OH)_2$ vitamin D3, which normalized plasma levels of 24,25-$(OH)_2$ vitamin D, was unable to cure or prevent worsening of symptomatic hyperparathyroidism, probably because it increased hypocalcemia. The association of 24,25-$(OH)_2$ vitamin D3 to calcitriol, which had induced hypercalcemia in two patients, decreased plasma calcium concentrations but had no additional bone effect. The only interesting effect noted by Muirhead et al. was decreased plasma phosphate, which was difficult to interpret since aluminic phosphate binders were also given.

In 1983, Hodsman et al.[151] reported that 24,25-$(OH)_2$ vitamin D3 had a hypocalcemic effect in 15 patients with osteomalacia (of probable aluminic origin since resistant to calcitriol) who became hypercalcemic with calcitriol. In 1985, Dunstan et al.[152] also reported that 24,25-$(OH)_2$ vitamin D3 at 2 to 10 μg/day had no PTH suppressive effect but a hypophosphatemic effect. The same year, Van Diemen-Steevorde et al.[153] showed that 24,25-$(OH)_2$ vitamin D3 added to DHT in children with uremia induced decreased plasma concentration of DHT and plasma calcium, which led to an increased dose of DHT, decreased osteoclastic resorption, and increased bone mineralization assessed with X-rays and biphotonic absorptiometry. More recently Mortensen et al.[154] showed on bone biopsy specimens from patients with uremia treated with calcitriol and 24,25-$(OH)_2$ vitamin D3, alone or in combination, that the increase in adenylate cyclase activity induced by PTH was abolished only with 24,25-$(OH)_2$ vitamin D3. Furthermore at the Singapore Symposium on renal bone disease, Evans et al. reported a new statistical analysis of data published in 1985 by Dunstan et al.[152] This analysis showed that 24,25-$(OH)_2$ vitamin D3 has an effect, since for the same decrease in PTH levels, the decrease in bone resorption is higher when 24,25-$(OH)_2$ vitamin D3 is associated with calcitriol than with calcitriol alone. At the same symposium. Popovtzer[155] presented a clinical trial with comparative histomorphometric data in patients with uremia receiving dialysis, 19 treated with 1α-OH vitamin D3 alone and 22 receiving 1α-OH vitamin D3 and 24,25-$(OH)_2$ vitamin D3 at a fixed dose of 10 μg/day. Bone biopsy specimens obtained before and after 1 year of treatment showed decreased osteoclastic resorption and double tetracycline-labeled surfaces in the group treated by the association. Although doses of 1α-OH vitamin D3 had been variable since adjusted to plasma calcium levels, mean plasma concentration of calcitriol and 25-OH vitamin

D were similar in both groups. Plasma 24,25-$(OH)_2$ vitamin D3 levels were low in control subjects (0.5 ± 0.3 ng/mL normal at 2 to 4 ng/mL), but high in the experimental group (5.1 ± 4 ng/mL). Plasma PTH did not vary significantly. No precise information was given on $Al(OH)_3$ and $CaCO_3$ doses. The extent of surfaces stained with Aluminon increased similarly up to 30%; no deferoxamine test or measurement of bone aluminum content is available however. Therefore some doubt persists as to the exclusive role of 24,25$(OH)_2$ vitamin D3 in the greater reduction of the resorptive surface and of the tetracycline double-labeled surfaces since the similarity in aluminum overload of the parathyroid glands and of bone is not certain. Furthermore since 24,25-$(OH)_2$ vitamin D3 increases calcitriol catabolism, it is likely that the dose of 1α-OH vitamin D3 had been higher in the group receiving 24,25-$(OH)_2$ vitamin D3 since plasma levels of calcitriol were similar. Thus a study comparing $CaCO_3$ alone to $CaCO_3$ + 24,25-$(OH)_2$ vitamin D3 seems now to be required to precisely define the role of 24,25-$(OH)_2$ vitamin D3 in the treatment of renal osteodystrophy, without the interference of different doses of 1α-OH vitamin D3 and of aluminum phosphate binder.

Use of 22-Oxacalcitriol (OCT)

Since study of its toxicity in animals is not yet completed, 22-oxacalcitriol cannot yet be studied in humans. However its suppressive effect on PTH synthesis shown in vivo in the rat by Brown et al.[155a] is of interest for the clinician because after 4 days no hypercalcemia was observed. Suppression was observed with 0.5 μg/day, a dose at which calcitriol always induces hypercalcemia (from 8.4 to 11.4 mg/L). In vitro, OCT suppresses PTH secretion by parathyroid cells in culture at the same dose as for calcitriol (10 nmol), which induces a 33% decrease in PTH secretion. As for calcitriol, suppression of PTH synthesis is linked to blockade of PTH gene transcription, which is 80% suppressed within 48 hours. OCT will probably replace with advantage calcitriol in the treatment of hyperparathyroidism secondary to renal insufficiency, in association with oral intake of alkaline salts of calcium as phosphate binder, since the risk of hypercalcemia will be greatly diminished.

Use of Osteoclastic Resorption Blocking Agents: Calcitonin and Biphosphonates

Calcitonin is well known to normalize plasma calcium, and is widely used for emergency treatment of severe hypercalcemia of primary hyperparathyroidism or of malignancies. It can also be used transiently in treating symptomatic hypercalcemia of tertiary hyperparathyroidism in uremia to prepare the patient for parathyroidectomy. Its long-term use in uremia has however been a failure, since osteitis fibrosa actually worsened.[156]

Biphosphonates block osteoclastic resorption. In contrast to etidronate, which also blocks bone mineralization, APD (amino hydroxypropylene biphosphonate or sodium pamidronate) and clodronate are biphosphonates that block only resorption. Thus their therapeutic profile is adequate for treating uremic hyperparathyroidism especially when hypercalcemia occurs spontaneously or with low doses of $CaCO_3$ or 1α-OH vitamin D3 derivatives. Clinical experience with these drugs in uremia is still limited. Yap et al.[157] reported that 15 or 30 mg APD corrected hypercalcemic episodes occurring in a patient receiving CAPD while immobilized because of infections and vascular problems. Hene et al.[158] were unsuccessful in treating hypercalcemia in five patients with uremia (three receiving dialysis) due to hyperparathyroidism as diagnosed with elevated plasma levels of PTH and alkaline phosphatases and, on the first bone biopsy specimen, on an increased number of osteoblasts while the number of osteoclasts was paradoxically normal. The dose was 15 mg IV at each of three weekly dialyses and 200 mg/day orally in the two patients not yet receiving dialysis. After 9 months of treatment, the second biopsy specimen showed worsening of osteitis fibrosa parameters (fibrosis, number of osteoblasts and osteoclasts, osteoclastic surface) with a curious increase in osteoclast-like cells in the medullary space, while plasma PTH and alkaline phosphatases levels remained unchanged. Hamdy et al.[159] were more successful with clodronate given in nine patients receiving chronic hemodialysis, 300 to 600 mg, five times at the end of dialysis; they obtained decreased plasma concentrations of calcium, phosphate, and hydroxyproline while plasma levels of PTH and alkaline phosphatases increased. After treatment discontinuation, hypercalcemia recurred and was again normalized with 1,100 mg/day oral clodronate during 2 weeks.

Although etidronate also inhibits bone mineralization, it was used in patients with renal insufficiency by Zuccheli et al.[160] because of potential beneficial effects on bone resorption and soft tissue calcifications. Since in an initial study these authors had found that the beneficial effect on metastatic calcification was counterbalanced by worsening of bone mineralization, they used in their second study 300 mg/day etidronate in association with 100 μg 25-OH vitamin D3 in nine patients receiving chronic dialysis, and compared this treatment to 100 μg 25-OH vitamin D3 alone given to control subjects. After 9 months they observed a similar improvement in all bone histomorphometric parameters with the exception of the osteoclastic resorption surfaces, which were more reduced in the group receiving etidronate. Soft tissue calcifications remained unchanged in both groups.

In conclusion, these preliminary results with biphosphonates in uremia are interesting but conflicting, and justify complementary studies. For the present, they are mainly interesting for the acute treatment of symptomatic hypercalcemia due to autonomous hyperparathyroidism. They would be, of course, contraindicated when hypercalcemia is associated with a low bone turnover disease.

Treating severe hypercalcemia in a patient receiving dialysis in whom hyperparathyroidism was unsuccessfully treated with parathyroidectomy, Zingraf et al.[161] used the chemoprotective and radiation protective drug WR

24-21, which has a hypocalcemic effect by blocking bone resorption and PTH secretion. After transient but constant efficacy of twice weekly administrations of the drug during 3 months, plasma levels of Ca and PTH before perfusion remained elevated and treatment was discontinued.

Practical Advice for Medical Treatment of Hyperparathyroidism in Adults With Renal Insufficiency

While awaiting the clinical availability of 24,25-$(OH)_2$ vitamin D3 and 22-oxacalcitriol, it seems useful to summarize practical advice in 1991 for treating hyperparathyroidism in the adult with uremia while excluding, in accordance with our proposition of 1981, prolonged administration of even low doses of aluminum-phosphate binders. As shown in the latest edition of the *The Kidney* by Brenner and Rector and in the editorial of the *New England Journal of Medicine* by Sherrard,[32] a consensus is also emerging in the United States to exclude these agents. This attitude is justified by our experience in the years before 1981, which showed that the association of $CaCO_3$ and moderate doses of $Al(OH)_3$ prevented aluminic osteomalacia but not aluminic adynamic bone disease,[95,166a] a finding recently confirmed in the children on CAPD by Salusky et al. [166b]

Before dialysis, early treatment of hyperparathyroidism is important because hyperparathyroid hyperplasia is better prevented than cured. In our experience,[160] 70% of patients receiving dialysis who ultimately underwent parathyroidectomy had severe osteitis fibrosa with subperiosteal resorption and/or increased plasma alkaline phosphatases at the beginning of dialysis. Most authors now recommend starting preventive measures when GFR decreases below 60 mL/min in the adult and below 80 mL/min in children. At this stage the choice is between low doses of 1α-hydroxylated vitamin D derivatives (0.25 μg/day calcitriol or 0.5 μg/day alfacalcidol) or 3 g $CaCO_3$ associated with good vitamin D repletion by vitamin D2, D3, or 25-OH vitamin D3 to bring plasma 25-OH vitamin D levels to 30 $\pm$ 5 ng/mL. Doses of calcitriol or $CaCO_3$ can be modulated to maintain urinary calcium at 100 $\pm$ 20 mg/24 hours while plasma calcium and phosphate levels remain normal. Concomitantly, protein intake is reduced to 1 g/kg/day when GFR remains above 40 mL/min and to 0.70 g/kg/day when GFR is 20 to 40 mL/min. Below 20 mL/min, protein intake can be further reduced to 0.4 g/kg/day with a vegetarian diet containing 3 to 5 mg/kg phosphate and 35 kcal/kg/day provided supplements of essential amino acids or ketoanalogs are given. We have seen that calcic ketoanalogs can also complex phosphate. These diets have been proved to be effective not only on the rate of renal function decline but also on hyperparathyroidism as assessed with PTH levels and bone histomorphometry.[163–166] Thus renal function and improvement of hyperparathyroidism are correlated, but it is not known which of these parameters comes first in the causal relationship. Diets very poor in phosphate would perhaps allow toleration of small doses of calcitriol in the case in which diet, ketoanalogs, and oral calcium would not prevent increased plasma intact PTH above twice the upper limit of normal. The recent experience of Aparicio and Lefage has however shown that this kind of diet in very compliant patients was able to cure hyperparathyroidism (assessed not only on intact PTH levels but also on bone histomorphometry) while low plasma calcitriol did not increase, demonstrating in man (as in dog, according to Lopez Hilker) that strict control of phosphate retention can decrease PTH secretion in spite of constant low synthesis of calcitriol and stable normal plasma calcium levels (personal communication)

In patients receiving chronic dialysis, the first measure is use of oral calcium with meals in order to complex phosphate. If the $CaCO_3$ dose is below 3 g/day, DCa concentration would be better kept at 7.0 mg/dL. When it is 3 to 6 g/day, decreasing DCa to the neutral concentration of 6.5 mg/dL is advised. If the dose of $CaCO_3$ is above 6 g/day, DCa can be decreased to 5.0 mg/dL or less to keep predialysis plasma concentrations of calcium at 2.5 ± 0.2 mmol/L and of phosphate at 1.7 ± 0.2 mmol/L. Vitamin D depletion is prevented by adequate exposure to sun and/or adequate supplement of vitamin D2, D3, or 25-OH vitamin D3 to maintain plasma 25-OH vitamin D at about 30 ng/mL. 1α hydroxylated vitamin derivatives are introduced only secondarily (preferentially as intermittent oral or intravenous bolus at each dialysis under medical supervision) when plasma concentrations of intact PTH increase above twice the upper limit of normal. Control of hyperphosphatemia will still rely on oral $CaCO_3$, but DCa concentration will be eventually decreased to prevent hypercalcemia.

Indications and Modalities of Parathyroidectomy for Hyperparathyroidism Secondary to Renal Insufficiency

Despite preventive treatment, severe forms of hyperparathyroidism are still not rare in patients with renal insufficiency, and in some cases, surgical parathyroidectomy may be the only effective treatment.[53, 167]

The high prevalence of parathyroidectomy in the dialyzed population is due to extended life expectancy by dialysis treatment. After 15 years of dialysis, prevalence is about 400 for 1,000 patients (Fig 4)[168] and still higher in our experience after 20 years of dialysis. Median survival time without parathyroidectomy in the population of dialyzed patients in the Amiens Center between 1974 and 1988 was 13 years; i.e., after 13 years of dialysis, 50% of patients are likely to undergo parathyroidectomy.[162] These figures agree with the prevalence calculated by the European Dialysis Transplantation Association (EDTA) registry.

The main reasons for failure of medical treatment are the delay in its application before dialysis and poor patient compliance to phosphate binders. More rarely, insufficient dialysis treatment, mainly because of vascular access problems, is at fault. Occasionally hypercalcemia and soft tissue calcifications associated with hyperphosphatemia prevent the use of $CaCO_3$

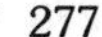

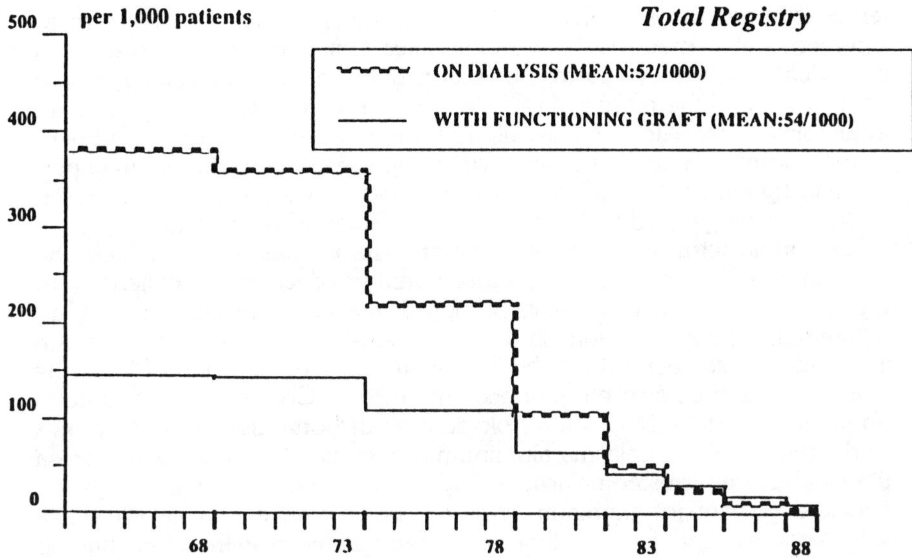

FIG 4.
Prevalence of parathyroidectomy (From Brunner, et al: *Nephrol Dial Transplant* 1991; 6(suppl 3):28–31. Used by permission.)

and calcitriol. In a few patients, previously well-controlled hyperparathyroidism abruptly escapes without obvious explanation.

Surgical Parathyroidectomy

Surgical removal of the parathyroid glands remains the treatment of choice in severe hyperparathyrodism. Its indications are not easy to define precisely. There is no consensus among nephrology centers as to the degree of hyperparathyroidism for which medical treatment is still worthwhile.

Indications and Contraindications

Schematically, parathyroidectomy is necessary when medical treatment of severe hyperparathyroidism has been pushed to its ultimate or when medical treatment is too late, i.e., in case of an emergency such as fractures, cutaneous necrosis by calciphylaxis, and symptomatic hypercalcemia.

Whatever the situation, the diagnosis of severe hyperparathyroidism must be safely ascertained mainly on biologic parameters: increased plasma alkaline phosphatases not explained by cholestasis; and frank elevation of plasma PTH concentrations interpreted according to the nature of the antibody used and to the upper limit of normal. To give some reference points, severe hyperparathyroidism is diagnosed on the basis of an increase above ten times the upper limit of normal with a C terminal antibody, above 15 to 20 times the upper limit of normal with a midregion antibody and above five times this limit when an antibody against the N terminal fragment or against the intact molecule is used (the latter measurement being made with two antibodies taking the PTH molecule in sandwich). Clinical symptoms such as pruritus or osteoarticular pain are nonspecific and therefore not reliable, the pain being even more prevalent in aluminic osteopathy and usually not improved by surgery.[162] Subperiosteal resorption is related specifically to hyperparathyroidism but may persist after hyperparathyroidism has been replaced by aluminic osteomalacia.

Bone histologic study with quantitative evaluation of static and dynamic (after double tetracycline labeling) parameters is considered by Malluche and Faugère[53] to be required before parathyroidectomy in patients with uremia. The deferoxamine test, proposed initially by Milliner et al.[169] to differentiate aluminic osteomalacia from osteitis fibrosa in severe aluminum intoxication, has been proven by the recent multicentric study of Malluche et al.[53,171a] and by a recent monocentric study of Chazan et al.[170] to be of no value for establishing the histologic type of bone disease. In Chazan's study, the increase in plasma aluminum is even greater with osteitis fibrosa than with aluminic osteomalacia and adynamic bone disease, although histologic deposition of aluminum is much less in osteitis fibrosa. We agree with Malluche and Chazan that the deferoxamine test therefore has no value for establishing histologic diagnosis of bone disease in a patient with uremia, but we question the superiority of bone biopsy over the deferoxamine test for excluding the aluminum overload and therefore deciding without after thoughts on parathyroidectomy in a patient with uremia, bone pain, and hypercalcemia.

Parathyroidectomy promotes aluminum deposition at the interface of the osteoid and calcified tissues and favors aluminic osteomalacia in patients with aluminum overload even when they had typical histologic osteitis fibrosa before parathyroidectomy.[56,171b] Therefore even if bone biopsy shows typical osteitis fibrosa, we think that parathyroidectomy should not be decided on before a deferoxamine test has been performed and the patient has been treated with long-term deferoxamine in case of positive results. The difficult question is that of the positivity criterion. Since M.C. de Vernejoul et al.[171] found that patients with significant bone aluminum overload (defined not only on histologic aluminum staining [Aluminon positive surfaces $>$ 0.8 mm/mm2], but also on increased bone aluminum content [$>$ 25 μg/g of bone]) could be differentiated with 100% sensitivity and specificity by increased plasma aluminum of 50 μg/L while the basal aluminemia was 43 $\pm$ 31 μg/L, we propose to take this increase as the positivity criterion. When deferoxamine treatment has been decided on, close monitoring of plasma alkaline phosphatases and plasma PTH levels is mandatory; osteitis fibrosa may worsen considerably[171c] because of the lack of aluminum inhibition of osteoblast[166a] and PTH secretion.[102] In a few cases, aluminum-induced hypercalcemia may disappear and 1α-OH vitamin D3 may be tried again.

On what criteria is failure of medical treatment of hyperparathyroidism recognized? In 1991, failure is usually recognized only after having tried 1α-OH vitamin D3 derivatives (perhaps given preferentially as intermittent oral or intravenous bolus) in association with oral calcium as exclusive phosphate binder while DCa concentration has been decreased if necessary. Persistence of elevated plasma levels of PTH, osteocalcin, and alkaline phosphatases while plasma calcium concentration is above 2.7 mmol/L and phosphate is above 2 mmol/L is an indication for parathyroidectomy. When cutaneous necrosis and metastatic calcifications or fracture are present, we recommend performing parathyroidectomy without delay. When the radiobiologic picture of hyperparathyroidism is severe with subnormal plasma calcium and hyperphosphatemia, it is wise not to extend medical treatment too long, even with its new modalities, given the risk of fractures and soft tissue calcification, but rather to perform parathyroidectomy, which entails only minor risks.

Hypercalcemia with hyperphosphatemia and metastatic calcifications are thus the limiting factors of medical treatment. However, before deciding to operate for hypercalcemia, causes of hypercalcemia other than hyperparathyroidism must be carefully excluded. As previously stated, aluminum intoxication must first be excluded. Classical causes of hypercalcemia in nonuremic patients must also be excluded: granulomatous diseases secreting (sarcoidosis, tuberculosis) or not secreting calcitriol (dialysis-related granulomatosis, induced by silicone from tubing crushed by the blood pump), cancer and malignant hemopathies, immobilization, thyroid disorders, hypocortisolism, and rare hypophosphatemia and vitamin A intoxication.[36, 172]

Surgical Contraindications

Local and general contraindications should be considered. Anatomic condition and/or particular diseases may make neck extension hazardous or even impossible. Attention should be paid to the possibility of erosive spondylarthropathy associated or not to $\beta 2$ microglobulin, and a profile x-ray or, better, a magnetic resonance image of the neck should always be examined (especially for a lysis of the odontoid aprophysis of the axis). Previous neck surgery may make new surgery difficult and hazardous with increased risk of damage to recurrent and phrenic nerves. Cardiorespiratory insufficiency may be incompatible with long anesthesia. In such cases invasive but nonsurgical parathyroidectomy may be a useful alternative.

Preoparative Localization of the Parathyroid Glands

Ultrasonography.—Parathyroid gland visualization with ultrasonography may be useful before neck exploration for hyperparathyroidism. In the experience of F. Moreau et al.[173] with primary hyperparathyroidism the sonographic localization of primary adenomas can be made with a sensitivity of 73% and a specificity of 99%. Such a high rate of success reflects a long, dedicated experience with a large number of patients. Teams with less experience have sometimes similar[174] but also lower[175, 176] success rates. The main factors decreasing sensitivity are small size of the gland

and thyroid disease.[173] Advanced age of the patient and recent change of apparatus also contribute to decreased sensitivity. A few negative results are explained by ectopic localization of parathyroid glands in the mediastinum or behind the esophagus. In case of hyperparathyroidism secondary to renal insufficiency, a good correlation has been found between the size measured by sonography and the weight of the glands removed.[177, 178] However, experienced surgeons consider that especially in patients with renal failure, the four parathyroid glands should be identified in any case during the neck exploration. Preoperative sonography is therefore mainly appreciated in case of persistence or recurrence of hyperparathyroidism after a previous surgery.[179] Hyperplasia of the parathyroid grafts in the forearm after total parathyroidectomy may also be evaluated with sonography.[180]

Cervical Tomodensitometry and Parathyroid Scintigraphy.—In our experience, these two examinations are also useful only for localizing abnormal parathyroid glands after unsuccessful parathyroidectomy when ultrasonographic examination is negative. Tomodensitometry can localize a parathyroid gland behind the sternum or the oesophagus; the number of false-positive results is quite high in some series,[175] but modest in others.[178,179] In our experience and that of others,[175] double subtractive scintigraphy with thalium 201 and technetium 99m is rarely informative. Arteriography of the internal mammary artery may sometimes be the only means to localize a gland in the lower mediastinum.

Fine Needle Cytoaspiration.—With sonographic control, this method allows distinction between a thyroid and a parathyroid mass.[177, 183, 183a] In our hands, cytoaspiration is also useful for localization of the parathyroid glands before alcoholization, in particular after persistance or recurrence of hyperparathyroidism.

Surgical Techniques

We will describe these techniques and discuss their advantages and disadvantages only briefly. Success depends more on the experience of the surgeon than on the technique. The critical issue is to find all the parathyroid glands. If the four parathyroid glands (or even more in case of supernumerary glands) are not found, correction of hyperparathyroidism will be necessarily incomplete. Great experience is required to localize ectopic glands situated inside the thyroid, behind the sternum or behind the esophagus. Because of frequent localization behind the sternum, systematic bilateral thymectomy from the neck is recommended.[185] When doubt as to total ablation of pathologic glands persists, ultrarapid measurement of intact immunoreactive PTH can be made during surgery. Such extemporaneous dosage is, however, reserved to a small number of centers.

Subtotal Parathyroidectomy.—After identification of the four glands, all are removed except half of one, which is marked by a silk thread or a clip. Vascularization of the gland left in situ should be carefully maintained to prevent necrosis. According to Kaye et al.,[186] this technique would be associated paradoxically to less recurrence of hyperparathyroidism than total parathyroidectomy with reimplantation. In his general review, Kaye notes recurrence in respectively 6.6% (of 503 cases) and 10.7% (of 755 cases). It should be pointed out, however, that these estimations are based on evaluation of parathyroid function by unreliable PTH radioimmunoassays. In our experience[186a] recurrence or persistence of hyperparathyroidism in patients with uremia is more frequent after subtotal parathyroidectomy than after total parathyroidectomy followed by reimplantation. This estimation is, however, also based on a retrospective study without prior randomization of the two surgical techniques and with evaluation of parathyroid function with an unreliable assay.

Total Parathyroidectomy Followed Immediately by Reimplantation.—After removal of all the parathyroid glands, a few fragments of parathyroid tissue (usually 10 to 20 microcubes of 1 mm of side) are reimplanted into the forearm flexor muscles (preferably in the forearm without the arterioveinous fitula). If the surgeon discovers both hyperplastic and adenomatous tissue, the fragments for reimplantation will be taken only from the hyperplastic tissue because risk of recurrence seems higher when adenomatous tissue is reimplanted.[187, 188] Secretion of PTH by the autografts is almost constant. Nevertheless, it is wise to cryopreserve a few fragments in case of nonviable grafts.

This technique has been popularized on the basis that in case of recurrence it would be easier to remove, with simple local anesthesia, a part of the hypertrophied graft than to undertake a new neck exploration. Actually removal of hyperplastic grafts is often difficult because of diffuse infiltration of the muscle by parathyroid cells. A few authors have even suggested that a reimplanted graft could have undergone malignant transformation.[189–192] This was suspected on the persistence or recurrence of hypercalcemia and on the histologic finding of nuclear abnormalities of the parathyroid cells and of neovascular formations around the parathyroid islets. Doubt persists regarding the certainty of malignancy because the histologic diagnosis of parathyroid cancer is very difficult. In any case, such observations are rare. In the experience of Necker Hospital[192a] on more than 80 total parathyroidectomies with reimplantation during the past 15 years, such an unfavorable course was never observed. The same is true with a larger Japanese experience on 196 cases.[193]

Total Parathyroidectomy Followed by Delayed Reimplantation.—When the surgeon is not sure that all the parathyroid glands have been removed, he may prefer to wait for the decrease in plasma calcium and PTH levels before deciding to reimplant the parathyroid fragments. During the interval it is obviously necessary to cryopreserve the parathyroid fragments. Cryopreserved tissue is however more fragile than fresh tissue, and successful function of the graft is less certain than that after immediate reimplantation.[194, 195]

Total Parathyroidectomy Without Reimplantation.—This procedure was preferred in the 1960s.[196] It was later abandoned because of the difficulty of maintaining normocalcemia in some patients, which was poorly tolerated in patients with successful kidney transplantation since large amounts of oral calcium and vitamin D were necessary.

It is noteworthy that, in 1989, Kaye et al. proposed to choose this technique[197] because in their experience total parathyroidectomy does not remove all parathyroid tissues. These may remain dispersed in the neck and undergo hyperplasia after surgery so that after a few months or years of hypoparathyroid state, a normal or even a hyperparathyroid state may emerge. This technique would be associated with a lower risk of early recurrence (with a frequency of 6.9% in 116 cases according to Kaye et al.[186]). Results published as a letter by another group in 1987 support this approach.[198] We remain opposed to total parathyroidectomy without autograft, however, for two reasons. The first is that a hypoparathyroid state is not compatible with normal bone turnover and predisposes to adynamic bone disease, which may become clinically significant because osteopenia may develop in the patient with uremia secondarily to aluminum exposure or to immunosuppressive drugs when he has a kidney graft.[8] The second reason is the difficulty previously mentioned of maintaining normocalcemia after successful kidney transplantation. In our experience, most patients who have undergone subtotal or total parathyroidectomy with reimplantation remain in a euparathyroid state.

Complications

Serious complications are rare. Hematoma or infections are rare even in the patient with uremia despite the hemostasis problems. Hyperkalemia remains a potentially serious complication and may sometimes necessitate emergency administration of chelators or even a dialysis. Hayes et al.[199] have suggested that this hyperkalemia would be more frequent after parathyroidectomy because parathyroidectomy and plasma calcium interfere with potassium homeostasis. Interaction of these factors is not unidirectional however so it is dubious that parathyroidectomy actually favors hyperkalemia more than other surgery. On the one hand, it is established that PTH rapidly releases calcium from the exchangeable pool around the osteocytes in exchange with potassium.[39] Therefore, the decrease in circulating levels of PTH after parathyroidectomy would decrease bone uptake of potassium and increase plasma potassium. On the other hand, other works suggest that the cellular uptake of potassium (specially by the erythrocytes) is inhibited by PTH.[200, 201] Therefore parathyroidectomy would improve the cellular uptake of potassium and decrease the risk of hyperkalemia.

Hypocalcemia is not an actual complication since it is a marker of parathyroidectomy efficacy. However, if not corrected, it may induce tetany or generalized convulsions with a risk of fracture of a fragile skeleton from renal osteodystrophy.

Recurrent and phrenic palsies occur mainly after new cervical exploration.

Clinical Follow-Up After Parathyroidectomy

Plasma calcium concentration usually decreases rapidly after surgical removal of all the parathyroid glands. The higher the activity of alkaline phosphatases before surgery, the greater the decrease.[201a] Plasma PTH concentrations also decrease rapidly to normal levels within a few days. In contrast, plasma alkaline phosphatase activity increases in the first 2 weeks and decreases to normal only after several weeks or months. The initial increase in plasma alkaline phosphatase is more marked in patients without aluminum intoxication.[201a] Treatment to maintain plasma calcium in the normal range is usually necessary the day after parathyroidectomy. It consists of calcium supplements, either oral or intravenous (according to degree of hypocalcemia) and administration of 1α-OH vitamin D3 derivatives. Usually we give 12 to 24 g oral $CaCO_3$ in fractionated doses every hour or 2 hours and up to 3 μg calcitriol or 6 μg of 1α-OH vitamin D3. If plasma calcium decreases below 1.75 mmol/L (70 mg/L) or if symptoms of tetany occur, 8 to 12 g/day calcium gluconate is given IV diluted in 500 mL isotonic glucose. Hypophosphatemia usually accompanies hypocalcemia. Both reflect the avidity of remineralizing bone (hungry bone syndrome). In case of protracted hypophosphatemia resistant to dietary or pharmacologic phosphate supplement, it may be necessary to add phosphate to the dialysate. Hypocalcemia and hypophosphoremia are more profound with more severe osteitis fibrosa. This stresses the usefulness of treatment with IV 1α-OH vitamin D3 derivatives during the week preceding parathyroidectomy when hypercalcemia or hyperphosphatemia do not preclude such treatment.[167]

Other Nonsurgical but Invasive Parathyroidectomies

Alcoholization of the Parathyroid Glands

Sonographically guided injection of alcohol into the parathyroid glands is still experimental. The technique consists of injecting absolute alcohol into parathyroid glands localized by echography. The volume of alcohol must not be greater than that of the gland to be destroyed. Only detected and accessible glands can be destroyed. Glands close to major vessels should not be injected.

Experience of Other Teams.—Few teams have experience with this method.[202–204] The largest is that of the Milano group, based on 80 patients. Most patients had secondary hyperparathyroidism, but this group also has experience with primary hyperparathyroidism. In a recent paper, these authors report most consistent success in moderately severe secondary hyperparathyroidism with repeated injections. Severe hyperthyroidism does not usually regress.

Personal Experience.—At Necker Hospital, with the collaboration of J.F. Moreau and B. Page, preliminary experience was gained in five adult patients with severe hyperparathyroidism despite transiently successful parathyroidectomy in two. Quantities injected were lower than those of the Milano group. Results depended on the number of glands to treat; hyperparathyroidism regressed only in two men with recurrent hyperparathyroidism after previous subtotal parathyroidectomy. Figure 5 shows the decrease in plasma intact PTH levels after alcoholization in one. Interestingly, plasma calcium decreased to 1.75 mmol/L as early as the day after alcoholization. On the contrary, hyperparathyroidism was practically unchanged in the three others (women) despite repeated injections in one. Recurrent palsy occurred in these three and did not completely regress in

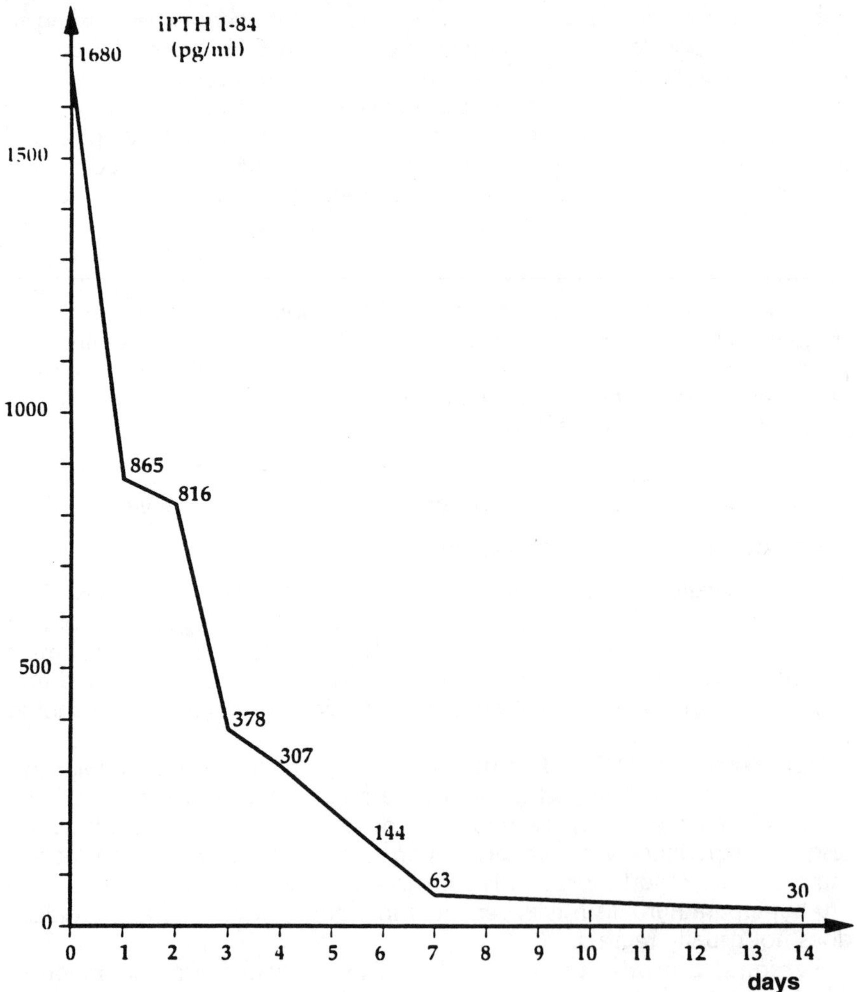

FIG 5.
Plasma levels of 1 to 84 PTH after alcoholization of a parathyroid gland.

one. Two subsequently underwent successful surgical parathyroidectomy. Surgery was relatively difficult because of tissue sclerosis, probably provoked by the injections.

Considering the poor result of our limited experience, we are presently reserved regarding the indication of alcoholization of parathyroid glands. However ever-increasing progress in sonographic localization of the glands make percutaneous reduction of hyperparathyroidism very attractive. Use of other necrotizing agents is currently being evaluated.

Embolization of the Parathyroid Glands

Another way to destroy a parathyroid gland is to embolize its artery to induce ischemic necrosis. After localization of the glands by arteriography, embolization is performed with injection of contrast media. This method has been reported in 18 patients with primary adenoma.[205] In 12, embolization was successful with a follow-up of 35 months. Because of technical difficulties, the authors recommend reserving this method for patients with recurrent hyperparathyroidism and to the rare nonoperable case.

Particularities of Treatment of Hyperparathyroidism in the Child With Uremia

Hyperparathyroidism is especially severe in children because of its impact on skeleton maturation and growth, bone remodeling in the first years of age being 50% of bone mass whereas it is only 3% to 5% in the adult.

In Children Not Yet Receiving Dialysis

Although renal rickets is the term for renal osteodystrophy in children, implying the same mineralization defect as in osteomalacia, histological study of the skeleton shows that lamellar osteoid tissue is rarely not calcified but that severe osteitis fibrosa is present.[206] Noncalcified woven bone is in fact the explanation of the metaphysal radiolucent zones (comparable to those of rickets) and of the slipped epiphysis, responsible for major skeletal deformities (coxa vara, genu valgum). Therefore in severe cases the child's small size is explained both by deformities and growth stunting. In moderate forms, it is not sure that renal osteodystrophy per se is responsible for growth retardation since treatment of renal osteodystrophy is not regularly followed by growth catching-up as in patients with vitamin D-dependent rickets type I after treatment with 1α-OH vitamin D3 derivatives. Bone growth of the child with uremia actually appears more dependent on sodium and water balances (which may sometimes necessitate nocturnal hydration with intestinal tubing), on good correction of acidosis (plasma bicarbonate must be maintained above 22 mmol/L by alkali supplement without citrates if aluminum salts are still used) and on adequate protein and caloric intake according to the Recommended Diet Allowance (RDA).

These measures must be taken earlier than in the adult, as soon as GFR has decreased below 80 mL/min/1.73 m^2

Early phosphate restriction is theoretically indicated as in the adult but is impossible if optimal RDA protein intake is respected. This stresses the greater importance of phosphate binder in the child.[206, 206a] Aluminum phosphate binders should be more scrupulously excluded in children than in adults because children and especially infants need proportionally higher doses (related to body weight) of $Al(OH)_3$ to control hyperphosphatemia, and intestinal absorption of aluminum is greater.[207] This is why a few months of treatment with $Al(OH)_3$ can induce fatal encephalopathy and osteomalacia.[54] Disastrous intellectual prognosis of children who develop renal insufficiency in the first years of life was related by Polinsky et al.[208] to aluminum intoxication. In 32 patients studied, aluminum intoxication was certain in 13 and highly probable in 15. This contrasts with the experience of Loirat et al.[209] who found an acceptable intellectual quotient of 89 ± 10% in 13 uremic children, five of whom had never taken $Al(OH)_3$ and six only moderate doses.

Priority should therefore be given to oral calcium taken with meals. The most widely used salt so far is $CaCO_3$. The successful experience of Alon et al.[210] in 12 children with plasma creatinine of 3.7 to 5.1 mg/dL suggests beginning with a dose of 0.1 g/kg/day and introducing 1α-OH vitamin D3 only when plasma phosphate has decreased below 5.5 mg/dL. The dose of $CaCO_3$ can then be increased to 0.3 g/kg/day to maintain normal plasma calcium (10.3 mg/dL) and plasma phosphate (4.2 mg/dL). Urinary calcium must be regularly monitored to prevent hypercalciuria keeping Ca/Cr (mg/mg) <0.21. This experience from Israel is more satisfactory than that of the group Chanlter et al.,[26, 211, 212] who controlled the hyperphosphatemia of 12 children (age 5 to 15 years) with moderate-to-severe renal insufficiency (GFR between 10 and 45 mL/min/1.73 m^2) during 6 months with $Al(OH)_3$ and then with $CaCO_3$ during 6 months or according to the reverse sequence. This study showed that if hyperparathyroidism was effectively controlled (assessed on plasma N terminal PTH levels and bone histomorphometry), the price was aluminic osteomalacia. Therefore these authors conclude their study by recommending to exclude definitively $Al(OH)_3$ and to replace it by $CaCO_3$. In a more recent study, the same team reported its experience with $CaCO_3$ given for 6 to 54 months (mean, 24 months) as exclusive phosphate binder at 97 ± 46 mg/kg/day in 45 children with severe renal failure.[213] Plasma concentrations of PTH and phosphate decreased significantly and GFR remained stable. Side effects were independently reported in a paper by Clark et al.[211] They found that the incidence of hypercalcemia (>2.8 mmol/L) (expressed per 100 patient months) increased with the severity of renal insufficiency: 1.4 when GFR was >15 mL/min, 4 when GFR was between 10 and 15 mL/min, 8.8 when GFR was <10 mL/min, and 48 for patients receiving chronic hemodialysis. Reversible degradation of renal function was observed 29 times during the 47 hypercalcemic episodes. Screening for ectopic calcification with ^{99}Tc pyrophosphate showed only two cases of nephrocalcinosis without other soft tissue calcifications.

When the association of oral 1α-OH vitamin D3 derivatives and $CaCO_3$ induces hypercalcemia, 1α-OH vitamin D3 may be given intramuscularly. This has been tried with success by Trachtman et al.[213a] in two cases of severe renal osteodystrophy in a child of 2½ years and another of 13 years, with GFR of 25 and 16 mL/min, respectively. Doses were 0.3 to 0.6 μg (10 to 20 ng/kg) three times a week in the first and 0.75 to 1.2 μg (10.5 ng/kg and 17 ng/kg) in the second, while both took 1,200 mg of elemental calcium per day.

In Children Receiving Dialysis

In children receiving hemodialysis or CAPD, the principles of treatment of renal osteodystrophy are the same as those in adults.

In dialyzed children, Salusky et al.[214] showed that 5 ± 2.5 g/day (384 ± 315 mg/kg) $CaCO_3$ (i.e., comparable to that in adults) alone kept plasma phosphate at 1.57 ± 0.2 mmol/L and plasma calcium at 2.6 ± 0.12 mmol/L while plasma aluminum decreased from 90 to 34 μg/L. Similar results were obtained in ten children by Andreoli et al.,[214] with a mean dose of 7.4 g/day $CaCO_3$ (318 mg/kg/day). Hypercalcemia occurred in both series (8.8 and 3.1 episodes per 100 patient months) but disappeared after discontinuation or decrease of 1α-OH vitamin D3 derivatives given in association.

As in the adult, decrease in the DCa may be necessary to prevent hypercalcemia with the association of $CaCO_3$ and 1α-OH vitamin D3 derivatives, the latter being given perhaps preferably by intravenous route.[215] The recent long-term experience of Salusky et al.[216] with oral calcitriol in children receiving CAPD is much less optimistic than his first publication.[69] In 13 cases with osteitis fibrosa, the bone lesion persisted in 10. On the other hand, histologic improvement was frank in 4 of 6 cases with initially mild lesions. These observations stress the importance of early treatment.

Let us recall that in children receiving dialysis, predialysis plasma phosphate should be maintained between 4.5 and 5.5 mg/dL if the patient is over 2 years of age and between 5.0 and 6.0 mg/dL if he is under 2 years. This has to be achieved without any aluminum binder since the recent study by Salusky et al.[166b] has definitely shown that even the moderate doses recommended by Sedman[207] induce within one year not only significant aluminum overload but also histological adynamic bone disease, confirming our earlier observations in the adult.[63, 165]

Parathyroidectomy is rarely performed in children because they undergo rapid transplantation. There is no consensus regarding the choice between subtotal parathyroidectomy and total parathyroidectomy with reimplantation. Whatever the technique, a fragment of parathyroid tissue should always be cryopreserved for reimplantation should hypoparathyroidism occur.

Surgical correction of deformities should not be made until hyperparathyroidism is controlled. Children with crippling deformities should be given priority for kidney transplantation because corrective surgery is more reliably performed after transplantation.

Hyperparathyroidism After Kidney Transplantation

Changes in Phosphocalcic Metabolism and Skeleton After Successful Kidney Transplantation

Allowing normalization of phosphate and aluminum retention and restoring the capacity of calcitriol synthesis,[216a] kidney transplantation is theoretically the therapy of choice for renal osteodystrophy. However, although renal function may return to normal, abnormalities of phosphocalcic metabolism may persist and even worsen or appear. Immunosuppressive drugs interfering with bone metabolism complicate the analysis of this complex situation for which no simple experimental model is available.

Hypophosphatemia is the most frequent ionic abnormality encountered after successful kidney transplantation.[216b] In fact mild hypophosphatemia is almost constant in the first month. It is usually transient and explained by high plasma levels of PTH. However one fourth to one third of patients keep hypophosphatemia after the first year, although 20% of them have plasma PTH levels not different from those with no hypophosphatemia.[217] One frequent cause of PTH-independent hypophosphatemia is high doses of corticosteroids, which decrease intestinal absorption of phosphate and, to prevent gastrointestinal ulceration, lead to prescription of antacids, which are all phosphate binders with the exception of aluminum phosphate. However, a renal leak of phosphate with a low reabsorption rate not corrected by calcium infusion has been reported by several authors suggesting a PTH-independent renal phosphate leak.[218] This phosphate diabetes may be functional, related to high doses of steroids or may be part of a complex proximal tubulopathy Fanconi syndrome with associated glycosuria, hyperphosphaturia.[219] Tubular leak of magnesium has been reported in association with cyclosporine and has been incriminated as promoting hyperphosphaturia.[219a] However the persistence of hypophosphatemia after the first year is always associated with high plasma levels of PTH.

Hypercalcemia is also very frequent after kidney transplantation and may be transient or persistent, of early or delayed onset. Initial transient hypercalcemia is usually explained by hypophosphatemia, the mechanisms of which have just been discussed.

The efforts made in patients receiving dialysis to control hyperparathyroidism have decreased the frequency of severe posttransplantation hypercalcemia, seen previously in patients having florid hyperparathyroidism at the time of transplantation. However moderate hypercalcemia related to some degree of parathyroid hyperplasia is usual when steroid dose is decreased. This hypercalcemia subsides spontaneously with gradual normalization of plasma PTH. After successful kidney transplantation, plasma levels of C terminal PTH decrease very rapidly in the first weeks because of normalization of C terminal fragment catabolism whereas plasma levels of intact PTH decrease more slowly. One year after kidney transplantation, plasma levels of intact PTH are still increased in most patients although plasma concentrations of Ca and PO_4 are normal in 50% of cases.[37] The frequency of this residual hyperparathyroidism varies among series. For Ulmann et al.,[220] using a C terminal PTH assay in 1981, it was 100% in a series of 44 patients with transplants for 2 to 238 months.

Several mechanisms are responsible for persistence of hyperparathyroidism:

1. degree of hyperplasia of the parathyroid glands at time of transplantation
2. steroid therapy—steroids reduce calcium intestinal absorption which indirectly stimulates PTH secretion; a recent work on parathyroid cells in culture showed that steroids (dexamethasone) directly stimulate transcription of the prepro-PTH gene, which on the other hand is depressed by calcitriol[221]
3. relative deficiency of calcitriol may also be implicated. Although plasma levels of calcitriol normalize after kidney transplantation for most authors,[218, 222–224] they remain lower than the optimal levels necessary to correct hypophosphatemia. Lucas et al.[224] found that in patients treated with cyclosporine, 25-OH vitamin D3 does not normalize low calcitriol plasma levels. This was confirmed by Graziani et al.[225] in a study comparing two groups of patients with transplants, one receiving cyclosporine, the other azathioprine, since levels of calcitriol were lower in the cyclosporine group. This author found an inverse correlation between plasma concentrations of cyclosporine and variations in plasma calcitriol after an oral load of calcidiol, suggesting direct inhibition of 1α hydroxylase activity by cyclosporine.
4. Finally, successful renal transplantation is never accompanied by recovery of a quite normal GFR and we have seen that a GFR of 60 mL/min may be responsible for a certain degree of hyperparathyroidism.

Plasma alkaline phosphatases decrease rapidly during the month following transplantation because of correction of hyperparathyroidism and of inhibition of osteoblastic activity by steroids. They usually increase again when steroids are decreased.[226] Several authors have reported higher plasma alkaline phosphatases in patients receiving cyclosporine than in those not treated with the drug.[222] This is confirmed by the increase in plasma alkaline phosphatases when cyclosporine is secondarily introduced. The significance of this increase, probably of bone origin since it is correlated with osteocalcin, remains uncertain.[227]

Radiologic bone changes after successful transplantation have been reported to be similar in patients treated with cyclosporine and in those given azathioprine. Since plasma alkaline phosphatases are higher with cyclosporine, it was suggested that this increase was not related to hyperparathyroidism but could indicate accelerated bone repair with cyclosporine. This hypothesis is supported by numerous in vitro studies showing a powerful inhibiting effect of cyclosporine on bone resorption, induced either by lymphokines[228] or by PTH and calcitriol.[229] However the results of in vivo studies on rat skeleton are far from confirming a bone protective effect of cyclosporine. In a first study Movsowitz et al.[230] showed that bone loss with cyclosporine alone is dose-dependent and related to increased bone turnover, whereas in a second study they showed that this deleterious effect of cyclosporine alone is unexpectedly prevented by association of high doses of steroids, probably because of the decrease in bone turnover induced by steroids. These experimental data should be related to comparative histomorphometric data reported by Aubia et al.,[231] showing that patients receiving cyclosporine have higher osteoblastic and osteoclastic activity than those given azathioprine.

Therapeutic Approach

Faced with hypophosphatemia, associated or not with hypercalciuria and hypercalcemia, it is first necessary to exclude iatrogenic causes of phosphate depletion; i.e., gastric antacids that are phosphate binders (Maalox, Ulcar, etc.) with the exception of aluminum phosphate (Phosphalugel). If hypomagnesemia without sufficient hypomagnesuria is present (as seen with cyclosporine), this magnesium depletion must be corrected because it may favor tubular phosphate leak.

Other measures to correct hypophosphatemia are phosphate supplement or administration of calcitriol. The first has the advantage of decreasing frequently associated hypercalciuria and hypercalcemia but may stimulate PTH secretion. It seems to us logical to use it when plasma levels of intact PTH are not frankly elevated (<three times the upper limit of normal), when no ultrasonographic hyperplasia of the parathyroid glands exists, and when renal insufficiency is not related to hypercalcemia. The use of calcitriol seems to us logical when hypophosphatemia is not associated with hypercalciuria or hypercalcemia and when plasma intact PTH levels are elevated.

When hypercalcemia exists with high plasma levels of PTH, the risk with calcitriol is to increase hypercalcemia by increasing calcium intestinal absorption. However we have seen that in the patients receiving dialysis IV calcitriol can decrease transiently plasma calcium by directly suppressing PTH synthesis and thereby decreasing the release of calcium from bone to a greater extent than increasing intestinal calcium absorption. Such an approach has been unsuccessfully tried by Gardin and Foucray,[232] who gave IV calcitriol at 2 μg/day for 2 days and then 4 μg/day for 2 days and observed a decrease in plasma PTH levels from 108 to 70 pg/mL but at the price of an increase in plasma calcium (from 2.79 to 2.93 mmol), (explaining 85% of the decrease in plasma PTH levels).

Thus in practice, surgical parathyroidectomy sometimes remains the only possible treatment for hyperparathyroid hypercalcemia for which phosphate repletion was ineffective or dangerous (increase in plasma creatinine). The prevalence of parathyroidectomy in patients with transplants is however much less than that in patients who continue to receive chronic dialysis: 150 vs. 400 per 1,000 patients after 15 years of renal replacement therapy.[168] The main reason not to postpone parathyroidectomy is to decrease the risk of nephrocalcinosis, lithiasis, and aseptic bone necrosis for which severe hyperparathyroidism is now a well-recognized risk factor.[233]

Conclusion

During the past 10 years, treatment of hyperparathyroidism secondary to renal insufficiency has been marked mainly by recognition of the iatrogenic pathologic conditions induced by aluminum phosphate binders. To respect the adage *Primum non nocere,* this has led us, according to the proposition we made in 1981,[1] to recommend the use of oral calcium not only to counterbalance calcium dietary restriction but also to complex the phosphate thanks to its administration at higher doses during meals. The use of 1α-OH vitamin D3 derivatives is therefore no longer justified by stimulation of active calcium absorption but by their direct suppressive effect on PTH synthesis. This use is however limited by the frequent occurence of hypercalcemia because of the high doses of oral calcium used as phosphate binder. This had led to administering them intermittently as intravenous or oral boluses and to decreasing dialysate calcium concentration in order to induce a negative intradialytic calcium balance. The practical difficulties of such treatment limit, for the present time, its use to severe hyperparathyroidism. On the other hand, oral calcium alone remains the basis of preventive treatment. Much hope is now placed in the future use, in association with oral calcium, of vitamin D derivatives that have no hypercalcemic or hyperphosphatemic effect but have either a direct suppressive effect on PTH secretion as 22-oxacalcitriol or a direct osteoclastic resorption protective effect as 24,25-$(OH)_2$ vitamin D3.

References

1. Fournier A, Moriniere Ph, Coevoet B, et al: Prevention and medical treatment of hypoparathyroidism secondary to renal insufficiency in the adult, in Grunfeld JP (ed): *Advances in Nephrology.* Chicago, Year Book Medical Publishers, 1981.
2. Silver J, Naveh-Many T, Mayer H, et al: Regulation by vitamin D metabolites of parathyroid hormone gene transcription in vivo in the rat. *J Clin Invest* 1986; 78:1296–1301.
3. Naveh-Many T. Friedlander M, Mayer H, et al: Calcium regulates PTH mRNA but not calcitonin mRNA in vivo in the rat. Dominant role of 1,25 (OH)2 vitamin D3. *Endocrinology* 1989; 25:275–280.
4. Naveh-Many T, Silver J: Regulation of parathyroid hormone gene expression by hypocalcemia, hypercalcemia and vitamin D in the rat. *J Clin Invest* 1990; 86:1313–1316.
5. Lambrey G, N'Guyen TM, Sebert JL, et al: Possible link between 24,25

(OH)2 vitamin D3 and healing of bone resorption in dialysis osteodystrophy. *Metab Bone Dis Related Res* 1982; 4:25–30.
6. Morinière Ph, Sebert JL, Sandler L, et al: Plasma levels and biological effects of 25,26(OH)2 vit D3 in uremic patients, in Norman AW (ed): *Vitamin D, Chemical, Biochemical and Clinical Endocrinology of Calcium Metabolism.* Berlin, Walter de Gruyter, 1982, pp 889–892.
7. Lopez Hilker S, Dusso A, Rapp N, et al: Phosphorus restriction reverses hyperparathyroidism in uremia independent of changes in calcium and calcitriol. *Am J Physiol* 1990; 259:432–437.
8. Fournier A, Moriniere PH, Cohen Solal ME, et al: Adynamic bone disease in uremia: May it be idiopathic? Is it an actual disease (editorial). *Nephron* 1991; 58:1–12.
9. Van de Vyver FL, Visser WJ, D'Haese C, et al: Iron overload and bone disease in chronic dialysis patients. *Nephrol Dial Transplantation* 1990; 5:781–787.
10. Cohen Solal ME, Sebert JL, Boudailliez B, et al: Non aluminic adynamic bone disease in non dialyzed uremic patients: A new type of osteopathy due to overtreatment? *Bone,* in press.
11. Slatopolsky E, Lopez-Hilker S, Delmez J, et al: The parathyroid calcitriol axis in health and chronic renal failure. *Kidney Int* 1990; 38:41–47.
12. Delmez JA, Tindra C, Grooms P, et al: Parathyroid hormone suppression by intravenous 1,25 (OH)2 vitamin D. A role for increased sensitivity to calcium. *J Clin Invest* 1989; 83:1349–1355.
13. Dunlay R, Rodriguez M, Felsenfeld MJ, et al: Direct inhibitory effect of calcitriol on parathyroid function (sigmoidal curve) in dialysis. *Kidney Int* 1989; 36:1093–1098.
14. Korkor AB: Reduced binding of ^{3}H 1,25 dihydroxyvitamin D3 in the parathyroid glands of patients with renal failure. *N Engl J Med* 1987, 316:1573–1577.
15. Merke J, Hügel U, Zlotkowski A, et al: Diminished parathyroid 1, 25-$(OH)_2$ vitamin D3 receptors in experimental uremia. *Kidney Int* 1987; 32:350–353.
16. Szabo A, Merke J, Beier E, et al: 1,25(OH)2 vitamin D3 inhibits parathyroid cell proliferation in experimental uremia. *Kidney Int* 1989; 35:1045–1056.
17. Adler AJ, Berlyne GM: Phosphate retention and the genesis of secondary hyperparathyroidism. *Am J Nephrol* 1986; 6:417–421.
18. Bonjour JP: 1,25 dihydroxyvitamin D and phosphate homeostasis in early chronic renal failure: The trade off theory revisited, in Davison AM (ed): *Nephrology.* London, Baillère Tindall, 1988, pp 1059–1066.
19. Ritz E, Seidel A, Szabo A: Disturbed calcium metabolism in early renal failure. Recent progress. *J Nephrol* 1989; 2:229–236.
20. Prince RL, Hutchinson BG, Kent JC, et al: Calcitriol deficiency with retained synthetic reserve in chronic renal failure. *Kidney Int* 1988; 33:722–728.
21. Llach F, Coburn JW: Renal osteodystrophy and maintenance dialysis, in *Replacement of Renal Function by Dialysis.* JF Maher (ed): Dordrecht, Kluwer Academic Publishers, 1989, pp 911–952.
22. Llach F, Massry SG: On the mechanism of secondary hyperparathyroidism in moderate renal failure. *J Clin Endocrinol Metab* 1985; 61:601–606.
23. Portale A, Halleran BP, Morris RC: Physiologic regulation of serum concentration of 1,25 dihydroxyvitamin D by phosphorus in normal men. *J Clin Invest* 1989; 83:1494–1499.

24. Seidel A, Stein O, Ritz E: Do changes in phosphate balance modulate 1,25(OH)2 levels? (abstract). *EDTA Proc Wien* 1990; 281.
25. Portale A, Booth B, Halloran B, et al: Effect of dietary phosphate on circulating concentration of 1,25 dihydroxy vitamin D and immunoreactive parathyroid hormone in children with moderate renal insufficiency. *J Clin Invest* 1984; 73:1580–1589.
26. Turner C, Compston J, Mak RHK, et al: Bone turnover and 1,25 dihydroxycholecalciferol during treatment with phosphate binders. *Kidney Int* 1988; 33:989–995.
27. Lucas PA, Brown RC, Woodhead JS, et al: 1,25 dihydroxycholecalciferol and parathyroid hormone in advanced chronic renal failure: Effect of simultaneous protein and phosphorus restriction. *Clin Nephrol* 1986; 25:7–10.
28. Takamoto S, Onishi T, Morimoto S, et al: Serum phosphate, parathyroid hormone and vitamin D metabolites in patients with chronic renal failure: Effect of aluminium hydroxyde administration. *Nephron* 1985; 40:286–291.
29. Dabbaugh S, Chesney R, Gusowski V, et al: Aminoaciduria of vitamin D deficiency is independent of PTH levels and urinary cyclic AMP. *Min Electrolyte Metab* 1989; 15:221–232.
30. Hsu CH, Patel S: Factors influencing calcitriol metabolism in renal failure. *Kidney Int* 1990; 37:44–50.
31. Hsu CH, Patel S: Effects of polyamines, methylguanidine and guanidinosuccinic acid on calcitriol synthesis. *J Lab Clin Med* 1990; 115:69–73.
32. Sherrard DJ: Aluminum, much ado about something. *N Engl J Med* 1991; 324:558–559.
33. Cohen Solal ME, Boudailliez B, Sebert JL, et al: Comparison of intact, mid region and carboxyterminal assays of parathyroid hormone for the diagnosis of bone disease in hemodialyzed patients. *J Clin Endocrinol Metab,* in press.
34. Morinière Ph, Cohen Solal ME, Belbrik S, et al: Disappearance of aluminic bone disease in a long term asymptomatic dialysis population restricting Al(OH)3: Emergence of an idiopathic adynamic bone disease. *Nephron* 1989; 56:93–101.
35. Clair F, Leenhardt L, Bourdeau A, et al: Effect of calcitriol in the control of plasma calcium after parathyroidectomy. *Nephron* 1987; 46:18–22.
36. Coburn JW, Slatopolsky E: Vitamin D, parathyroid hormone, and the renal osteodystrophies, in Brenner, Rector (eds): *The Kidney*. Philadelphia, WB Saunders, 1991, pp 2036–2120.
37. Fournier A, Boudailliez B, Moriniere Ph, et al: Osteodystrophie rénale in Fournier A, Garabedian M, Sebert JL, et al (eds): Vitamine D et maladie des os et du métabolisme minéral. Paris, Masson, 1984, pp 200–246.
38. Fournier A, Moriniere Ph, Sebert JL: Renal osteodystrophy: General concepts and current issues, in Robinson R (ed): *Nephrology,* New York, Springer Verlag, 1985, pp 1357–1373.
39. Reeves J, Zanelli JM: Parathyroid hormone and bone. *Clin Sci* 1986; 71:231–238.
40. Gordeladze JO, Gautvik KM: Hydroxycholecalciferols modulate parathyroid hormone and calcitonin sensitive adenylcyclase in bone and kidneys in rats. *Biochem Pharmacol* 1986; 35:899–902.
41. Gordeladze JO, Mortensen B, Nordal K, et al: The effect of parathyroid hormone and 24-25 (OH)2 vitamin D3 on adenylcyclase of iliac crest biopsies:

Diagnostic and prognostic interest for evaluation and treatment of uremic patients. *Scand J Clin Lab Invest* 1987; 47:13–20.
42. Malluche M, Faugère MC, Ritz E: Endogenous calcitonin does not protect against hyperparathyroid bone disease in renal failure. *Min Electrolyte Metab* 1984; 12:113–120.
43. Canterbury JM, Lerman S, Clafin AS, et al: Inhibition of parathyroid hormone secretion by 25 hydroxycholecalciferol and 24,25 dihydroxycholecalciferol in the dog. *J Clin Invest* 1978; 61:1375–1383.
44. Canterbury JM, Gavellas G, Reiss A: Effect of dietary calcium on the suppressive effects of 24,25 (OH)2 vitamin D3 on PTH secretion in hyperparathyroid dogs (abstract). *Clin Res* 1982; 30:566.
45. Olgaard K, Finio D, Schwartz J, et al: Effect of 24,25 (OH)2 D3 on PTH levels and bone histology in dogs with chronic uremia. *Kidney Int* 1984; 26:791–797.
46. Main J, Velasco N, Heves SD, et al: The effect of the dihydroxylated metabolites of vitamin D and dietary phosphate restriction on bone disease in uraemic rats. *Clin Sci* 1986; 71:539–543.
47. Mortensen B, Gordeladze JO, Aksnes L, et al: Long term administration of vitamin D3 metabolites alters PTH responsive osteoblastic adenylate cyclase in rats. *Calcif Tissue Int* 1990; 46:339–345.
47a. Klem KH, Jablonski G, Saether O, et al: 1,25 dihydroxyvitamin D3 and 24, 25 dihydroxyvitamin D3 affect parathormone sensitive adenyl cyclase activity and alkaline phosphatase secretion of osteoblactic cells through different mechanisms of action. *Biochem Biophys Acta* 1990, 1054:304–310.
48. Tatsumi J, Kurihara N, Nakashima K: 24 R, 25(OH)2 D3 inhibits fusion of committed precursors for human osteoclast like cells. Eighth workshop on Vitamin D, Paris, July 1991, abstract 325.
49. Rubinger O, Krause I, Popovtzer M: 24,25 (OH)2 D3 blunts the hypercalcemic effect of 1,25(OH)2 D3 by a mechanism independent of intestinal calcium absorption. (abstract). *Kidney Int* 1990; 33:343.
50. Lefebvre A, de Vernejoul MC, Gueris J, et al: Optimal correction of acidosis changes progression of dialysis osteodystrophy. *Kidney Int* 1989; 36:1112–1118.
51. Morinière PH, Boudailliez B, Westeel PF, et al: Place du carbonate de calcium dans le traitement de l'ostéodystrophie rénale. *Nephrologie* 1991; 12:831–841.
52. Fournier A, Idrissi A, Sebert JL, et al: Preventing renal bone disease in moderate renal failure with CaCO3 and 25(OH) vitamin D3. *Kidney Int* 1988; 33(suppl 18):S178–S179.
53. Malluche H, Faugère MC: Renal bone disease 1990: An unmet challenge for the nephrologist. *Kidney Int* 1990; 38:193–211.
54. Andreoli SP, Bergstein JM, Sherrard DJ: Aluminum intoxication from aluminum-containing phosphate binders in children with azotemia not undergoing dialysis. *N Engl J Med* 1984; 310:1079–1084.
55. Fournier A, Moriniere PH, Boudailliez B: 1,25 (OH)2 vit D3 deficiency and renal osteodystrophy: Should its well-accepted pathogenetic role in secondary hyperparathyroidism lead to its systematic preventive therapeutic use? *Nephrol Dial Transplantation* 1987; 2:498–503.
56. Fournier A, Moriniere Ph, Boudailliez B, et al: Recent advances in the treatment of renal osteodystrophy. in Andreucci A (ed): *International Year Book of Nephrology*. Boston, Kluwer, 1990, pp 185–214.

57. Llach F, Felsenfeld AJ, Coleman MD: The natural course of dialysis osteomalacia. *Kidney Int* 1986; 29:74–79.
58. Coburn JW: Use of oral and parenteral calcitriol in the treatment of renal osteodystrophy. *Kidney Int* 1990; 38(suppl 29):S14–S21.
59. Adler AJ, Berlyne GM: Duodenal aluminum absorption in the rat. Effect of vitamin D. *Am J Physiol* 1985; 249:209–213.
60. Demontis R, Westal PF, Morinière Ph, et al: 1alpha (OH) vitamin D3 increases plasma aluminum in hemodialysed patients taking Al(OH)3. *Kidney Int* 1988; 33(suppl 24):S175–S177.
61. Demontis R, Reissi D, Noel C, et al: Indirect clinical evidence that 1αOH vitamin D3 increases the intestinal absorption of aluminum. *Clin Nephrol* 1989; 31:123–127.
62. Morinière Ph, Roussel A, Tahiri Y, et al: Substitution of Al(OH)3 by high doses of CaCO3 in patients on chronic hemodialysis: Disappearance of hyperaluminemia and equal control of hyperparathyroidism. *Proc EDTA* 1982; 19:784–787.
63. Sebert JL, Fournier A, Leflon P, et al: Comparative evaluation of bone aluminium content and bone histology in patients on chronic hemodialysis and hemofiltration. *Nephron* 1986; 42:34–40.
64. Merke J, Lucas P, Szabo A, et al: 1,25(OH)2 D3 receptors and end organ response in experimental aluminium intoxication. *Kidney Int* 1987; 32:204–211.
65. Cannata Audia J, Diaz Lopez JB: The diagnosis of aluminum toxicity, in de Broe ME, Coburn JW (eds): *Aluminum and Renal Failure.* Dordrecht, Kluwer Academic Publishers, 1990, pp 287–308.
66. Zins B, Petitclerc T, Basile C: Tumoral calcinosis in hemodialysis patients: Role of aluminum (abstract). *Kidney Int* 1989; 35:267.
67. Roullet JB, Haluska M, Morchoisne O, et al: 1,25 (OH)2 vitamin D3 induced alteration of lipid metabolism in human monocyte macrophage. *Am J Physiol* 1989; 257:290–295.
68. Milliner DS, Zinsmeister AR, Lieberman L, et al: Soft tissue calcification in pediatric patients with end stage renal disease. *Kidney Int* 1990; 38:931–936.
69. Salusky IB, Fine R, Kangarlov H, et al: High dose calcitriol for control of renal osteodystrophy in children on CAPD. *Kidney Int* 1987; 32:89–95.
70. Clarkson EM, McDonald SJ, de Wardener HE: The effect of high intake of calcium carbonate in normal subjects and patients with chronic renal failure. *Clin Sci* 1966; 30:425–438.
71. Fournier A, Idrissi A, Sebert JL, et al: Prévention de l'ostéodystrophie rénale des insuffisants rénaux modérés par le CaCO3 à des doses non hypercalcémiantes et le calcifédiol, in Legrain M (ed): *Séminaires d'Uronéphrologie.* Paris, Masson, 1985, pp 166–181.
72. Fournier A, Moriniere Ph, Sebert JL: Calcium carbonate, an aluminum free agent for control of hyperphosphatemia, hypocalcemia and hyperparathyroidism in uremia. *Kidney Int* 1986; 18:114–119.
73. Bordier PJ, Tunchot S, Eastwood JD: Lack of histological evidence of vitamin D abnormality in the bones of anephric patients. *Clin Sci* 1973; 44:33–41.
74. Schiller LR, Santa Ana C, Sheikh MS, et al: Effect of the time of administration of calcium acetate on phosphorus binding. *N Engl J Med* 1989; 320:1110–1113.

75. Deleted in proofs.
76. Morinière Ph, Fournier A, Leflon A, et al: Comparison of 1 α OH vitamin D3 and high doses of calcium carbonate for the control of hyperparathyroidism and hyperaluminemia in patients on maintenance dialysis. *Nephron* 1985; 39:309–315.
77. Addison JF, Foulks CG: Calcium carbonate: An effective phosphate binder in patients with chronic renal failure. *Curr Ther Res* 1985; 38:241–249.
78. Monnier N, Bournerias F, Reveillaud RJ: Hemodialyse à long terme sans aluminium. in Traeger J (ed): *Survie à Long Terme des Hémiodalyés*. Paris, Gambro Publisher, 1986, pp 155–158.
79. Slatopolsky E, Weerts C, Lopez-Hilker S, et al: Calcium carbonate as a phosphate binder in patients with chronic renal failure undergoing dialysis. *N Engl J Med* 1986; 315:157–161.
80. Hercz G, Kraut J, Andress DA: Use of calcium carbonate as a phosphate binder in dialysis patients. *Miner Electrolyte Metab* 1981; 12:314–319.
81. Mactier RA, Vanstone M, Twaroowski Z: Calcium carbonate is an effective phosphate binder when dialyzate calcium concentration is adjusted to control hypercalcemia. *Clin Nephrol* 1987; 28:222–226.
82. Sawyer N, Noonan K, Altman P: High dose calcium carbonate with stepwise reduction in dialysate calcium concentration: effective phosphate control and aluminium avoidance in haemoidialysis patients. *Nephrol Dial Transplantation* 1989; 4:105–109.
83. Slatopolsky E, Windus D, Norwood K, et al: Short term comparison of calcium carbonate and calcium acetate in hemodialysis patients treated with 2.5 mEq/L calcium dialysate (abstract). *J Am Soc Nephrol* 1990; 1:378.
84. Malberti F, Montoli A, Surian M: Long term effect of low calcium dialysate on parathyroid activity in dialysis patients treated with calcium carbonate as a phosphate binder. *Nephrol Dial Transplantation* 1989; 4:758–759.
85. Nolan CR, Califano JR, Butzin CA: Influence of calcium acetate or calcium citrate on intestinal aluminum absorption. *Kidney Int* 1990; 38:937–941.
86. Schaefer K, Von Herrath D, Asmus G, et al: The beneficial effect of ketoacid on serum phosphate and parathyroid hormone in patients with chronic uremia. *Clin Nephrol* 1988; 30:93–96.
87. Schaefer K, Von Herrath D, Erley CM, et al: Calcium ketovaline as new therapy for uremic hyperphosphatemia. *Miner Electrolyte Metab* 1990; 16:362–364.
88. Sheikh MS, Maguire JA, Emmett M, et al: Reduction of dietary phosphorus absorption by phosphate binders: A theoretical in vitro and in vivo study. *J Clin Invest* 1989; 83:66–73.
89. Mai L, Emmett M, Sheikh M: Calcium acetate an effective phosphorus binder in patients with renal failure. *Kidney Int* 1989; 36:690–695.
90. Morinière Ph, Djerad M, Boudailliez B, et al: Control of predialytic hyperphosphatemia by oral calcium carbonate: Comparable efficacy for half the dose elemental calcium given as acetate without lower incidence of hypercalcemia. *Nephron,* in press.
91. Schaefer K, Scheer J, Asmus G: The effect of calcium acetate and calcitriol on the calcium and phosphorus metabolism in hemodialysis patients (abstract). *J Am Soc Nephrol* 1990; 1:581.
92. Tielemans C, Knoop C, Doutrelemont JM, et al: Superiority of calcium acetate over carbonate to bind phosphorus in hemodialysis patient (abstract). *Proceed ISN* 1990; 219.

93. Meric F, Yap P, Bia MJ: Etiology of hypercalcemia in hemodialysis patients on calcium carbonate therapy. *Am J Kidney Dis* 1990; 16:459–464.
94. Morinière Ph, Fournier A, Westeel PF, et al: Calcium Carbonate and magnesium hydroxide in the prevention of renal osteodystrophy or the demise of aluminium toxicity in uremia, in de Broe (ed): *Bone and Renal Insufficiency. Contrib Nephrol* 1988; 64:58–73.
95. Morinière PH, Boudailliez B, Hocine Ch, et al: Prevention of osteitis fibrosa, aluminium bone disease and soft tissues calcification in dialysis patients: A long term comparison of moderate doses of oral calcium ± Mg(OH)2 versus Al(OH)3 ± 1 alpha OH vitamin D3. *Nephrol Dial Transplantation* 1989; 4:1045–1053.
96. O'Donnovan R, Monitz C, Baldwin D, et al: Control of hyperphosphatemia by oral magnesium carbonate on zero magnesium dialyzate without aluminium binders. *Lancet* 1986; 1:880–881.
97. Morinière P, Vinatier I, Westeel PF, et al: Magnesium hydroxide as a complementary aluminum free phosphate-binder of high doses of oral calcium in uremic patients on chronic hemodialysis. Lack of deleterious effect on bone mineralization. *Nephrol Dial Transplantation* 1988; 3:651–656.
98. Slatopolsky E, Weerts C, Norwood K: Long-term effects of CaCO3 and 2.5 mEq/L calcium dialysate on mineral metabolism in haemodialysis patients. *Kidney Int* 1989; 36:897–903.
99. Hutchinson AJ, Gokal R: Low calcium dialysis fluid and oral calcium carbonate in control of serum calcium and phosphate in CAPD (abstract). Proceedings, Singapore Symposium on Renal Bonde Disease, July 1990.
100. Kaye M, Barber E, Vasilevsky M, et al: Calcium-free dialyzate: Development and application. *Clin Nephrol* 1989; 31:132–138.
101. Kaye M, Barber B: Maintenance of a negative calcium balance during hemodialysis by the use of a calcium free dialysate and a low calcium infusion rate (abstract). *J Bone Miner Res* 1990; 5:102.
102. Berland Y, Charbit M, Henry JF, et al: Aluminum overload of parathyroid glands in haemodialyzed patients with hyperparathyroidism: Effect on bone remodeling. *Nephrol Dial Transplantation* 1988; 3:417–422.
103. Morinière Ph, Maurouard C, Boudailliez B, et al: Prevention of hyperparathyroidism in patients on maintenance dialysis by intravenous 1 α OH vitamin D3 in association with Mg (OH)2 as sole phosphate binder. A randomized comparative study with the association CaCO3 ± Mg(OH)2. *Nephron,* in press.
104. Morinière Ph, Hocine C, Boudailliez B, et al: Long term efficacy and safety of oral calcium as compared to Al(OH)3 as phosphate binders. *Kidney Int* 1989; 36:(suppl 27):S133–S135.
105. Curtis JR, de Wardener HE, Gower PE: The use of CaCO3 and phosphate without vitamin D in the management of renal osteodystrophy. *Proceed EDTA* 1970; 7:141–145.
106. Deleted in proofs.
107. Deleted in proofs.
108. Meyrier A, Marsac J, Richet G: The influence of a high Ca CO3 intake on bone disease in patients undergoing haemodialysis. *Kidney Int* 1973; 4:146–153.
109. Renaud H, Atik A, Hervé M, et al: Evaluation of vascular calcinosis risk in patients on chronic haemodialysis. Lack of influence of CaCO3 doses. *Nephron* 1988; 48:28–32.

110. Nichols P, Owen JP, Ellish A, et al: Parathyroidectomy in chronic renal failure: A nine year follow-up study. *Q J Med* 1990; 77:1175–1193.
111. Fournier A, Bordier Ph, Gueris J, et al: Comparison of 1α hydroxycholecalciferol and 25 OH cholecalciferol in the treatment of renal osteodystrophy: greater effect of 25 OH cholecalciferol on bone mineralization. *Kidney Int* 1979; 15:196–204.
112. Hollis BW, Jacob AI, Salman A, et al: Circulating vitamin D and its photoproduction in uremia, in Norman AW (ed): *Vitamin D, Chemical, Biochemical and Clinical Endocrinology of Calcium Metabolism.* Berlin, Walter de Gruyter, 1982; pp 1157–1160.
113. Lambert PW, de Oreo PB: Urinary and plasma vitamin D3 metabolites in the nephrotic syndrom. *Metab Bone Dis Related Res* 1982; 4:7–15.
114. Bucciani G, Bianchi MR, Valenti G, et al: Effect of calcifidiol treatment on the progression of renal osteodystrophy during continuous ambulatory peritoneal dialysis. *Nephron* 1990; 56:353–356.
115. Gokal R, Ramos JM, Ellis HA, et al: Histological renal osteodystrophy and 25 OH cholecalciferol and aluminum levels in patients on CAPD. *Kidney Int* 1983; 23:15–21.
116. Delmez JA, Fallon MD, Bergfeld MA, et al: Continuous ambulatory peritoneal dialysis and bone. *Kidney Int* 1986; 30:379–384.
117. Pierides AM, Ellis HA, Ward M, et al: Barbiturate and anticonvulsant treatment in relation to osteomalacia with haemodialysis and renal transplantation. *Br Med J* 1976, i:190–193.
118. Christiansen C, Rodbro P, Christensen MS, et al: Deterioration of renal function during treatment of chronic renal failure with 1,25 (OH)2D3 *Lancet* 1978; i:700–703.
119. Massry SG: Assessment of 1,25(OH)2 D3 in the correction and prevention of renal osteodystrophy in patients with mild to moderate renal failure, in Norman, Schaefer, Grigoleit (eds): *Vitamin D, Chemical Biochemical and Clinical Update.* Berlin, de Gruyter, 1985, pp 936–937.
119a. Coen G, Mezzaferro S, Bonucci E, et al: Treatment of secondary hyperparathyroidism of predialysis chronic renal failure with low doses of 1,25(OH)2 D3: Humoral and histomorphometric results. *Miner Electrolyte Metab* 1986; 12:375–382.
120. Baker LRJ, Abram S, Roe C, et al: 1,25 (OH)2 vitamin D3 administration in moderate renal failure: A prospective double blind trial. *Kidney Int* 1989; 35:661–669.
121. Nordal KP, Dalh E: Low dose calcitriol versus placebo in patients with predialysis renal failure. *J Clin Endocrinol Metab* 1988; 67:929–936.
122. Bertoli M, Luisetto G, Ruffati A, et al: Renal function during calcitriol therapy in chronic renal failure. *Clin Nephrol* 1990; 33:98–102.
123. Reichel H, Ritz E: Workshop on vitamin D and analogues in the treatment of renal osteodystrophy (videotape). EDTA, Vienna, 1990.
124. Coburn JW: Use of oral and parenteral calcitriol in the treatment of renal osteodystrophy. *Kidney Int* 1990; 38(suppl 29):S54–S61.
125. Deleted in proofs.
126. Peacock M (ed): The clinical use of 1α hydroxy vitamin D3. *Clin Endocrinol* 1977; 7(suppl).
127. Berl T, Berns AS, Huffer WE, et al: 1,25(OH)2D3 effects in chronic dialysis. *Ann Intern Med* 1978; 88:774–780.
128. Fournier A, Bordier Ph, Bedrossian J, et al: Effects of phosphate binders on

bone formation and resorption in patients on chronic hemodialysis with and without kidneys, in Norman-Schaeffer-Grigoleit (ed): *Vitamin D and Problems to Uremic Bone Disease.* Berlin, Walter de Gruyter Publishers, 1975, pp 576–584.

129. Slatopolsky E, Weerts C, Thielan J, et al: Marked suppression of secondary hyperparathyroidism by intravenous administration of 1,25(OH)2D3 in uremic patients. *J Clin Invest* 1984; 74:2136–2143.
130. Hamdy NAT, Brown CB, Kanis JA: Intravenous calcitriol lowers serum calcium concentration in uraemic patients with severe hyperparathyroidism and hypercalcemia. *Nephrol Dial Transplantation* 1989; 4:545–548.
130a. Andress DL, Norris KC, Coburn JW, et al: Intravenous calcitriol in the treatment of refractory osteitis fibrosa of chronic renal failure. *N Engl J Med* 1989; 321:274–279.
131. Fournier A, Moriniere PH, Boudailliez B, et al: Calcitriol for osteitis fibrosa. *N Engl J Med* 1989; 321:1831–1832.
132. Gallieni M, Brancaccio O, Padovese P, et al: Clinical effects of low dose intravenous calcitriol in 83 hemodialysis patients with mild to severe hyperparathyroidism (abstract). Proceedings, Singapore symposium on renal bone disease, July 1990.
133. Laut J, Dressier R, Lynn R, et al: Intravenous calcitriol therapy for secondary hyperparathyroidism in patients with ESRD (abstract). Proceedings, Singapore symposium on renal bone disease, July 1990.
134. Brandi L, Daugaard H, Tvedegaard E, et al: Effect of intravenous 1 alpha hydroxyvitamin D3 on secondary hyperparathyroidism in chronic uremic patients on maintenance dialysis. *Nephron* 1989; 53:194–200.
135. Ljunghall S, Althoff Y, Fellström B, et al: Effects on serum parathyroid hormone of intravenous treatment with alpha calcidiol in patients on chronic hemodialysis. *Nephron* 1990; 55:380–385.
136. Morinière PH, Viron B, Judith D, et al: New approach of the treatment of secondary hyperparathyroïdism in haemodialyzed patients combining IV 1 alpha OH vitamin D3, calcium carbonate and low calcium dialysate (abstract). Eighth Workshop on Vitamin D, Paris, 1991.
137. Brandi L, Daugaard H, Egsmose C, et al: Oral treatment of secondary hyperparathyroidism in patients on chronic hemodialysis after marked suppression of PTH secretion by previous intravenous administration of 1 α OHD3 (abstract). Proceedings, Singapore Symposium on renal bone disease, July 1990.
138. Fukagawa M, Okazaki R, Takanu K, et al: Regression of parathyroid hyperplasia by calcitriol pulse therapy in patient on long term dialysis. *N Engl J Med* 1990; 323:421.
139. Tsukamoto Y, Nomura M, Takahashi Y, et al: The oral 1,25-Dihydroxyvitamin D3 pulse therapy in hemodialysis patients with severe secondary hyperparathyroidism. *Nephron* 1991; 57:23–28.
140. Akaziwa T, Koshikawa S, Ogura Y, et al: Oral pulses of 1αOHD suppresses PTH in refractory patients with secondary hyperparathyroidism (abstract). Proceedings, Singapore symposium on renal blood disease, July 1990.
141. Van der Merwe WH, Rodger RS, Grant AC, et al: Low calcium dialysate and high dose oral calcitriol in the treatment of secondary hyperparathyroidism in haemodialysis patients. *Nephrol Dialy Transplantation* 1990; 5:874–877.
142. Memmos DE, Eastwood JB, Talner LB, et al: Double blind trial of oral 1,25

(OH)2 vitamin D3 versus placebo in asymptomatic hyperparathyroidism in patients receiving maintenance haemodialysis. *Br Med J* 1981; 282:1919–1924.

143. Coburn, JW, Di Domenico NC, Byrce CF, et al: Use of calcitriol in prophylaxis of bone disease in dialysis patients: A prospective double blind study (abstract). *Kidney Int* 1983; 23:145.
144. Baker LRJ, Muir JW, Sharman VL, et al: Controlled trial of calcitriol in hemodialysis patients. *Clin Nephrol* 1986; 26:185–191.
145. Sebert JL, Fournier A, Gueris J, et al: Limit by hyperphosphatemia of the usefulness of vitamin D metabolites (1 α OH calcitriol and 25 OH calcitriol) in the treatment of renal osteodystrophy. *Metab Bone Dis Related Res* 1980; 2:217–222.
146. Coevoet B, Morinière Ph, Sebert JL, et al: 1,25 dihydroxycholecalciferol in infraradiological dialysis osteodystrophy: Cure of osteomalacia variable response to resorption depending on phosphate control, in Cohn DV (ed): *Hormonal Control of Calcium Metabolism.* Amsterdam, Excerpta Medica, 1981.
147. Ruedin P, Rizzoli R, Slosman D, et al: Bone mineral density in patients with terminal chronic renal failure: A prospective controlled study on the effects of calcitriol therapy (abstract). *Am Soc Nephrol* 1990; 1:573.
148. Deleted in proofs.
149. Okada K, Takamashi S, Yanai M, et al: Treatment of secondary hyperparathyroidism in patients with chronic renal failure at the predialytic stage and while on dialysis. Proceedings, Singapore Symposium on Renal Bone Disease, July 1990.
150. Muirhead N, Adami S, Sandler LM, et al: Long term effects of 1,25 dihydroxy vitamin D3 and 24,25 dihydroxy vitamin D3 in renal osteodystrophy. *Q J Med* 1982; 51:427–444.
151. Hodsman AB, Wong EGG, Sherrard DJ: Preliminary trial with 24,25 dihydroxy vitamin D3 in dialysis osteomalacia. *Am J Med* 1983; 74:407–417.
152. Dunstan CR, Mills E, Norman AW, et al: Treatment of haemodialysis bone disease with 24,25(OH)2D3 and 1,25(OH)2D3 alone or in combination. *Miner Electrolyte Metab* 1989; 11:358–368.
153. Van Diemen-Steenvoorde R, Donckerwolcke RA, Bosch R, et al: Treatment of renal osteodystrophy in children with dihydrotrachysterol and 24,25(OH)2 vitamin D3. *Clin Nephrol* 1985; 24:292–299.
154. Mortensen B, Klein KH, Jablonski G, et al: A permissive role of 24,25(OH)2 vitamin D3 in treatment of renal osteodystrophy (abstract). *Calcif Tissue Int* 1990; 46:56.
155. Popovtzer M: The future of 24,25(OH)2 D in the treatment of uremic bone disease (abstract). Proceedings, Singapore Symposium on Renal Bone Disease. July 1990.

155a. Brown AJ, Ritter CR, Finch JL, et al: The noncalcemic analogue of vitamin D 22-oxacalcitriol suppresses parathyroid hormone synthesis and secretion. *J Clin Invest* 1989; 84:728–732.

156. Cundy T, Kanis JA, Heynen C, et al: Deterioration of renal bone disease in patients treated with salmon calcitonin. *Clin Endocrinol* 1982; 16:29–37.
157. Yap AS, Hockings GI, Flemming SJ, et al: Use of amino-hydroxypopylidene biphosphate (APD) for the treatment of hypercalcemia in patients with renal impairment. *Clin Nephrol* 1990; 34:225–229.
158. Hené RJ, Visser WJ, Duursma A, et al: No effect of APD (Aminohydroxy-

prolene Biphosphonate) on hypercalcemia in patients with renal osteodystrophy. *Bone* 1990; 11:15–20.
159. Hamdy NAT, Mc Closkey EU, Brown CB, et al: Effects of clodronate in severe hyperparathyroid bone disease in chronic renal failure. *Nephron* 1990; 56:6–12.
160. Zucchelli P, Catizone L, Casanovas S, et al: Therapeutic effects of 25 OH cholecalciferol and sodium etidronate on renal osteodystrophy. *Min Electrolyte Metab* 1982; 7:86–96.
161. Zingraf J, Bourdeau A, Clais F, et al: Hypocalcaemic effect of WR 2721, 5-2 63-Aminopropylaminol Ethyl-phosphorothioic acid in an anuric haemodialysis patient. *Nephrol Dial Transplantation* 1987; 2:48–52.
162. Saksi S: Parathyroidectomie pour hyperparathyroïde des hémodialysés. Mémoire pour le DIS de Néphrologie, Université de Lille II, 1991.
163. Aparicio M, Gin H, Merville P, et al: Parathormone activity and rate of progression of chronic renal failure in patients on low protein diet. *Nephron* 1990; 56:333–334.
164. Aparicio M, Lafage MH, Combe C, et al: Low protein diet and renal osteodystrophy. *Nephron,* in press.
165. Fröhling PT, Kokot F, Schmicker R, et al: Influence of ketoacids on serum parathyroïd hormone levels in patients with chronic renal failure. *Clin Nephrol* 1983; 20:212–217.
166. Lindenau K, Benoroth K, Kokot F, et al: Therapeutic effect of ketoacids on renal osteodystrophy. *Nephron* 1990; 55:133–135.
166a. Sebert JL, Marie A, Gueris J, et al: Assessment of the aluminum overload and of its possible toxicity in asymptomatic uremic patients: Evidence for a depressive effect on bone formation. *Bone* 1985; 6:373–375.
166b. Salusky IB, Foley J, Nelson P, et al: Aluminum accumulation during treatment with aluminum hydroxide and dialysis in children and young adults with chronic renal failure. *N Engl J Med* 1991; 324:527–531.
167. Llach F: Parathyroidectomy in chronic renal failure: indications, surgical approach and the use of calcitriol. *Kidney Int* 1990; 38:62–68.
168. Brunner FP: Combined report on regular dialysis and transplantation in Europe. *Nephrol Dial Transplant* 1991; 6(suppl 1):28–31.
169. Milliner DS, Nebeker HG, Ott JM, et al: Use of the deferoxamine infusion test in the diagnosis of aluminum related osteodystrophy. *Ann Intern Med* 1984; 101:775–780.
170. Chazan JA, Libbey NP, London MR, et al: The clinical spectrum of renal osteodystrophy in 57 hemodialysis patients: A correlation between biochemical parameters and bone pathology findings. *Clin Nephrol* 1991; 35:78–85.
171. De Vernejoul MC, Marchais S, London G, et al: Deferoxamine test and bone disease in dialysis patients with mild aluminum accumulation. *Am J Kidney Dis* 1989; 14:124–130.
171a. Malluche H, Smith AJ, Abeo K, et al: The use of deferoxamine in the management of aluminum accumulation in bone in patients with renal failure. *N Engl J Med* 1984; 311:140–144.
171b. Johnson WJ, McCarthy JT, Van Meerden JA, et al: Results of subtotal parathyroidectomy in hemodialysis patients. *Am J Med* 1988; 84:23–32.
171c. Felsenfeld AJ, Rodriguez M, Coleman M, et al: Deferrioxamine therapy in hemodialysis patients with aluminum-associated bone disease. *Kidney Int* 1989; 35:1371–1378.

172. Frame B, Jackson CE, Reynolds WA, et al: Hypercalcemia and skeletal effects in chronic hypervitaminosis A. *Am J Med* 1974, 80:44–48.
173. Moreau JF, Chigot JP, de Feraudy MN, et al: Ultrasonographie parathyroidienne Pré-opératoire. *Presse Med* 1987; 16:804–807.
174. Edis AJ, Evans Jr TC: High resolution realtime ultrasonography in the preoperative location of parathyroid tumors. *N Engl J Med* 1979; 301:532–534.
175. Roses DF, Sudarsky LA, Sanger J, et al: The use of preoperative localization of adenomas of the parathyroid glands by thallium-technicium subtraction scintigraphy, high-resolution ultrasonography and computed tomography. *Surg Gynecol Obstet* 1989; 168:99–106.
176. Scheible W, Deutsch AL, Leopold GR: Parathyroid adenoma: accuracy of preoperative localization by high-resolution real-time sonography. *J Clin Ultrasound* 1981; 9:325–330.
177. Brzac HT, Pavlovic D, Halbauer M, et al: Parathyroid sonography in secondary hyperparathyroidism: Correlation with clinical findings. *Nephrol Dial Transplantation* 1989; 4:45–50.
178. Morinière Ph, Tyan P, Fournier A, et al: Exploration ultrasonographique à haute résolution en temps réel de 60 hémodialysés chroniques. Résultats préliminaires et comparaison avec les autres indices d'hyperparathyroïdie secondaire. *Nephrologie* 1983; 4:135–140.
179. Moreau JF, Chenesseau B, Horviller S, et al: Hyperparathyroïdies persistantes ou récurrentes des hémodialysés périodiques. Intérêt de l'échographie cervicale pré-opératoire. Six observations. *Presse Med* 1986; 15: 1920–1923.
180. Karsenty G, Petraglia A, Bourdeau A, et al: Evaluation of parathyroid autograft growth and function in hemodialysis patients. *Am J Kidney Dis* 1986; 8:43–50.
181. Gooding GAW, Okerlund MD, Stark DD: Parathyroid imaging: Comparison of double tracer (T1-201, Tc-99m) scintigraphy and high-resolution US. *Radiology* 1986; 161:57–61.
182. Stark DD, Gooding GAW, Moss AA: Parathyroid imaging: Comparison of high resolution CT and high-resolution sonography. *AJR* 1983; 141:633–638.
183. Charboneau JW, Grant SC, James EM, et al: High resolution ultrasound-guided percutaneous needle biopsy and intraoperative ultrasonography of a cervical parathyroid adenoma in a patient with persistent hyperparathyroidism. *Mayo Clin Proc* 1983; 58:497–500.
183a. Solbiati L, Montali G, Croce F, et al: Parathyroid tumors detected by fine-needle aspiration biopsy under ultrasonic guidance. *Radiology* 1983; 148:793–797.
184. Mincione Borelli D, Cicchi P, Ipponi LP, et al: Fine-needle aspiration cytology of parathyroid adenoma, a review of seven cases. *Acta Cytol* 1986; 30:65–69.
185. Proye C, Carnaille B, Sanher A: Hyperparathyroïdie chez l'insuffisant rénal: PTX sub-totale ou PTX totale avec autotransplantation. Expérience suivie de 121 observations. *J Chir* 1990; 127:136–140.
186. Kaye M: Parathyroid surgery in renal failure. A review. *Semin Dialy* 1988; 3:86–92.
186a. Dubost C, Drüeke T: Comparison of subtotal PTX with total PTX and autotransplantation, in Kaplan EL (ed): *Clinical Surgery International. Surgery of*

the Thyroid and Parathyroid Glands. Edinburgh, Churchill Livingstone, 1983, pp 253–261.

187. Ellis HA: Fate of long-term parathyroid autografts in patients with chronic renal failure treated by parathyroidectomy: a histopathological study of autografts, parathyroid gland and bone. *Histopathology* 1988; 13:289–309.
188. Wallfelt Ch, Larsson R, Gylfe E, et al: Secretory disturbance in hyperplastic parathyroid nodules of uremic hyperparathyroidism: Implication for parathyroid autotransplantation. *World J Surg* 1988; 12:431–438.
189. Klempa I, Rottger P, Schneider M, et al: Transplantat-Hyperparathyreoidismus: Tumorähnliches Wachstum und autonome Funktion menschlicher Autotransplantate von hyperplastischen Epithelkörperchen. Naligus. *Arch Chir* 1982; 356:191–204.
190. Korzets Z, Magen H, Kraus L, et al: Total parathyroidectomy with autotransplantation: Should it be abandoned? *Nephrol Dial Transplantation* 1987; 2:341–346.
191. McKeown PP, McGarity WC, Sewell LW: Carcinoma of the parathyroid gland: Is it overdiagnosed? *Am J Surg* 1984; 147:292–298.
192. White JV, Lo Gerfo P, Feind C, et al: Autologous parathyroid transplantation. *Lancet* 1983; 2:461.
192a. Dubost C, Zingraff J, Drüeke TB: Total parathyroidectomy with autotransplantation in haemodialysed patients: Should it be abondoned (letter)? *Nephrol Dial Transplantation* 1988; 3:356.
193. Tagagi H, Tominaga Y, Yanaka Y, et al: Treatment of renal hyperparathyroidism by total parathyroidectomy with forearm autografts. Proceedings, Singapore Symposium on renal bone disease (abstract). July 1990.
194. Basile C, Drüeke T, Lacour B, et al: Total parathyroidectomy and delayed parathyroid autotransplantation using a simplified cryopreservation technique: Human and animal studies. *Am J Kidney Dis* 1984; 3:366–370.
195. Wells SA, Christiansen C: The transplanted parathyroid gland: Evaluation of cryopreservation and other environmental factors which affect its function. *Surgery* 1974; 75:49–55.
196. Ogg CS: Total parathyroidectomy in the treatment of secondary (renal) hyperparathyroidism. *Br Med J* 1967; 4:331–334.
197. Kaye M, D'Amour P, Henderson J: Elective total parathyroidectomy without autotransplant in end-stage renal disease. *Kidney Int* 1989; 35:1390–1399.
198. Farrington K, Varghese Z, Chan MK, et al: How complete is total parathyroidectomy in uraemia? *Br Med J* 1987; 294:743.
199. Hayes JF, Cross GF, Schuman ES: Surgical management of renal hyperparathyroidy in the dialysis patient. *Am J Surg* 1982; 143:569–571.
200. Diez J, Fernandes J, Lacour B, et al: Increased potassium permeability in erythrocytes from patients with hyperparathyroidism. *Horm Metab Res* 1986; 18:642–646.
201. Soliman AR, Akmal M, Massry SG: Parathyroid hormone interferes with extrarenal disposition of potassium in chronic renal failure. *Nephron* 1989; 52:262–267.
201a. Urena P, Basile C, Grateau G, et al: Short-term effects of parathyroidectomy on plasma biochemistry in chronic uremia: A prospective study. *Kidney Int* 1989; 36:120–126.
202. Charboneau JW, Hay ID, van Heerden JA: Persistent primary hyperparathyroidism: Successful ultrasound-guided percutaneous ethanol ablation of an occult adenoma. *Mayo Clin Proc* 1988; 63:913–919.

203. Giangrande A, Castiglioni A, Solbiati L, et al: US-guided percutaneous fine-needle ethanol injection into parathyroid glands in secondary hyperparathyroidism (soumis pour publication).
204. Solbiati L, Giangrande A, De Pra L, et al: Percutaneous ethanol injection of parathyroid tumors under US guidance: Treatment for secondary hyperparathyroidism. *Radiology* 1985; 155:607–610.
205. Pallota JA, Sacks BA, Moller DE: Arteriographic ablation of cervical parathyroid adenomas. *J Clin Endocrinol Metab* 1989; 69:1249–1255.
206. Mehls O, Salusky B: Recent advances and controversies in childhood renal osteodystrophy. *Pediatr Nephrol* 1987; 1:212–223.
206a. Boudaillez B, Bony H, Berquin P, et al: Osteódystrophie rénale de l'enfant; Rôle pathogénique et modalités de contrôle de la rétention phosphatée. *Arch Pediatr* 1991; 48:279–286.
207. Sedman AB, Miller NL, Warady BA: Aluminum loading in children with chronic renal failure. *Kidney Int* 1984; 26:201–204.
208. Polinsky MS, Kaiser BA, Stover JB: Neurological development of children with severe renal failure from infancy. *Pediatr Nephrol* 1987; 1:157–165.
209. Loirat C, Guillemont G, Pillion G, et al: Intellectual development of children with severe chronic renal insufficiency in infancy (abstract). *Pediatr Nephrol* 1988; 2:121.
210. Alon U, Davidai G, Bentur L: Oral calcium carbonate as phosphate binder in infants and children with chronic renal failure. *Miner Electrolyte Metab* 1986; 12:320–325.
211. Clark AG, Ward G, Turner C, et al: Safety and efficacy of calcium carbonate in children with chronic renal failure. *Nephrol Dial Transplantation* 1989; 4:539–544.
212. Mak RHK, Turner C, Thompson T, et al: Suppression of secondary hyperparathyroidism in children with chronic renal failure by high dose phosphate binders: Calcium carbonate versus aluminum hydroxide. *Br Med J* 1985; 291:623–627.
213. Tamanaha K, Mak RHK, Rigden SPA, et al: Long term suppression of hyperparathyroidism by phosphate binders in uremic children. *Pediatr Nephrol* 1987; 1:145–149.
213a. Trachtman H, Gauthier B: Parenteral calcitriol treatment of severe renal osteodystrophy in children with chronic renal insufficiency. *J Pediatr* 1987; 110:9666–9670.
214. Saluski IB, Coburn JW, Foley J, et al: Effects of oral calcium carbonate on control of serum phosphorus and changes in plasma aluminum levels after discontinuation of aluminum-containing gels in children receiving dialysis. *J Pediatr* 1986; 108:767–780.
215. Salusky IB, Goodman WG, Horst R, et al: Pharmacokinetics of calcitriol in continuous ambulatory and cycling peritoneal dialysis patients. *Am J Kidney Dis* 1990; 16:126–132.
216. Salusky IB, Foley J, Goodman WG: Progression of secondary hyperparathyroidism despite oral calcitriol therapy in pediatric patients on CAPD/CCVD (abstract). *J Am Soc Nephrol* 1990; 1:573.
216a. Riancho JA, De Francisco ALM, Del Arco C, et al: Serum levels of 1,25 dihydroxyvitamin D after renal transplantation. *Miner Electrolyte Metab* 1988; 14:332–337.
216b. Felsenfeld AJ, Gutman RA, Drezner M: Hypophosphatemia in long-term re-

nal transplant recipients; Effects on bone histology and 1,25-dihydroxycholecalciferol. *Miner Electrolyte Metab* 1986; 12:333–341.

216c. De Francisco AM, Riancho JA, Amado JA: Calcium, hyperparathyroidism and vitamin D metabolism after kidney transplant. *Transplantation Proc* 1987; 19:3721–3723.

217. Parfitt AM: Hypercalcemic hyperparathyroidism following renal transplantation: Differential diagnosis, management and implications for cell population control in the parathyroid gland. *Miner Electrolyte Metab* 1982; 8:92–112.

218. Pabico RC, McKenna BA: Metabolic problems in renal transplant patients. Persistent hyperparathyroidism and hypophosphatemia. Effects of intravenous calcium infusion. *Transplantation Proc* 1988; 20:438–442.

219. Rosenbaum RW, Kruska KA, Krobar A, et al: Decreased phosphate absorption after renal transplantation. Evidence for a mechanism independent of calcium and parathyroid hormone. *Kidney Int* 1981; 19:568–578.

219a. Caine Y (European Multicentre Trial Group): Cyclosporin in cadaveric renal transplantation: 5 years followup of a multicentre trial. *Lancet* 1987; 2:506–507.

220. Ulmann A, Chkoff N, Lacour B: Anomalies du métabolisme phosphocalcique après transplantation rénale réussie, in Grünfeld JP (ed): *Actualités Néphrologiques.* Paris, Flammarion, 1981, pp 99–107.

221. Peraldi MN, Rondeau E, Jousset V, et al: Dexamethasone increases prepro-parathyroid hormone messenger RNA in human hyperplastic parathyroid cells in vitro. *Eur J Clin Invest* 1990; 20:392–397.

222. Alsina J, Gonzalez MT, Bonnin R, et al: Long-term evolution of renal osteodystrophy after renal transplantation. *Transplantation Proc* 1989; 21:2151–2158.

223. Garabedian M, Silve C, Levy-Bentolila D, et al: Changes in plasma 1,25 and 24,25 dihydroxyvitamin D3 after renal transplantation in children. *Kidney Int* 1981; 20:403–410.

224. Lucas PA, Woodhead JS, Brown RC: Vitamin D3 metabolites in chronic renal failure and after renal transplantation. *Nephrol Dial Transplantation* 1988; 3:70–76.

225. Graziani G, Castelnovo C, Aroldi A, et al: Response of renal transplanted patients to oral calcium load. *Nephrol Dial Transplantation* 1990; 5:531–534.

226. Cundy T, Kanis JA: Rapid supression of plasma alkaline phosphatase activity after renal transplantation in patients with osteodystrophy. *Clin Chim Acta* 1987; 164:285–291.

227. Schmidt H, Stracke H, Scheuermann EH, et al: Osteocalcin serum levels in patients following renal transplantation. *Klin Wochenschr* 1989; 67:297–303.

228. Orcel P, Denne MA, de Vernejoul MC: Cyclosporin A decreases the fusion of osteoclast precursors in vitro (abstract). *Calcif Tissue Int* 1990; 46:43–166.

229. Stewart PJ, Green OC, Stern PH: Cyclosporin A inhibits calcemic hormone-induced bone resorption in vitro. *J Bone Miner Res* 1986; 1:285.

230. Movsowitz C, Epstein S, Fallon M, et al: Cyclosporin A in vivo produces severe osteopenia in the rat: effect of dose and duration of administration. *Endocrinology* 1988; 123:2571–2577.

231. Aubia J, Masramon J, Serrano S, et al: Bone histology in renal transplant patients receiving cyclosporin. *Lancet* 1988; 1:1408.
232. Gardin JP, Foucray, Paillard M: Traitement de l'hyperparathyroidie du transplanté rénal par Calcitriol intraveineux. Personal communication.
233. Nehme D, Rondeau E, Paillard F, et al: Aseptic necrosis of bone following renal transplantation: Relation with hyperparathyroidism. *Nephrol Dial Transplantation* 1989;4:123–128.

Treatment of Chronic Viral Hepatitis

Patrick Marcellin, M.D.

Service d'Hépatologie and Unité de Recherches de Physiopathologie Hépatique (INSERM), Hôpital Beaujon, Clichy, France

Françoise Degos, M.D.

Service d'Hépatologie and Unité de Recherches de Physiopathologie Hépatique (INSERM), Hôpital Beaujon, Clichy, France

Jean-Pierre Benhamou, M.D.

Service d'Hépatologie and Unité de Recherches de Physiopathologie Hépatique (INSERM), Hôpital Beaujon, Clichy, France

There have been recent advances in the treatment of chronic viral hepatitis, mainly since recombinant α interferon was introduced. However, the present treatment of chronic viral hepatitis is not entirely satisfactory, mainly because the efficiency is inconstant and/or incomplete.

Chronic viral hepatitis can be the consequence of infection with hepatitis B virus (HBV), or infection with HBV and hepatitis delta virus (HDV), or infection with hepatitis C virus (HCV).

Chronic Viral Hepatitis B

Natural History of Chronic Viral Hepatitis B

The natural history of chronic viral hepatitis B consists of three successive phases that have in common the permanent presence of hepatitis B surface antigen (HBsAg) in serum (Fig 1). In the first phase, there is a marked replication of HBV. This phase is characterized by the presence of markers of HBV replication in serum: HBV-deoxyribonucleic acid (HBV-DNA) and hepatitis B e antigen (HBeAg). During this phase, the activity of chronic hepatitis is intense or moderate. The level of activity is indicated biochemically by the increased serum aminotransferases, in particular alanine aminotransferase (ALT), and histologically by the presence of hepatocyte necrosis and infiltration with mononuclear cells in the periportal area. The degree of activity seems to be determined by the degree of immune response to HBV infection: if the immune response is vigorous, hepatocyte necrosis is marked; if the immune response is weak, hepato-

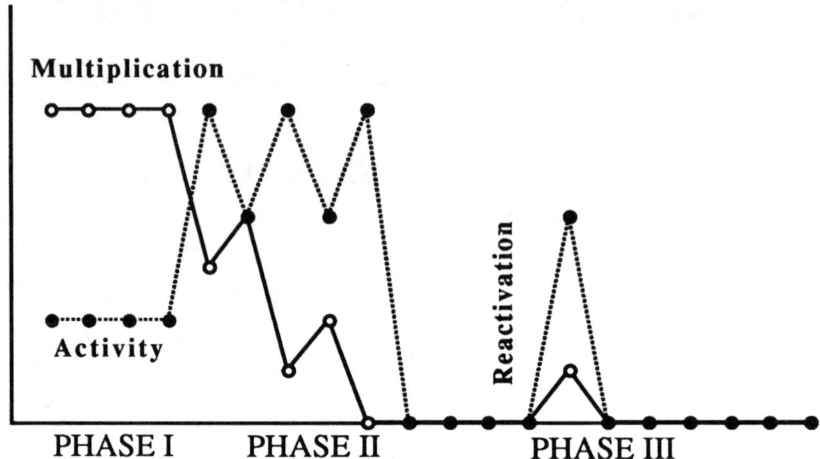

FIG. 1.
Natural history of chronic hepatitis B. During phase I, the activity of chronic hepatitis is low and the viral multiplication is high. During phase II, the activity of chronic hepatitis increases and the viral multiplication decreases (seroconversion). During phase III, the activity of chronic hepatitis disappears with the viral multiplication. Note during phase II the possible occurrence of episodes of exacerbation of the chronic hepatitis (abortive seroconversion hepatitis). Note during phase III the possible occurrence of episodes of reactivation of the chronic hepatitis.

cyte necrosis is limited. This phase of marked HBV replication lasts 1 or several years.

The second phase of seroconversion is determined by exaggeration of the immune response to HBV infection. During this phase of seroconversion, the markers of HBV replication, i.e., HBV-DNA and HBeAg, diminish and disappear. During this phase of seroconversion, the activity of chronic hepatitis is very marked; as a consequence, severe lesions of the liver, in particular cirrhosis, can be produced. This phase of seroconversion may be short, lasting several weeks, or prolonged, lasting several months or 1 or 2 years. When the phase of seroconversion is prolonged, there are often several episodes of abortive seroconversion characterized by severe exaggeration of the activity of chronic hepatitis. In a few patients, seroconversion induces clinical and biochemical manifestations resembling those of acute hepatitis or even fulminant hepatitis.

It is noteworthy that seroconversion is an almost constant event in the natural history of chronic viral hepatitis B. The annual incidence of spontaneous seroconversion is 5% to 10%. This relatively high incidence must be taken into consideration in the evaluation of the treatment of chronic viral hepatitis B.

Seroconversion is followed by a third period of low or absent HBV replication. This phase is characterized by the disappearance of markers of HBV replication and appearance of antibody to HBeAg (anti-HBe). During this phase, the activity of chronic hepatitis is low or absent: serum ALT is normal or slightly increased; and hepatocyte necrosis and infiltration by mononuclear cells are limited or absent.

During this third phase, two types of events may occur. First, reactivation may take place. Reactivation is characterized by reappearance of markers of HBV replication and by reappearance of the activity of chronic hepatitis. Several successive episodes of reactivation can occur in some patients. Reactivation can develop spontaneously or can be induced by immunosuppressive drugs.[1]

Second, in very few patients, HBsAg disappears. This disappearance may take place early after seroconversion or several years after seroconversion. Disappearance of HBsAg is often definitive, perhaps reflecting complete recovery from HBV infection. In some cases, especially in patients receiving immunosuppressive drugs, HBsAg reappears, indicating persistence of HBV in tissue despite disappearance of serum HBsAg.[2] In some patients with chronic hepatitis B in whom HBsAg is not detectable in serum, the presence of HBV-DNA sequences can be demonstrated with amplification by polymerase chain reaction in serum and in liver.[3]

Treatment of Chronic Viral Hepatitis B

The present treatment of chronic viral hepatitis B is based on two notions. The first notion is that the main effect of the two therapeutic agents presently available, i.e., adenine arabinoside and α interferon, is to interrupt HBV replication and thus bring forward the time of seroconversion; in other words, these therapeutic agents can be used only at the phase of HBV replication and can induce only the interruption of HBV replication (with, as a consequence, disappearance of the markers of HBV replication; i.e., HBV-DNA and HBeAg) and the diminution or disappearance of the activity of the liver disease (i.e., normalization of aminotransferase levels). In most of the patients, HBsAg persists; in only very few of the treated patients, HBsAg disappears.

The second notion is that these therapeutic agents exert their effect by inducing seroconversion. This therapeutically induced seroconversion, as spontaneous seroconversion, can be associated with exacerbation of the activity of chronic hepatitis. This exacerbation is marked in patients treated with α interferon, but less marked in those treated with adenine arabinoside. Because of the exacerbation, treatment with α interferon or adenine arabinoside is contraindicated in patients with severe liver disease (ascites, spontaneous bacterial peritonitis, gastrointestinal bleeding, jaundice, prothrombin less than 50% of normal).

The responses to adenine arabinoside or alpha interferon can be classified into three types. Type I response is characterized by disappearance of HBV-DNA, without disappearance of HBeAg; the activity of the liver disease diminishes, but does not disappear; type I response is often transient, followed by reappearance of HBV-DNA and re-increase in aminotransferase levels. Type II response is characterized by the disappearance of HBV-DNA and HBeAg; the activity of the liver disease diminishes and often disappears completely; the recurrence is less common than after type I response. Type III response is characterized by the disappearance of HBV-DNA, HBeAg, and HBsAg; type III response is associated with complete disappearance of the activity of chronic hepatitis in most cases.

Adenine arabinoside (ARA-A, Vidarabine), an analogue of adenosine, which inhibits HBV-DNA polymerase, is administered via continuous intravenous infusion, at a dose of 15 mg/kg body weight per day for 7 days, then at a dose of 7.5 mg/kg body weight per day for 14 days. Three controlled studies of ARA-A in patients with chronic hepatitis B have been reported [4–6] (Table 1); only one of these studies showed a difference of the seroconversion rate in the treated patients and in the untreated patients.[4] The pooled results of these three studies show that a type II response is obtained in 25% of the patients who received ARA-A.

The monophosphate derivative of ARA-A (ARA-AMP) is more water soluble and can be administered by intramuscular injections. Plasma concentration of the drug is higher in patients treated with ARA-AMP than in those treated with ARA-A. The therapeutic schedule consists of two daily intramuscular injections at a dose of 10 mg/kg body weight per day for 5 days, and then at a dose of 5 mg/kg body weight per day for 23 days. Five controlled studies of ARA-AMP in patients with chronic viral hepatitis B have been reported (Table 2); three of these studies showed a difference in treated and untreated patients, with a type II response in 33% to 55% of the former patients[8, 9, 11]; two of these studies showed no significant difference in the treated and untreated patients.[7, 10] The discrepancy between these studies is likely to be due to differences in the populations of the patients included in these trials. In the two studies in which there was no significant difference in treated and untreated patients, 70% and 75% of the patients were male homosexuals[7, 10]; in one of these two studies,[10] 40% of the male homosexuals were human immunodeficiency virus (HIV) positive. In our study, we compared the response to treatment in heterosexuals and homosexuals (HIV negative); we observed no significant difference in these two groups of patients.[1–11] Therefore, infection with HIV might diminish the response to treatment and account, at least in part, for the discrepancy between the different studies. The pooled result of the five aforementioned studies shows that a type II response is obtained in 32% of the patients who received ARA-AMP.

α Interferon exerts an antiviral effect on infection with HBV through two mechanisms. First, α interferon has a direct antiviral effect by inhibiting synthesis of viral DNA and by activating antiviral enzymes. Second, α interferon exaggerates the cellular immune response against hepatocytes infected with HBV by increasing the expression of class I histocompatibility antigens and by stimulating the activity of helper T lymphocytes and natural killer lymphocytes.[12] Thus, α interferon induces an early diminution of HBV replication (reflected by a diminution of HBV-DNA in serum) and a late (about 2 months later) increase in aminotransferase levels (Fig 2). Several controlled studies of α interferon in patients with chronic viral hepatitis B have been reported (Table 3). In some studies, recombinant α inter-

TABLE 1.
Controlled Trials of Adenine Arabinoside in Chronic Hepatitis B

		Treatment		Treated Patients		Untreated Patients	
First Author	**Date of Publication**	**Dosage (mg/kg/day)**	**Duration (days)**	**Number**	**Percentage with Type II Response***	**Number**	**Percentage with Type II Response***
Bassendine[4]	1981	10–15	10	7	57	6	0
Yokosuka[5]	1985	10	28–56	10	10	10	20
Ouzan[6]	1987	15–7.5	21	15	20	15	7
Total				32	25†	31	10†

*Loss of serum HBV-DNA and HBeAg with appearance of anti-HBe.
†Totals represent the mean.

TABLE 2.
Controlled Trials of Adenine Arabinoside Monophosphate in Chronic Hepatitis B

		Treatment		Treated Patients		Untreated Patients	
First Author	Date of Publication	Dosage (mg/kg/day)	Duration (days)	Number	Percentage With Type II Response*	Number	Percentage With Type II Response*
Hoofnagle[7]	1984	5–10	28	10	30	10	20
Weller[8]	1985	5–10	28	15	40	14	0
Ouzan[9]	1986	5–10	28	20	55	20	15
Garcia[10]	1987	5	3×38	24	8	27	15
Marcellin[11]	1989	5	49	24	33	19	9
Total				93	32†	90	11†

*Loss of serum HBV-DNA and HBeAg with appearance of anti-HBe.
†Totals represent the mean.

TABLE 3.
Controlled Trials of α Interferon in Chronic Hepatitis B

		Treatment					Treated Patients		Untreated Patients	
First Author	Date of Publication	Type*	Dosage (MU)†	Route‡	Schedule§	Duration (wk)	Number	Percentage with Type II Response¶	Number	Percentage with Type II Response¶
Dusheiko[13]	1985	R 2a	18-50	IM	3/wk	9	14	43	11	0
Alexander[14]	1987	Lb	6–10/m^2	IM	3/wk	24	32	26	23	0
Pastore[15]	1988	Ld	0.07–0.1/kg	IM	2/wk	12	14	57	14	14
Hoofnagle[16]	1988	R 2b	5–10	IM or SC	3/wk	16	31	32	14	14
Lok[17] ‖	1988	R 2a	2.5,5 or 10	IM	3/wk	12–24	54	11	18	6
Saracco[18]**	1989	Lb	5/m^2	IM	3/wk	24	33	79	31	39
Brook[19]††	1989	R 2a	2.5,5 or 10	IM	3/wk	24	45	27	15	0
Total							223	34‡‡	126	13‡‡

*Type of α interferon: R 2a = recombinant α 2a; Lb = lymphoblastoid; Ld = leukocyte derived; R 2b = recombinant α 2b.
†MU = million units.
‡Route of administration: IM = intramuscular; SC = subcutaneous.
§Schedule of administration: number of injections per week.
¶Loss of serum HBV-DNA and HBeAg with appearance of anti-HBe.
‖ Preliminary results of this study have been published in reference 20.
**Preliminary results of this study have been published in reference 21.
††Preliminary results of this study have been published in reference 12.
‡‡Totals represent the mean.

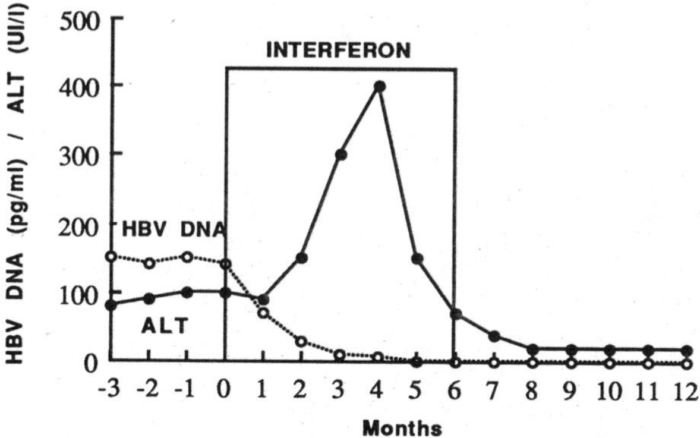

FIG. 2.
Response to α interferon in a patient with chronic hepatitis B. The viral multiplication starts to decrease during the first month of treatment. Serum ALT increases after 2 or 3 months of treatment (immune response).

feron, mainly α-2a (Roferon) and α-2b (Introna) were used; in other studies, lymphoblastoid (Wellferon) interferon was used. In these studies, the dose ranged from 2.5 to 50 million units (MU), administered by subcutaneous or intramuscular injections, either daily or thrice a week, for 9 to 24 weeks. The percentage of treated patients with type II response ranges from 11% to 79%. The discrepancy in the results of the different studies could be due, in part, to the different therapeutic schedules, but is mainly due to the population of patients included in these trials. The difference in the populations of patients studied is illustrated by the wide range in the percentages of spontaneous HBeAg to anti-HBe seroconversion (equivalent to type II response) in the untreated patients, which are parallel to the percentages of type II response in the treated patients. A certain number of factors are predictive of response to α interferon (Table 4)[22]: (a) infection with HIV seems to diminish the antiviral effect of α interferon[23]; (b) the occurrence of infection with HBV at birth or early in the patient's life (as is often the case in countries where HBV infection is hyperendemic, such as

TABLE 4.
Predictive Factors of Poor Response to α Interferon in Chronic Hepatitis B

Associated HIV infection
Low level of serum aminotransferases
Low histologic activity
High level of viral multiplication

southeast Asia) is a factor of poor response to α interferon[17, 20]; in general, immune depression diminishes the response to treatment. In white patients infected with HBV as adults, α interferon induces a type II response in about 40% of the cases. A dosage of 5 MU to 10 MU thrice a week for 4 to 6 months allows an optimal efficacy with a satisfactory tolerance.

β Interferon and γ interferon were evaluated in a few pilot studies.[17, 18] Their efficacy was lower than that of α interferon, probably because the antiviral effect of the former interferons is smaller than that of the latter. Azidothymidine was shown to have no significant effect on HBV replication.[28]

A certain number of therapeutic combinations was studied. The efficacy of the combination of α interferon to β interferon or γ interferon was not higher than that of α interferon alone.[26, 27] Acyclovir does not increase the efficacy of α interferon.[29] The percentages of seroconversion were not different in patients receiving ARA-AMP combined with α interferon from those in patients receiving α interferon or ARA-AMP alone and in patients receiving placebo[10]; however, in this study, 70% of the patients were homosexuals and 40% were HIV positive. Two other studies report encouraging results in patients treated with corticosteroids and vidarabine.[5, 30] A French trial has shown the efficacy of the combination of corticosteroids, vidarabine, and α interferon.[31] α Interferon preceded by administration of corticosteroids seems to be more efficient than α interferon alone in a subgroup of patients with marked HBV replication and chronic mildly active hepatitis.[32] When suddenly interrupted, administration of corticosteroids is supposed to induce an immune rebound with increased necrosis of the hepatic cells, a phenomenon which adds to, or improves, the effect of α interferon. Administration of corticosteroids followed by its sudden interruption is hazardous in patients with severe cirrhosis in whom massive necrosis of hepatic cells may result in severe liver failure.

Chronic Viral Hepatitis B-D

Natural History of Chronic Viral Hepatitis B-D

In patients with chronic viral hepatitis B-D, i.e., chronic hepatitis due to infection with HBV and infection with HDV, there is HDV replication as reflected by the presence of IgM anti-HD in serum, and/or the presence of hepatitis D antigen (HDAg) in serum, and/or the presence of HDAg in the liver, and/or the presence of HDV-RNA in serum. In most of these patients, HBV replication is absent as indicated by the absence of HBeAg, the absence of HBV-DNA, and the presence of anti-HBe. Chronic viral hepatitis B-D is often severe and can rapidly result in cirrhosis.

Treatment of Chronic Viral Hepatitis B-D

Only α interferon has some efficiency in the treatment of chronic viral hepatitis B-D. Published studies are not numerous and are based on a limited

TABLE 5.
Therapeutic Trials of α Interferon in Chronic Hepatitis D

		Interferon					Treated Patients		Untreated Patients	
First Author	Date of Publication	Type*	Dosage (MU)†	Route‡	Schedule§	Duration (mo)	Number	Percentage With Remission¶	Number	Percentage With Remission¶
Rosina[33]	1987	R 2b	5 MU/m^2	SC	3/wk	12	12	64	12	19%
Hoofnagle[34]	1987	R 2b	5 MU	SC	3/wk	4 or 12	6	50	0	
Farci[35]	1990	R 2a	3 MU	IM	3/wk	12	14	28		
			9 MU	IM	3/wk	12	14	71	14	7
Total							46	56**		

*Type of α interferon: R 2b = recombinant α 2b; R 2a = recombinant α 2a.
†Million units.
‡Route of administration: IM = intramuscular; SC = subcutaneous.
§Schedule of administration = number of injections per wk.
¶Loss of serum HDV-RNA with normalization of serum ALT.
**Total represents the mean.

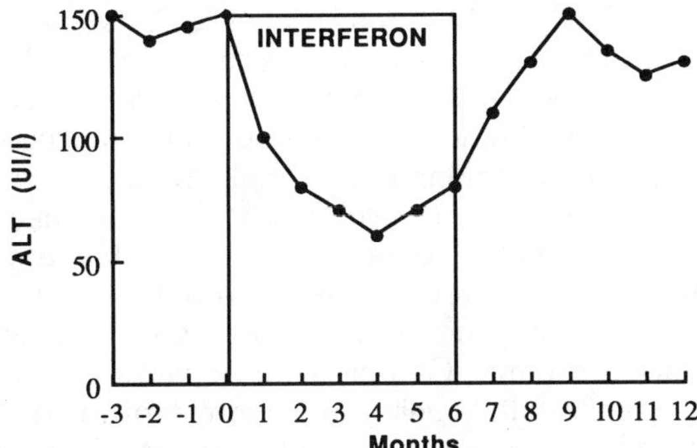

FIG. 3.
Response to α interferon in a patient with chronic hepatitis B-D. Serum ALT starts to decrease during the first month of treatment, but the decrease is incomplete and serum ALT re-increases after withdrawal of treatment.

number of patients, for two reasons: (a) chronic viral hepatitis B-D is less common than chronic viral hepatitis B; (b) chronic viral hepatitis B-D, in most countries, mainly affects drug addicts, i.e., patients in whom follow-up is often unsatisfactory. In addition, the results of any treatment are difficult to evaluate because associated infection with HIV or HCV infection is common. The serum markers of HDV replication, i.e., HDAg or HDV-RNA, are not routinely available. The response to α interferon is inconstant and often incomplete and transient (Fig 3).

The published controlled studies (Table 5) showed a significant diminution of HDV replication, as reflected by the disappearance of serum HDAg and/or serum HDV-RNA in about 50% of the patients.[33–35] This diminution of HDV replication is usually associated with normalization of ALT and reduced histologic activity. However, complete interruption of HDV replication is uncommon; in most of the patients, after interruption of α interferon administration, HDAg and/or HDV-RNA reappear in serum and ALT increases. A prolonged effect has been reported in 50% of the patients receiving a relatively high dose of α interferon, i.e., 9 MU thrice a week, for a relatively long period, i.e., 12 months.[35]

Chronic Viral Hepatitis Non-A Non-B (or C)

Natural History of Chronic Viral Hepatitis C

HCV is responsible for most of, and perhaps all, the cases of chronic viral hepatitis non-A non-B.[36] The first generation tests demonstrate that anti-HCV is present in 70% to 80% of the patients with chronic viral hepatitis non-A non-B.[37] The second generation tests are not fully evaluated yet, but would demonstrate anti-HCV in 90% of the patients with chronic viral hepatitis non-A non-B. Chronic viral hepatitis C is the most common chronic viral hepatitis in France, in Europe, and in North America. Themain source of infection with HCV is blood transfusion. The second source of infection with HCV is intravenous drug addiction. In 30% of the cases, the source of contamination remains unknown. The natural history of HCV infection is not well known. It is generally admitted that at least 50% of the patients contaminated with HCV are affected with chronic hepatitis; in 20%, chronic hepatitis would result in cirrhosis 10 to 30 years later. Cirrhosis due to HCV infection can be complicated by hepatocellular carcinoma. Chronic viral hepatitis C is often asymptomatic, the only manifestation being an intermittent increase in ALT; for periods lasting several weeks to several months, ALT may return to normal.

Treatment of Chronic Viral Hepatitis C

α Interferon is the only treatment of chronic viral hepatitis C. The effect of α interferon was described in 1986.[38] This first uncontrolled study showed a diminution of ALT in eight of the ten patients treated with α interferon with normalization of ALT in six. The effect of α interferon on ALT is rapid, within 2 to 3 weeks of administration (Fig 4). This rapid diminution of ALT, which is not preceded by an increase of ALT as in patients with chronic hepatitis B, suggests that the liver lesion induced by HCV results from a direct cytotoxicity rather than an immune mechanism. Since 1986, several controlled studies have confirmed that α interferon induced normalization of ALT in 33% of the treated patients and that this effect was associated with a decrease in histologic activity (Table 6).[39–41] It has been shown that the 3 MU dose was more efficient than the 1 MU dose. The therapeutic schedule usually used is 3 MU, subcutaneously, thrice a week, for 24 weeks. Studies are in progress for evaluation of a longer treatment (1 year or more) or a higher dose (5 to 10 MU). No factor predictive of a good response to the treatment has been identified; however, patients with cirrhosis seem to have a poor response and patients with recent infection a good response to α interferon. The response to α interferon is not different in patients with chronic hepatitis C due to blood transfusion, or due to intravenous drug injection or of unknown source.[41] The response to α interferon does not depend on the presence or absence of anti-HCV.[42] α Interferon should be used with caution in patients with severe cirrhosis: a rebound of the activity of chronic hepatitis at the interruption of α interferon can result in transient aggravation of liver dysfunction.[43] The long-term effect of α interferon in chronic viral hepatitis C is disappointing: after cessation of α interferon administration, in half of the patients in whom the ALT was normal at the end of the treatment, a re-increase in ALT is observed within 6 months.

TABLE 6.
Controlled Trials of α Interferon in Chronic Hepatitis C

		Interferon					Treated Patients		Untreated Patients	
First Author	**Date of Publication**	**Type***	**Dosage (MU)†**	**Route‡**	**Schedule §**	**Duration (wk)**	**Number**	**Percentage with Normal ALT¶**	**Number**	**Percentage with Normal ALT¶**
Di Bisceglie[39]	1989	R 2b	2 MU	SC	3/wk	24	21	48	20	0
Davis[40]	1989	R 2b	1 MU	SC	3/wk	24	57	16	51	4
		R 2b	3 MU	SC	3/wk	24	58	38		
Marcellin[41]	1991	R 2b	1 MU	SC	3/wk	24	20	45	19	0
		R 2b	3 MU	SC	3/wk	24	18	39		
Total							174	33**	90	2**

*Type of α interferon: R 2b = recombinant α 2b.
†MU = million units.
‡Route of administration: SC = subcutaneous.
§Schedule of administration = number of injections per wk.
¶At the end of interferon administration.
**Totals represent the mean.

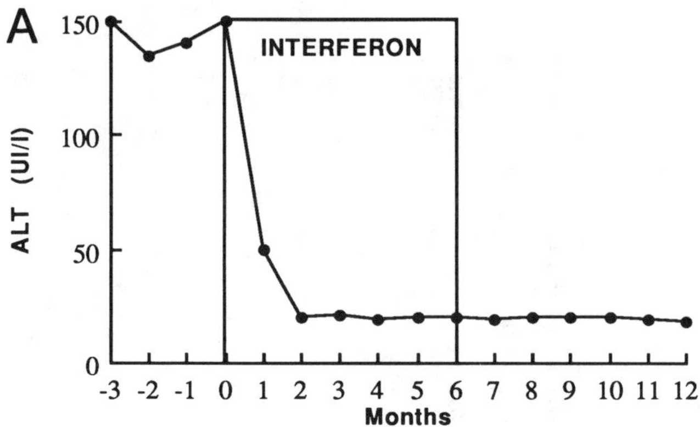

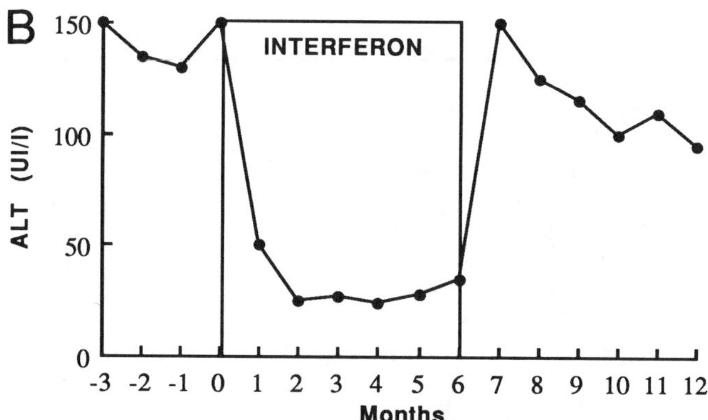

FIG. 4.
Response to α interferon in a patient with chronic hepatitis C. Serum ALT starts to decrease during the first month of treatment and normalizes. After withdrawal of treatment, serum ALT remains normal **(A)** or re-increases **(B).**

Treatment of Chronic Viral Hepatitis in Patients With Kidney Disease

Chronic Viral Hepatitis B

Hemodialysis

The prevalence of chronic infection with HBV is high in patients treated with hemodialysis. This high prevalence is due to two factors: first, the risk of exposure to HBV is high; second, the risk of chronic infection after exposure to HBV is especially high in patients treated with hemodialysis. The prevalence of chronic infection with HBV in the French hemodialysis centers was 50% or more before the introduction of vaccination against HBV.[44, 45] The prevalence of chronic infection with HBV was lower in British or American centers, probably because isolation of patients infected with HBV was much more strictly applied than in French centers. At present, in French hemodialysis centers, vaccination against HBV and isolation of patients infected with HBV in special centers have reduced the prevalence of chronic infection with HBV to 15%.[44, 65] This persistent relatively high prevalence despite vaccination results, at least in part, from an immune response to vaccination against HBV that is lower in patients with renal failure and/or treated with hemodialysis than that in healthy subjects[46]: the titer of antibodies to HBsAg is inversely correlated to the severity of renal failure as evaluated by creatinine clearance.[44]

The antiviral treatment of chronic viral hepatitis B should be similar in patients with or without hemodialysis. To our knowledge, there is no large study evaluating the therapeutic effect of α interferon in patients treated with hemodialysis. However, it can be anticipated that the efficiency of α interferon should be low in these patients with diminished immune response.

Renal Transplantation

In most cases, renal transplantation is performed in patients previously treated with hemodialysis, therefore often already infected with HBV. The immunosuppressive treatment alters the course of chronic infection with HBV: first, in patients with HBV infection at the replicative phase, serum concentration of HBV-DNA is often increased; second, in patients with chronic infection with HBV in the nonreplicative phase, HBV-DNA may reappear[47]; third, in a few patients without detectable HBsAg (but probably suffering from a latent infection with HBV), HBsAg may reappear.[2] In a series of patients, aggravation of histologic lesions of the liver was observed in 80% of HBsAg positive patients after a mean delay of 21 months after renal transplantation.[48] In another series, the prevalence of chronic hepatitis in HBsAg positive patients, which was 59% at renal transplantation, increased to 91% after a mean delay of 84.2 months after renal transplantation.[49] Thus, renal transplantation seems to aggravate chronic infection with HBV: it has been estimated that the annual rate of mortality directly related to liver disease in HBsAg positive patients would be 5% in those treated with renal transplantation and less than 1% in those treated with hemodialysis.

To our knowledge, there is no large study evaluating antiviral therapy in patients treated with renal transplantation. However, it can be anticipated that the efficacy of antiviral therapy should be relatively low in these patients receiving immunosuppressive drugs. In addition, there are serious reservations to the use of α interferon in renal transplant recipients because this agent may increase the risk of rejection.

Chronic Viral Hepatitis C

Hemodialysis

Chronic infection with HCV is common in patients treated with hemodialysis: in a Spanish hemodialysis center, the prevalence of anti-HCV was 36.6%, whereas the prevalence of HBsAG was 12.7%.[50] For the same duration, chronic infection with HCV induces less severe liver lesions than chronic infection with HBV. The efficiency of α interferon in the therapy of chronic infection with HCV in patients treated with hemodialysis has not been evaluated yet.

Renal Transplantation

Aggravation of chronic infection with HCV by immunosuppressive drugs has not been clearly demonstrated; if it was the case, this aggravation would be inconstant and moderate; thus, in HBsAg negative patients with chronic liver lesions (likely due to chronic infection with HCV) deterioration of the liver lesions has been observed in only 20% of the cases after a mean delay of 21 months after renal transplantation.[48] To our knowledge, antiviral therapy of chronic infection with HCV has not been evaluated in renal transplant recipients.

Glomerulonephritis Due to Chronic Infection With Hepatitis B Virus

Chronic infection with HBV can determine membranous or membranoproliferative glomerulonephritis due to deposits of immune complexes formed of HBeAg and anti-HBe, or HBcAg and anti-HBc, or less commonly, of HBsAg and anti-HBs.[51–54] Therefore, infection with HBV determining glomerulonephritis of this type is often associated with the production of HBeAg; i.e., the disease is at the replicative phase. Treatment with α interferon can interrupt HBV replication and thus induce dramatic improvement of glomerulonephritis.[54]

Side Effects of Antiviral Treatments

Vidarabine

Administration of ARA-A and ARA-AMP may induce peripheral neuropathy with dysesthesia and myalgia of the lower limbs (Table 7); this neuropathy is reversible if the treatment is immediately interrupted. An overdose of ARA-A or ARA-AMP can induce encephalopathy or cerebellar syndrome. ARA-A or ARA-AMP must be used with caution in patients with hepatic insufficiency. More rarely, these drugs can induce an increase of serum creatinine, neutropenia, and thrombocytopenia; all these disorders are reversible after interruption of the treatment.

TABLE 7.
Side Effects of Vidarabine and Vidarabine Monophosphate

Common Side Effects	Uncommon Side Effects
Extremity pain (myalgia)	Arthralgia
Diarrhea	Tremor (intention)
Nausea	Myoclonia
Abdominal pain	Depression
Weight loss	Encephalopathy (confusion, coma)
	Thrombocytopenia
	Neutropenia

α Interferon

α Interferon induces a flulike syndrome in most of the patients at the beginning of administration of the drug. The flulike syndrome consists of chills, fever, fatigue, myalgia, and headache. The intensity of the flulike syndrome progressively diminishes and frequently disappears within 2 to 4 weeks after the beginning of α interferon administration.

Other side effects (Table 8) are common: fatigue, irritability, partial alopecia, nausea, anorexia, weight loss, erythema, or pruritis at the site of injection. All these side effects are benign and do not require interruption of α interferon administration in most patients. These side effects rapidly disappear after cessation of α interferon administration.[55]

Severe side effects, which may require cessation of the treatment, are uncommon. Depression (affecting usually patients with previous history of depression) has been reported. Hypothyroidism or hyperthyroidism in relation to autoimmune thyroiditis is a well-recognized complication of treatment with α interferon: among 40 patients with chronic viral hepatitis C treated with α interferon, systematic measurement of thyroid stimulating hormone showed hypothyroidism or hyperthyroidism in six. Dysthyroidism induced by α interferon is often asymptomatic; however, in a few patients, dysthyroidism induces clinical manifestations, such as fatigue and weight loss, which are difficult to distinguish from other side effects of α interferon. Exacerbation of autoimmune disease can be induced by α interferon: au toimmune chronic active hepatitis, idiopathic thrombopenia, rheumatoid polyarthritis, and multiple sclerosis.[56]

TABLE 8.
Side Effects of α Interferon

Common Side Effects	Uncommon Side Effects
Fatigue	Depression
Fever	Epilepsy
Chills	Delirium
Myalgia	Exacerbation or induction of autoimmune disorder
Back pain	Hypothyroidism
Headache	Hyperthyroidism
Anorexia	
Weight loss	
Nausea	
Diarrhea	
Abdominal pain	
Loss of concentration	
Irritability	
Insomnia	
Alopecia	
Cutaneous rash	
Neutropenia	
Thrombopenia	

References

1. Levy P, Marcellin P, Martinot-Peignoux M, et al: Clinical course of spontaneous reactivation of hepatitis B virus infection in patients with chronic hepatitis B. *Hepatology* 1990; 12:570–574.
2. Marcellin P, Giostra E, Martinot-Peignoux M, et al: Redevelopment of hepatitis B surface antigen after renal transplantation. *Gastroenterology* 1991; 100:1432–1434.
3. Marcellin P, Martinot-Peignoux M, Loriot MA, et al: Persistence of hepatitis B virus DNA demonstrated by polymerase chain reaction in serum and liver after loss of HBsAg induced by antiviral therapy. *Ann Intern Med* 1990; 112:227–228.
4. Bassendine MP, Chadwick RG, Salmeron J, et al: Adenine arabinosine therapy in HBsAg positive chronic liver disease: A pilot study. *Gastroenterology* 1981; 80:1016–1022.
5. Yokosuka O, Omata M, Omazeki F, et al: Combination of short term prednisolone and adenine arabinoside in the treatment of chronic hepatitis B. *Gastroenterology* 1985; 89:246–251.
6. Ouzan D, Degos F, Marcellin P, et al: Traitement par la vidarabine de l'hépatite chronique active associèe à la multiplication du virus de l'hépatite B.

Etude multicentrique randomisée. *Gastroenterol Clin Biol* 1987; 11:568–573.
7. Hoofnagle JH, Hanson RG, Minuk GY, et al: Randomized controlled trial of adenine arabinoside monophosphate for chronic type B hepatitis. *Gastroenterology* 1984; 86:150–157.
8. Weller IVD, Lok ASF, Mindel A, et al: Randomized controlled trial of adenine arabinoside 5′-monophosphate (ARA-AMP) in chronic hepatitis B virus infection. *Gut* 1985; 26:745–751.
9. Ouzan D, Chevallier M, Laffranchi B, et al: Therapeutic efficacy of ARA-AMP in symptomatic HbeAg positive CAH: A randomized placebo control study in heterosexuals (abstract). *Hepatology* 1986; 6:1151.
10. Garcia G, Smith CI, Weissberg JI, et al: Adenine arabinoside monophosphate (vidarabine phosphate) in combination with human leucocyte interferon in the treatment of chronic hepatitis B. *Ann Intern Med* 1987; 10:278–285.
11. Marcellin P, Ouzan D, Degos F, et al: Randomized control trial of adenine arabinoside 5' monophosphate (ARA-AMP) in chronic active hepatitis: Comparison of the efficacy in heterosexual and homosexual patients. *Hepatology* 1989; 10:328–331.
12. Thomas HC, Scully LJ, McDonald JA: Lymphoblastoid and recombinant alpha-A interferon therapy of chronic hepatitis B virus infection. The Royal Free Hospital experience. *J Hepatol* 1986; 3:193–197.
13. Dusheiko G, Di Bisceglie A, Bowyer S, et al: Recombinant leukocyte interferon treatment of chronic hepatitis B. *Hepatology* 1985; 5:556–560.
14. Alexander GJ, Brahm J, Fagan EA, et al: Loss of HBsAg with interferon therapy in chronic hepatitis B virus infection. *Lancet* 1987; 2:66–68.
15. Pastore G, Santantonio T, Monno L, et al: Permanent inhibition of viral replication induced by low dosage of human leukocyte interferon in patients with chronic hepatitis B. *Hepatogastroenterology* 1988; 35:57–61.
16. Hoofnagle JH, Peters M, Mullen KD, et al: Randomized, controlled trial of recombinant human alpha interferon in patients with chronic hepatitis B. *Gastroenterology* 1988; 95:1318–1325.
17. Lok ASF, Lai CL, Wu PC, et al: Long-term follow-up in a randomized controlled trial of recombinant alpha2 interferon in chinese patients with chronic hepatitis B infection. *Lancet* 1988; 2:298–302.
18. Saracco G, Mazzella G, Rosina F, et al: A controlled trial of human lymphoblastoid interferon in chronic hepatitis B in Italy. *Hepatology* 1989; 10:336–341.
19. Brook MG, Mc Donald JA, Karayiannis P, et al: Randomised controlled trial of interferon alfa 2A (rbe) (Roferon-A) for the treatment of chronic hepatitis B virus (HBV) infection: Factors that influence response. *Gut* 1989; 30:1116–1122.
20. Lok ASF, Lai CL, Wu PC: Interferon therapy of chronic hepatitis B virus infection in Chinese. *J Hepatol* 1986; 3:209–215.
21. Barbara L, Mazzella G, Baraldini M, et al: A randomized controlled trial with human lymphoblastoid interferon versus no treatment in chronic hepatitis B virus infection. Preliminary results. *J Hepatol* 1986; 3:235–238.
22. Scully LJ, Lever AML, Yap I, et al: Identification of factors influencing response rate to antiviral therapy of chronic hepatitis B virus infection. *J Hepatol* 1986; 3:291–299.
23. Novick DM, Lok ASF, Thomas HC: Diminished responsiveness of homosexual men to antiviral therapy for HBsAg positive chronic liver disease. *J Hepatol* 1984; 1:29–35.

24. Di Bisceglie AM, Rustgi VK, Kassianides C, et al: Therapy of chronic hepatitis B with recombinant human alpha and gamma interferon. *Hepatology* 1990; 11:266–270.
25. Marcellin P, Loriot MA, Boyer N, et al: Recombinant human gamma interferon in patients with chronic active hepatitis: Pharmacokinetics, tolerance and biological effects. *Hepatology* 1990; 12:155–158.
26. Caselmann WH, Eisen burg J, Hofschneider PH, et al: Beta and gamma interferon in chronic active hepatitis B: A pilot trial of short-term combination therapy. *Gastroenterology* 1989; 96:449–455.
27. Gomez C, La Banda F, Porse J, et al: Combined recombinant alpha and gamma interferon treatment of chronic hepatitis B virus infection, in Zuckerman AJ (ed): *Viral Hepatitis and Liver Disease*. New York, Alan R. Liss, 1988, pp 872–874.
28. Marcellin P, Pialoux G, Girard PM, et al: Absence of effect of azidothymidine on hepatitis B virus replication in patients with chronic HIV and HBV infection (letter). *N Engl J Med* 1989; 321:1758.
29. A European Multicentre Study Group: A randomized controlled trial of acyclovir/interferon therapy in HbeAg-positive chronic hepatitis B: Assessment by quantitative HBe-Ag analysis (abstract). International Symposium on Viral Hepatitis and Liver Disease, Houston, 1990.
30. Perillo RP, Regenstein FG, Bodicky CJ, et al: Comparative efficacy of adenine arabinoside 5′ monophosphate and prednisone withdrawal followed by adenine arabinoside 5′ monophosphate in the treatment of chronic active hepatitis type B. *Gastroenterology* 1985; 88:780–786.
31. Brissot P, Jacquelinet C, David V, et al: Short term prednisolone followed by recombinant human alpha-interferon alone or combined with adenine-arabinoside in chronic hepatitis B: A prospective and randomised trial. Preliminary results. *J Hepatol* in press.
32. Perillo RP, Schiff ER, Davis GL, et al: A randomized controlled trial of interferon alfa-2b alone and after prednisone withdrawal for the treatment of chronic hepatitis B. *N Engl J Med* 1990; 323:295–301.
33. Rosina F, Saracco G, Lattore V, et al: Treatment of chronic delta hepatitis with alpha-2 recombinant interferon, in Zuckerman AJ, *Viral Hepatitis and Liver Disease*. New York, Alan R. Liss, 1988, p 857.
34. Hoofnagle JH, Di Bisceglie A: Therapy of chronic viral hepatitis: Chronic hepatitis D and non-A non-B hepatitis, in Zuckerman AJ (ed): *Viral Hepatitis and Liver Disease*. New York, Alan R. Liss, 1988, pp 823–830.
35. Farci P, Mandas A, Lai ME, et al: Treatment of chronic delta hepatitis with high and low doses of interferon alpha-2a. A randomized controlled trial (abstract). *Hepatology* 1990; 12:869.
36. Choo QL, Kuo G, Weiner AJ, et al: Isolation of a cDNA clone derived from a blood-borne non-A non-B viral hepatitis genome. *Science* 1989; 244:359–362.
37. Kuo G, Choo QL, Alter HJ, et al: An assay for circulating antibodies to a major etiologic virus of human non-A, non-B hepatitis. *Science* 1989; 244:362–364.
38. Hoofnagle JH, Mullen KD, Jones DB, et al: Treatment of chronic non-A, non-B hepatitis with recombinant human alpha interferon: A preliminary report. *N Engl J Med* 1986; 315:1575–1578.
39. Di Bisceglie AM, Martin P, Kassianides C, et al: Recombinant interferon alfa therapy for chronic hepatitis C: A randomized, double-blind, placebo controlled trial. *N Engl J Med* 1989; 321:1506–1510.
40. Davis GL, Balart LA, Schiff ER, et al: Treatment of chronic hepatitis C with recombinant interferon alfa. *J Engl J Med* 1989; 321:1501–1506.

41. Marcellin P, Boyer N, Giostra E, et al: Recombinant human alpha interferon in patients with chronic non-A, non-B hepatitis: A multicenter randomized controlled trial from France. *Hepatology* 1991; 13:393–397.
42. Marcellin P, Giostra E, Boyer N, et al: Is the response to recombinant alpha interferon related to the presence of antibodies to hepatitis C virus in patients with chronic non-A, non-B hepatitis ? *J Hepatol* 1990; 11:77–79.
43. Marcellin P, Hautekeete M, Giostra E, et al: Evolution of chronic non-A, non-B hepatitis after alpha interferon: Evidence for a rebound phenomenon (abstract). International Symposium on Viral Hepatitis and Liver Disease, Houston, 1990.
44. Crosnier J, Degos F, Jungers P: Dialysis associated hepatitis, in: Maher JF, (ed): *Replacement of Renal Function by Dialysis,* ed 3. Dordrecht, Kluwer Academic Publishers, 1989, pp 881–903.
45. Crosnier J, Jungers P, Courouсé AM, et al: Randomized placebo-controlled trial of hepatitis B surface antigen vaccine in French haemodialysis units. II. Haemodialysis patients. *Lancet* 1981; 1:797–800.
46. Degos F, Lugassy C, Degott C, et al: Hepatitis B virus and hepatitis B-related viral infection in renal transplant recipient. *Gastroenterology* 1988; 94:151–156.
47. Nagington J, Cossart YE, Cohen BJ: Reactivation of hepatitis B after transplantation operations. *Lancet* 1977; 2:558–560.
48. Pol S, Debure A, Degott C, et al: Chronic hepatitis in kidney allograft recipients. *Lancet* 1990; 335:878–880.
49. Degos F, Degott C: Hepatitis in renal transplant recipients. *J Hepatol* 1989; 9:114–128.
50. Bruguera M, Vidal L, Sanchez-Tapias JM, et al: Incidence and features of liver disease in patients on chronic hemodialysis. *J Clin Gastroenterol* 1990; 12:298–302.
51. Hattori S, Furuse A, Matsuda I: Presence of HBe-antibody in glomerular deposits in membranous glomerulonephritis is associated with hepatitis B virus infection. *Am J Nephrol* 1988; 8:384–387.
52. Lee HS, Koh HI: Hepatitis B e antigen-associated membranous nephropathy. *Nephron* 1989; 52:356–359.
53. Venkataseshan VS, Lieberman K, Kim DU, et al: Hepatitis B associated glomerulonephritis: Pathology, pathogenesis and clinical course. *Medicine* 1990; 69:200–216.
54. Lisker-Melman M, Webb D, Di Bisceglie A, et al: Glomerulonephritis caused by chronic hepatitis B virus infection: Treatment with recombinant human alpha-interferon. *Ann Intern Med* 1989; 111:479–483.
55. Renault PF, Hoofnagle JH: Side effects of alpha interferon. *Semin Liver Dis* 1990; 9:273—277.
56. Larrey D, Marcellin P, Freneaux E, et al: Exacerbation of multiple sclerosis after the administration of recombinant human interferon alfa. *JAMA* 1989; 261:2065.

Idiotypic Modulation of Autoimmunity by Therapeutic Human Immunoglobulin Preparations (IVIg)

Srinivas V. Kaveri, Ph.D.

INSERM U28 and Service d'Immunologie, Hôpital Broussais, Paris, France

Gilles Dietrich, M.B.

INSERM U28 and Service d'Immunologie, Hôpital Broussais, Paris, France

Denise Jobin, M.D.

INSERM U28 and Service d'Immunologie, Hôpital Broussais, Paris, France

Françoise Rossi, M.D.

INSERM U28 and Service d'Immunologie, Hôpital Broussais, Paris, France

Yvette Sultan, M.D.

Laboratoire d'Hemostase, Hôpital Cochin, Paris, France

C. Martin Lockwood, M.D.

Department of Medicine, School of Clinical Medicine, Addenbrooke's Hospital, Cambridge, United Kingdom

Michel D. Kazatchkine, M.D.

INSERM U28 and Service d'Immunologie, Hôpital Broussais, Paris, France

Polyspecific human immunoglobulin preparations for intravenous use (IVIg) were introduced in the early eighties in the treatment of autoimmune disease. IVIg are a preparation of intact immunoglobulins obtained from a pool of plasma of over 15,000 healthy donors. Intravenous administration of high-dose IVIg has been beneficial in the treatment of a variety of autoimmune diseases including autoimmune peripheral cytopenias, myasthenia gravis, chronic inflammatory demyelinating polyneuropathy, recurrent abortions associated with anti-cardiolipin autoantibodies, anti-factor VIII

Advances in Nephrology,® vol 21

autoimmune disease, and systemic vasculitis associated with anti-neutrophil cytoplasmic antigen (ANCA) autoantibodies (Table 1).[1–30]

Several mutually nonexclusive mechanisms of action of IVIg have been proposed. One of them is the reversible blockade and/or downregulation of Fc receptors on cells of the reticuloendothelial system by Fc fragments of injected immunoglobulins. The latter hypothesis, which could explain at least in part the effect of IVIg in peripheral autoimmune cytopenias, has been studied by determining the clearance of autologous erythrocytes coated with anti-rhesus D antibodies. The clearance was found to be decreased for about 4 weeks following treatment with IVIg,[31] which supports the hypothesis of a blockade of Fc receptors on the surface of macrophages and a subsequent reduction in phagocytic activity of cells of the

TABLE 1.
Reported Beneficial Effect of IVIg in Human Autoimmune Diseases

Diseases*	References
Idiopathic thrombocytopenic purpura	1–4
Autoimmune hemolytic anemias	5–8
Autoimmune neutropenia	6, 9, 10
Autoimmune erythroblastopenia	11, 12
Myasthenia gravis	13–16
Chronic inflammatory demyelinating polyneuropathy	17, 18
Systemic vasculitis†	
Guillain-Barré syndrome	19
Kawasaki's disease	20, 21
Birdshot retinopathy†	
Anti-cardiolipin antibodies and recurrent abortions	22
Anti-factor VIII autoimmune disease	23–29
Refractory polymyositis	30

*Autoimmune diseases in which a clinical improvement and/or decrease in autoantibody titer has been established or suggested.
†Unpublished results.

reticuloendothelial system. Other mechanisms of action that imply the role of Fc fragments of injected IVIg have been proposed, including feedback inhibition of autoantibody synthesis by B cells,[32–34] Fc-dependent modulation of the function of suppressor or helper T cells,[34–37] and inhibition of cytotoxic activity of natural killer (NK) cells.[38] These hypotheses fail, however, to explain the rapidly occurring inhibitory effect of IVIg on titers of autoantibodies observed within a few hours after infusion in patients with certain autoimmune disorders and long-term clinical responses that may persist for several years, far beyond the half-life of injected IgG.

We have proposed that the modulatory effect of IVIg on autoimmune responses depends on the interaction of IVIg with the elements of the idiotypic network that normally control the expression of the autoimmune repertoire.[39–43] An idiotypic regulation of immune responses has been proposed by Lindenmann[44] and Jerne.[45] According to their concept, antibody diversity allows an individual to recognize a large number of antigenic specificities as well as the idiotypic specificities expressed on his own antibodies. The network theory implies that the immune system has evolved toward the recognition of autoantigens, preferentially or in addition to that of the foreign antigens. Antiidiotypic antibodies include Ab2α antibodies that recognize idiotypic determinants located outside the paratopic site of the Ab1 and Ab2β antibodies that are complementary of the paratope of Ab1. Ab2β antibodies, which present the topographic copy or the internal image of the antigenic determinant, recognize the antibody binding site of the Ab1 antibodies in a similar fashion to the antigen. Some of the idiotopes expressed by antibody molecules are functionally associated with idiotopes carried by other antibody molecules in the idiotypic network. Thus, so-called regulatory idiotopes could interact with parallel sets within the idiotypic network.[46]

It is now well established that autoreactive antibodies and T cells are present in normal individuals and that the immune system uses its own diversity to select the actual B and T cell repertoires.[47] Natural autoantibodies of IgG and IgM isotypes are present in the circulation in the normally healthy human and mouse.[48–56] The natural autoantibodies are often polyreactive and are interconnected[57–63] in the sense that they are capable of recognizing—and of being recognized by—other autoantibodies of the same individual. Natural autoantibodies are germ-line encoded.[64–69] It is as yet unclear if autoantibodies that are detected in the serum of patients with autoimmune disorders represent an abnormal expansion of these natural autoreactive clones or the emergence of somatically mutated autoantibodies.[70] In either case, the emergence of pathologic autoimmunity could result from a primary or a secondary defect in the regulation of the expression of the autoimmune repertoire by the idiotypic network. Our current hypothesis is that IVIg interferes with the structure, function, and dynamics of the interactions of the idiotypic network, and the administration of IVIg restores physiologic control over the expression of the autoimmune repertoire in the treated patient.

IVIg Contain Antiidiotypes Directed Against Autoantibodies

The presence in IVIg of antiidiotypic antibodies directed against pathologic autoantibodies was first suggested during the course of the initial investigation carried out in two patients with autoantibodies to factor VIII. Infusion of 0.4 g/kg body weight/day of IVIg for 5 days resulted in a rapid and persistent decrease in autoantibody titer (Fig 1).[28] The prolonged suppressive effect of IVIg on autoantibody titer (now over 5 years) indicated that infused IgG had inhibited synthesis of autoantibodies. The occurrence of suppression within the first 30 hours after infusion indicated that infused

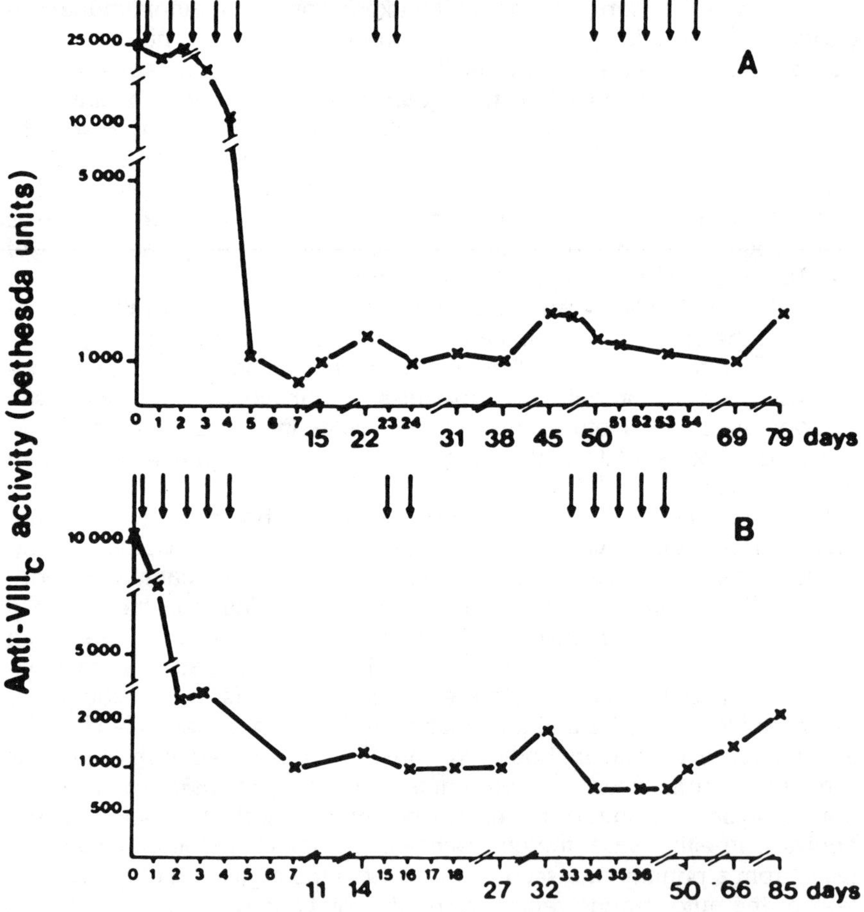

FIG 1.
Time course of antifactor VIII activity in plasma after infusion of IVIg in two patients with autoantibodies to factor VIII. *Arrows* indicate administration of IVIg (400 mg/kg/day). (From Sultan Y, Kazatchkine MD, Maisonneuve P, et al: *Lancet* 1984; ii:765–768. Used by permission.)

IVIg had also directly interacted with circulating autoantibodies (see Fig 1). This interaction could be demonstrated in vitro by incubating the patients' IgG or $F(ab')_2$ fragments of IgG with IVIg or $F(ab')_2$ fragments of IVIg, which resulted in a dose-dependent neutralization of autoantibody activity. These experiments suggested that IVIg could interact with variable regions of autoantibodies through idiotypic complementarity.

The presence in IVIg of antibodies directed against autoantibodies was then extended to a number of other disease-associated autoantibodies including antithyroglobulin autoantibodies from patients with Hashimoto's thyroiditis, antineuroblastoma antibodies from patients with Guillain-Barré syndrome, ANCA autoantibodies from patients with Wegener's granulomatosis, antiintrinsic factor autoantibodies from patients with megaloblastic anemia, anti-gp IIb IIIa autoantibodies from patients with idiopathic thrombocytopenic purpura,[71] and anti-DNA autoantibodies from patients with systemic lupus erythematosus. We have now gathered four lines evidence to demonstrate that IVIg contain antiidiotypes against autoantibodies:

1. $F(ab')_2$ fragments of IVIg neutralize the functional activity of autoantibodies and/or inhibit the binding of autoantibodies to autoantigens (Table 2).[72–75] Inhibition of antoantibody activity by IVIg is dose-dependent with a bell-shaped pattern of inhibition curves and a maximum inhibition being reached at a specific molar ratio of patient's IgG to IVIg (Fig 2).

TABLE 2.
Inhibition of Autoantibody Activity by $F(ab')_2$ Fragments Prepared From IVIg

Autoantibody	Inhibition (%)	Autoantibody (mol)/$F(ab')_2$ of IVIg (mol)*
Antifactor VIII	100	0.450
Antithyroglobulin	61	0.090
AntiDNA	96	2.900
Antiperipheral nerve†	82	0.001
Antiintrinsic factor	36	6.670
Antineutrophil cytoplasmic antigen	74	0.080

*$F(ab')_2$ fragments of IVIg (Sandoglobulin) were incubated with $F(ab')_2$ fragments, IgG, or IgM containing autoantibody activity for 1 hour at 37°C and overnight at 4°C. Residual antiDNA, antithyroglobulin, antiintrinsic factor, and antineutrophil cytoplasmic antigen activities were quantitated with enzyme-linked immunosorbent assay. Residual antifactor VIII activity was measured with a functional coagulation assay. Antiperipheral nerve activity was assessed with indirect immunofluorescence.

†Antibodies against the NBL 108 cc 15 cell line.

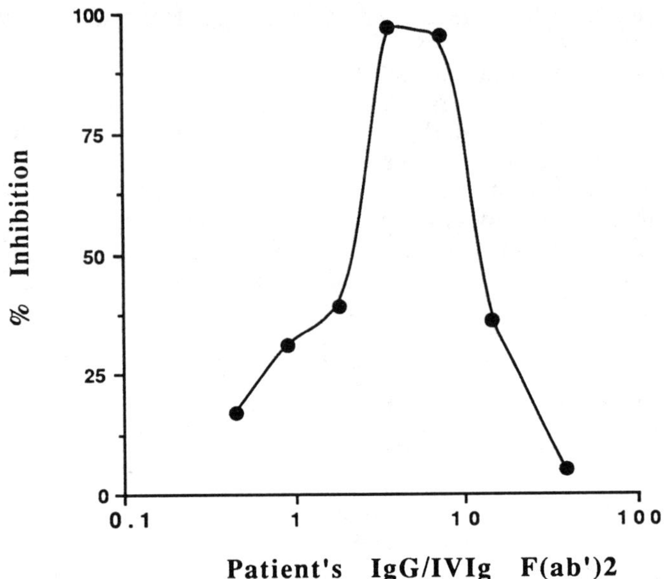

FIG 2.
Inhibition of antiDNA activity in the IgG fraction of the serum of a patient with systemic lupus erythematosus by $F(ab')_2$ fragments of IVIg. (From Rossi F, Kazatchkine MD: *J Immunol* 1989; 143:4104–4109. Used by permission.)

2. Autoantibody activity is specifically retained on affinity chromatography columns of $F(ab')_2$ fragments of IVIg coupled to sepharose. In these experiments, we loaded IgG or $F(ab')_2$ fragments of IgG with autoantibody activity onto columns of sepharose to which $F(ab')_2$ fragments of IVIg were coupled. IgG or $F(ab')_2$ fragments that bound to the column were eluted with an acidic buffer. Specific autoantibody activity expressed per milligram of protein was then measured in the acid eluates and compared with that of the material loaded on the columns. A 1.3- to 50-fold enrichment in specific activity was observed in the eluates, demonstrating that $F(ab')_2$ fragments of IVIg bind variable regions of autoantibodies with high affinity (Fig 3).

3. IVIg do not contain detectable antibodies against the most commonly expressed allotypes in the $F(ab')_2$ region of human IgG.[72]

4. IVIg share antiidiotypic specificities against autoantibodies with heterologous antiidiotypic antibodies. Thus, we found that IVIg compete with monoclonal or polyclonal antiidiotypic antibodies for the binding to idiotypes expressed by antifactor VIII[76] or antithyroglobulin autoantibodies.[77] We have obtained rabbit antiidiotypic antibodies, termed anti-T44, by immunization with affinity-purified antithyroglobulin $F(ab')_2$ fragments from a patient with autoimmune thyroiditis. We then showed that IVIg competes with anti-T44 antibodies for binding to the antithyroglobulin autoantibodies that served as immunogen, indicating that IVIg recognize the same id-

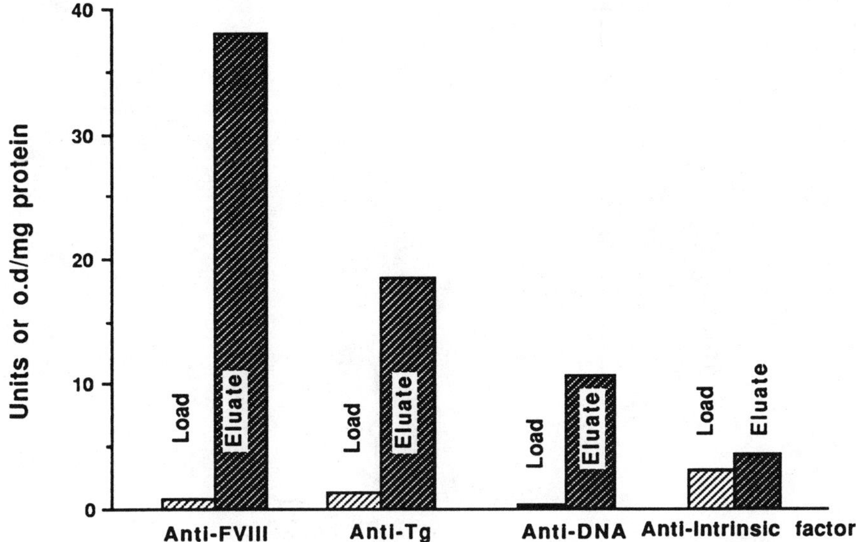

FIG 3.
Affinity chromatography: specific retention of autoantibody activity in the IgG fraction purified from the serum of patients with Hashimoto's thyroiditis, systemic lupus erythematosus, megaloblastic anemia, and antifactor VIII autoimmune disease, on a column of $F(ab')_2$ fragments of IVIg coupled to sepharose. Specific autoantibody activity expressed per mg of proteins was determined in the loaded material and in the acideluate from the column.

iotypic motifs on these autoantibodies as those identified with rabbit anti-T44 antibodies. Idiotype T44 was found to be expressed on antibodies of eight of nine patients with Hashimoto's thyroiditis, whereas it is not expressed by IgG from healthy individuals.[77]

The experiments demonstrated that IVIg recognize a cross-reactive idiotype that is a phenotypic marker of certain antithyroglobulin autoantibodies associated with Hashimoto's thyroiditis. The T44 idiotype is an α idiotype. Antithyroglobulin autoantibodies from patients that express the T44 idiotype recognize a specific epitopic domain of the thyroglobulin molecule that is not recognized by T44-antithyroglobulin autoantibodies from healthy individuals.[78] This antigenic region of thyroglobulin is the target of autoantibodies exclusively under pathologic autoimmune conditions.[78–80] In another set of experiments carried out with antifactor VIII autoantibodies, we found that an idiotype of β type defined by a mouse monoclonal antibody on antifactor VIII autoantibody from a patient was also recognized by IVIg and was expressed on autoantibodies from two of three patients that were investigated. Taken together, the results suggest that cross-reactive idiotypes expressed by disease-associated autoantibodies are recognized by IVIg. Such idiotypes would represent privileged target sites for therapeutic immunomodulation.

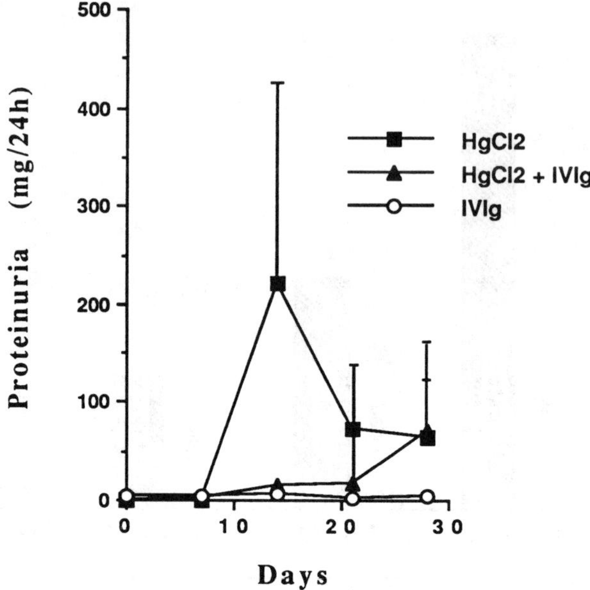

FIG 4.
Occurrence of proteinuria in Brown Norway rats treated with $HgCL_2$, or $HgCL_2$ and IVIg or IVIg alone. Animals received $HgCl_2$ from day 0. IVIg was administered from day 0 to day 4. Each point represents the mean protein concentration in the urine from ten experimental rats. (From Rossi F, Bellon B, Vial MC, et al: *Clin Exp Immunol* 1991; 84:129–133. Used by permission.)

Cross-reactive idiotypes among different species have been described.[82–84] We have recently observed that infusion of IVIg simultaneously with $HgCl_2$ in the susceptible strain of Brown Norway rats resulted in a significant decrease in the occurrence of proteinuria and a significant drop in increased serum IgE levels (Fig 4).[85] IVIg could thus have an immunoregulatory effect independent of species.

Remission or Recovery From Autoimmune Disease May Correlate With the Occurrence of Antiidiotypes Against Autoantibodies

Remission or recovery from certain autoimmune diseases is associated with autologous suppression of autoantibodies by auto-antiidiotypes. Antiidiotypic antibodies against prerecovery autoantibodies have been found in remission sera in myasthenia gravis,[86] systemic lupus erythematosus,[87] Guillain-Barré syndrome,[75] Wegener's granulomatosis,[73] antifactor VIII autoimmune disease,[88, 89] and antifibrinogen autoimmune disease.[90] In the case of a patient who spontaneously recovered from antifactor VIII autoimmune disease, we observed that $F(ab')_2$ fragments of the patients' postrecovery IgG inhibited antifactor VIII activity present in $F(ab')_2$ fragments of autologous IgG obtained during the acute phase of the disease. IgG obtained from plasma of the patient 4 years after recovery exhibited an inhibitory capacity against antifactor VIII autoantibodies similar to that of IVIg. Affinity chromatography experiments showed that an affinity column of $F(ab')_2$ fragments of postrecovery IgG specifically retained the acute-phase antifactor VIII autoantibodies.[88] Inhibition of autoantibody activity and the specific retention of autoantibodies on affinity columns by postrecovery IgG has also been found in the case of patients in remission from Wegener's granulomatosis[73] and who recovered from Guillain-Barré syndrome.[75] In the three disease categories previously mentioned, antiidiotypic antibodies that were present in remission serum of a particular patient were capable of recognizing both autologous autoantibodies and autoantibodies from other patients. Thus, an analogy may be drawn between the spontaneous remission from autoimmune disease associated with the occurrence of autoantiidiotypic antibodies and therapeutic recovery from autoimmune disease induced by IVIg, which contain antiidiotypes against autoantibodies.

The Origin of Autoantibody-Specific Antiidiotypic Activity of IVIg

The spectrum of the antiidiotypic activity of IVIg, which is directed against a large number of autoantibodies, is related to the fact that IVIg are prepared from plasma of a large number of donors. It is possible that each individual contributing to the pool accounts for a given antiidiotypic reactivity and that pooling individual plasmas results in a cumulative or synergistic expression of antiidiotypic activity in IVIg. Experiments by Tankersley have demonstrated that IVIg contain $F(ab')_2$-$F(ab')_2$ dimers and that the relative proportion of dimers in IVIg increases with the number of donors contributing to the pool. An IVIg preparation obtained from over 15,000 donors contains approximately 40% of dimers.[91, 92] Electron microscopic studies have directly demonstrated that dimers form as a result of complementary interactions between variable regions of immunoglobulins.[93] Thus, as the number of donors increases, the probability of finding antiidiotypic antibodies directed against an autoantibody of a given idiotypic specificity increases considerably in the pool.

It may be argued, however, that an antiidiotype contributed by a particular donor is subject to a high degree of dilution in the pool. Therefore, the spectrum of antiidiotypes in the IVIg pool depends on the number of donors and on the occurrence of idiotypes in the donor population. We have recently observed that combining IgG from two, three, or four individuals whose IgG does not express antiidiotypic activity may be sufficient for the expression of antiidiotypic activity against antifactor VIII autoantibodies in the pool. Mixing antibodies probably results in an increase in avidity for idiotypes.[94] Thus, the complementation of several individual antibodies has a synergistic effect on the expression of antiidiotypic activity in the pool.

An alternative hypothesis to explain the occurrence of antiidiotypes in the IVIg pool is that it contains IgG from privileged donors rich in antiidiotypes. Such donors could be patients having recovered spontaneously from autoimmune diseases, whose serum contains antiidiotypic antibodies against prerecovery autoantibodies; or the donors could also be healthy individuals over the age of 50 years. We have found that IgG of sera from donors of 50 to 60 years of age was two times more effective than IgG of 20- to 30-year-old donors in inhibiting antifactor VIII autoantibody activity.[94] The finding with increased frequency of antiidiotypes against autoantibodies in the serum of aged donors may reflect a progressive loosening of the network control of the expression of autoreactivity with aging.

A third hypothesis relating to the presence of antiidiotypes against autoantibodies in IVIg is that not all immunoglobulins in the pool have identical immunomodulatory capacity toward control of autoimmunity. The latter hypothesis would imply that there exists a subfraction of IVIg that is enriched in complementary antibodies against autoantibodies. This subfraction could represent the human counterpart of immunoglobulins that participate in the central compartment of the immune system in the mouse.[95–97] The central compartment comprises naturally activated, autoreactive, and highly connected B cells that are positively selected for their capacity to regulate the expression of autoreactive clones under physiologic conditions. A part of such a highly complementary subfraction of IVIg could be made up of antibodies capable of binding to themselves, called autobodies. The self-binding property of antibodies was first demonstrated in the case of a murine monoclonal antiphosphorylcholine antibody[98] but it has also been shown to be present in IVIg.[99] The locus of self-complexing of the antibodies lies in the CDR2/FR3 region, which is evidenced by the ability of the peptide T15H(50–73) derived from this region to inhibit self-complexing.[101, 102] The self-binding locus overlaps with the antigen combining site as demonstrated by the ability of hapten to inhibit self-complexing. IgG could be isolated from IVIg that were capable of binding to the self peptide on an affinity column of T15H(50–73) coupled to sepharose.[99] The self-binding potential of this subfraction of IVIg provides an enriched source of complementary antibodies. Although the precise role of this antibody population in IVIg is still unclear, it stands out as a possible basis for the immunoregulatory effect of IVIg in autoimmune diseases.

IVIg and the Idiotypic Network

Taken together, the data that have been summarized indicate that IVIg contain antibodies directed against idiotypes expressed by autoantibodies present in the serum of patients with various types of autoimmune diseases. The beneficial effect of IVIg in antibody-mediated autoimmune diseases is probably not, however, merely due to the passive transfer (transfusion) of neutralizing antiidiotypic antibodies against autoantibodies. We believe that IVIg interact with the basic structure, function, and dynamics, of the idiotypic network that ensure the physiologic control of autoimmunity. Thus, IVIg do not only recognize idiotypic determinants of pathologic autoantibodies but are also capable of interacting with idiotytpes expressed on natural, polyreactive autoantibodies that form the constitutive elements of the normal idiotypic network of healthy individuals. This was demonstrated by using autoreactive monoclonal IgM antibodies secreted by Epstein-Barr virus-transformed normal B lymphocytes. Twenty percent of IgM autoantibodies secreted by these cells bind to $F(ab')_2$ fragments of IVIg through idiotypic interaction.[100] By reacting with natural, polyreactive IgM that are components of the normal idiotypic network, IVIg could exert a selective pressure on the expression of the available immune repertoire of an individual. In addition to antiidiotypes against idiotypes of IgM antibodies, IVIg contains antiidiotypes against idiotypic determinants expressed by natural autoantibodies of the IgG isotype. Such idiotypic interactions can be demonstrated within IVIg by affinity chromatography experiments of IVIg on IVIg.[103]

The primary or secondary defects that lead to the emergence of pathologic autoimmunity most likely affect the function of the entire immune network even in the case of organ-specific autoimmune diseases. To investigate the function of the network in the healthy and autoimmune individual, we have compared the kinetics of expression of antiDNA and antithyroglobulin activity in IgG from serum of healthy donors and in patients with Hashimoto's thyroiditis.[104] In healthy individuals, autoantibody activity fluctuates in serum with a well-defined periodicity that is identical in all individuals. Dynamics of spontaneous fluctuations differ between healthy individuals and patients. Furthermore, the abnormal kinetic behavior of autoantibody activity in the serum of patients with Hashimoto's thyroiditis was not restricted to antithyroglobulin autoantibodies, but also extended to antiDNA autoantibodies. Thus, a basic defect in the regulation of the entire autoimmune repertoire may be present at the onset of an autoimmune disease, even when it apparently only affects a specific target organ.[104]

In this context, one may envisage that IVIg is effective beyond its ability to neutralize/suppress specific autoantibodies by altering the structure and the function of the defective idiotypic network of autoimmune patients. The use of IVIg therapy could hence be regarded as immunorestoration imposing a normal function onto the defective regulatory elements of the network in individuals with autoimmune disease. The regulatory effect of IVIg on the expression of the autoimmune repertoire could depend on the recognition of highly represented regulatory idiotopes that ensure the functional cohesion of the normal idiotypic network. Since such regulatory idiotopes would be located outside the paratope,[46] somatic mutations that could characterize pathologic autoantibodies would not interfere with the ability of IVIg in controlling the expression of autoimmune repertoire. IVIg thus offers a novel approach in the treatment of autoimmune diseases, related to the substitutive therapy of immune deficiencies rather than to nonspecific immunosuppression or to idiotypic suppression of autoantibodies with specific antiidiotypes.

Acknowledgments

The authors thank M. Algiman, B. Bellon, A. Brand, A. Coutinho, I. Lundkvist, U. Nydegger, and F. Varela for helpful suggestions and collaboration in this work.

References

1. Bierling P, Divine M, Farcet JP, et al: Persistent remission of adult chronic autoimmune thrombocytopenic purpura after treatment with high-dose intravenous immunoglobulin. *Am J Hematol* 1987; 25:271–275.
2. Bussel JB, Kimberly RP, Inman RD, et al: Intravenous gamma-globulin treatment of chronic idiopathic thrombocytopenic purpura. *Blood* 1983; 62:480.
3. Imbach P, Barandun S, d'Apuzzo V, et al: High-dose intravenous immunoglobulin for idiopathic thrombocytopenic purpura in childhood. *Lancet* 1981; i:1228–1229.
4. Newland AC, Treleaven JG, Minchinton RM, et al: High-dose intravenous IgG in adults with autoimmune thrombocytopenia. *Lancet* 1983; ii:84–87.
5. Bussel JB, Cunningham-Rundles C, Abraham C: Intravenous treatment of autoimmune hemolytic anemia with very high doses of gamma globulin. *Vox Sang* 1987; 51:264.
6. Hilgartner MW, Bussel J: Use of intravenous gamma-globulin for the treatment of autoimmune neutropenia of childhood and autoimmune hemolytic anemia. *Am J Med* 1987; 83:25–29.
7. McIntyre EA, Linch DC, Macey MG, et al: Successful response to intravenous immunoglobulin in autoimmune hemolytic anemia. *Br J Haematol* 1985; 60:287–292.
8. Schmidt RE, Budde V, Schäfer G, et al: High-dose intravenous gammaglobulin for idiopathic thrombocytopenic purpura. *Lancet* 1981; ii:475.
9. Bussel JB, Lalezari P, Hilgartner M, et al: Reversal of neutropenia with intravenous gammaglobulin in autoimmune neutropenia of infancy. *Blood* 1983; 62:398–403.
10. Pollack S, Cunningham-Rundles C, Smithwick EM, et al: High-dose intravenous immunoglobulin for autoimmune neutropenia. *N Engl J Med* 1982; 307:243–244.
11. Clauvel JP, Vainchenker W, Herrera A, et al: Treatment of pure red cell aplasia by high dose intravenous immunoglobulins. *Br J Haematol* 1983; 55:380–384.
12. McGuire WA, Yong HH, Bruno E, et al: Treatment of antibody mediated pure red cell aplasia with high-dose intravenous immunoglobulin. *N Engl J Med* 1987; 317:1004–1005.
13. Devathasan G, Kueh YK, Chong PN: High-dose intravenous gammaglobulin for myasthenia gravis. *Lancet* 1984; ii:809–810.
14. Fateh-Moghadam A, Wick M, Besinger U, et al: High-dose intravenous gammaglobulin for myasthenia gravis. *Lancet* 1984; i:848–849.

15. Gadjos PH, Outin H, Elkharrat D, et al: High-dose intravenous immunoglobulin for myasthenia gravis. *Lancet* 1984; i:406–407.
16. Ippoliti J, Cosi V, Piccolo G, et al: High-dose intravenous gammaglobulin for myasthenia gravis. *Lancet* 1984; ii:809.
17. Albala M, McNanara ME, Sokol M, et al: Improvement of neurologic function in chronic inflammatory demyelinating polyradiculoneuropathy following intravenous gammaglobulin infusion. *Arch Neurol* 1987; 44:248.
18. Vermeulen M, Van Der Mesche FGA, Speelman JD, et al: Plasma and immunoglobulin infusion in chronic inflammatory polyneuropathy. *J Neurol Sci* 1985; 70:317–326.
19. Kleyweg RP, Van Der Mesche FGA, Meulstee J: Treatment of Guillain-Barré syndrome with high-dose gammaglobulin. *Neurology* 1988; 38:1639–1641.
20. Furusho K, Kamiy T, Nakano H, et al: High-dose intravenous gammaglobulin for Kawasaki disease. *Lancet* 1984; i:1055–1058.
21. Leung DYM: The immunologic effects of IGIV in Kawasaki disease. *Int Rev Immunol* 1989; 5:197–202.
22. Carreras LO, Perez GN, Vega HR, et al: Lupus anti-coagulant and recurrent fetal loss: Successful treatment with gammaglobulin. *Lancet* 1988; ii:393–395.
23. Gianella-Borradore A, Hirt A, Luthy A, et al: Haemophilia due to factor VIII inhibitors in a patient suffering from an autoimmune disease. Treatment with intravenous immuno-globulin. *Blut* 1984; 48:403–407.
24. Green D, Kwaan HC: An acquired factor VIII inhibitor responsive to high-dose gammaglobulin. *Thromb Haemost* 1987; 58:1005.
25. Heyman MR, Chakravarthy A, Edelman BB, et al: Failure of high-dose intravenous gammaglobulin in the treatment of spontaneously occurred factor VIII inhibitor. *Am J Hematol* 1988; 28:191–194.
26. Newland AC, Macey MG, Moffat EH, et al: Effect of intravenous immunoglobulins on a spontaneous inhibitor to factor VIII. *Clin Lab Hematol* 1988; 10:435–442.
27. Moffat EH, Furlong AH, Daannatt A, et al: Anti-idiotypes to factor VIII antibodies and their possible role in the pathogenesis and treatment of factor VIII inhibitors. *Br J Haematol* 1989; 71:85–90.
28. Sultan Y, Kazatchkine MD, Maisonneuve P, et al: Anti-idiotypic suppression of autoantibodies to factor VIII by high-dose intravenous immunoglobulin. *Lancet* 1984; ii:765–768.
29. Zimmerman R, Kommerell B, Harenberg J, et al: Intravenous IgG for patients with spontaneous inhibitor to factor VIII. *Lancet* 1985; i:273.
30. Sherin P, Heros S, Wechsler B, et al: Interest of intravenous gammaglobulin therapy in refractory polymyositis and dermatomyositis: Open study with 20 adult patients. *Am J Med,* in press.
31. Fehr J, Hoffman V, Kappeler V: Transient reversal of thrombocytopenic purpura by high-dose intravenous immunoglobulin. *N Engl J Med* 1987; 306:1254–1258.
32. Dammacco F, Iodice G, Campobasso N: Treatment of adult patients with idiopathic purpura with intravenous immunoglobulins: Effects on circulating T cell subsets and PWM-induced antibody synthesis in vitro. *Br J Haematol* 1986; 62:125–135.
33. Stohl W: Cellular mechanisms in the in vitro inhibition of pokeweed mitogen-induced B cell differentiation by immunoglobulin for intravenous use. *J Immunol* 1986; 136:4407–4413.
34. Tsubakio T, Kurata Y, Katagiri S, et al: Alteration of T cell subsets and immu-

noglobulin synthesis in vitro during high-dose gammaglobulin therapy in patients with idiopathic thrombocytopenic purpura. *Clin Exp Immunol* 1983; 53:697–702.

35. Delfraissy JF, Tchernia G, Laurian Y, et al: Suppressor cell function after intravenous gammaglobulin treatment in adult idiopathic thrombocytopenic purpura. *Br J Haematol* 1985; 60:315–322.
36. Durandy A, Fiscer A, Griscelli C: Dysfunctions of poke-weed mitogen stimulated T and B lymphocyte responses induced by gammaglobulin therapy. *J Clin Invest* 1981; 67:867–877.
37. Leung DYM, Burns JC, Newburger JW, et al: Reversal of lymphocyte activation in vivo in the Kawasaki syndrome by intravenous gammaglobulin. *J Clin Invest* 1987; 79:468–472.
38. Engelhard D, Waner JL, Kapoor N, et al: Effect of intravenous immune globulin on natural killer cell activity: Possible association with autoimmune neutropenia and idiopathic thrombocytopenia. *J Pediatr* 1986; 108:77–81.
39. Batchelor JR, Lombardi G, Lechler RI: Speculations on the specificity on the suppression. *Immunol Today* 1989; 10:37–40.
40. Chen PP, Soto-gil RW, Carson DA: The early expression of some human autoantibody-associated heavy chain variable region genes is controlled by specific regulatory elements. *Scand J Immunol* 1990; 31:673–678.
41. Dietrich G, Rossi F, Sultan Y, et al: IVIg and regulation of autoimmunity through the idiotypic network, in Imbach P, Morell A (eds): *Clinical Use of Intravenous Immunoglobulins.* New York, Academic Press, 1991, pps 3–14.
42. Kaveri SV, Dietrich G, Kazatchkine M: Can intravenous immunoglobulin (IVIg) treatment regulate autoimmune responses? *Semin Hematol,* in press.
43. Zanetti M: Idiotypic regulation of autoantibody production. *CRC Crit Rev Immunol* 1986; 6:151.
44. Lindenmann J: Speculations on idiotypy and homobodies. *Ann Immunol* 1973; 124:12.
45. Jerne NK: Towards a network theory of the immune system. *Ann Immunol* 1974; 125:373–389.
46. Bona CA: Regulatory idiotopes, in Kohler H, Urbain J, Cazenave PA (eds): *Idiotypy in Biology and Medicine.* New York, Academic Press, 1984, pp 29–42.
47. Martinez-AC, Pereira P, Toribio ML, et al: The participation of B cells and antibodies in the selection and maintenance of T cell repertoires. *Immunol Rev* 1988; 101:191.
48. Algiman M, Dietrich G, Nydegger U, et al: Antibodies to factor VIII in healthy individuals, *J Clin Invest,* submitted.
49. Avrameas S, Guilbert B, Dighiero G: Natural antibodies against tubulin, actin, myoglobin, thyroglobulin, fetuin, albumin and transferrin are present in normal human sera and monoclonal immunoglobulins from multiple myeloma and Waldenström's macroglobulinemia may express similar antibody specificities. *Ann Immunol* 1981; 132:231–236.
50. Guilbert B, Dighiero G, Avrameas S: Naturally occurring antibodies against nine common antigens in normal human sera. I. Detection, isolation, and characterization. *J Immunol* 1982; 128:2779–2787.
51. Karounos DG, Gruder JP, Pisetsky DS: Spontaneous expression of antibodies to DNA of various species origin in sera of normal subjects and patients with SLE. *J Immunol* 1988; 140:451–455.

52. Madaio MP, Schattner A, Shattner M, et al: Lupus serum and normal human serum contain anti-DNA antibodies with the same idiotypic marker. *J Immunol* 1986; 137:2535–2540.
53. Pfueller SL, Logan D, Tran TT, et al: Naturally occurring human IgG antibodies to intracellular and cytoskeletal components of human platelets. *Clin Exp Immunol* 1990; 79:67–73.
54. Ross C, Hansen MB, Schyberg T, et al: Autoantibodies to crude human leucocyte intereferon (IFN), native human IFN, recombinant human IFN alpha 2b and human IFN gamma in healthy blood donors. *Clin Exp Immunol* 1990; 82:57–62.
55. Seigneurin MJ, Guilbert B, Bourgeat MJ, et al: Polyspecific natural antibodies and autoantibodies secreted by human lymphocytes immortalized with Epstein-Barr virus. *Blood* 1988; 3:581.
56. Yadin O, Sarov B, Naggan L, et al: Natural autoantibodies in the serum of healthy women a five year follow up. *Clin Exp Immunol* 1989; 75: 402–406.
57. Coutinho A, Forni L, Holmberg D, et al: From an antigen-centered, clonal perspective of immune response to an organism-centered, network perspective of autonomous activity in a self-referential immune system. *Immunol Rev* 1984; 79:151.
58. Holmberg D, Coutinho A: Natural antibodies and autoimmunity. *Immunol Today* 1985; 6:356–357.
59. Holmberg D, Wennerstrom G, Andrade L, et al: The high idiotypic connectivity of natural newborn antibodies is not found in adult mitogen-reactive B cell repertoires. *Eur J Immunol* 1986; 16:82–87.
60. Huetz F, Jacquemart F, Pena-Rossi C, et al: Autoimmunity: The moving boundaries between physiology and pathology. *J Autoimmunity* 1988; 1:507–511.
61. Stewart J, Varela FJ: Exploring the meaning of connectivity in the immune network. *Immunol Rev* 1989; 110:37–61.
62. Vakil M, Kearney JF: Functional characterization of monoclonal auto-anti-idiotypic antibodies isolated from the early B cell repertoire of Balb/c mice. *Eur J Immunol* 1986; 16:1151–1158.
63. Lundkvist I, Coutinho A, Varela F, et al: Evidence for a functional idiotypic network among natural antibodies in normal mice. *Proc Natl Acad Sci (USA)* 1989; 86:5074–5078.
64. Baccala R, Vo Quang T, Gilbert M, et al: Two murine natural polyreactive autoantibodies are encoded by nonmutated germ-line genes. *Proc Natl Acad Sci (USA)* 1989; 86:4624–4628.
65. Dermisonian H, Schwartz RS, Barrett KJ, et al: Relationship of human variable region heavy chain germ-line genes to genes encoding anti-DNA autoantibodies. *J Immunol* 1987; 139:2496–2501.
66. Harttman AB, Mallett CP, Srinivasappa J, et al: Organ-reactive autoantibodies from non-immunized adult Balb/c mice are polyreactive and express nonbiased Vh gene usage. *Mol Immunol* 1989; 26:359–370.
67. Sanz I, Capra JD: The genetic origin of human autoantibodies. *J Immunol* 1988; 140:3283.
68. Sanz I, Dang H, Takei M, et al: Vh sequence of a human anti-Sm autoantibody: Evidence that autoantibodies can be unmutated copies of germline genes. *J Immunol* 1989; 142:883–887.
69. Siminovitch KA, Misener V, Kwong PC, et al: A natural autoantibody is en-

coded by germline heavy and lambda light chain variable region genes without somatic mutation. *J Clin Invest* 1989; 84:1675–1678.
70. Schwartz RS: Autoantibodies and normal antibodies, in Cinader B, Miller RG (eds): *Progress in Immunology*. New York, Academic Press, 1986, pp 478–482.
71. Berchtold P, Dale GL, Tani P, et al: Inhibition of autoantibody binding to platelet glycoprotein IIb/IIIa by anti-idiotypic antibodies in intravenous immunoglobulins. *Blood* 1989; 74:2414–2417.
72. Rossi F, Sultan Y, Kazatchkine MD: Anti-idiotypes against autoantibodies and alloantibodies to factor VIIIc (anti-hemophilic factor) are present in therapeutic polyspecific normal immunoglobulins. *Clin Exp Immunol* 1988; 74:311–317.
73. Rossi F, Jayne DR, Lockwood CM, et al: Antiidiotypes against anti-neutrophil cytoplasmic antigen autoantibodies in normal human polyspecific IgG for therapeutic use and in the remission serum of patients with systemic vasculitis. *Clin Exp Immunol* 1991; 83:298–303.
74. Rossi F, Kazatchkine MD: Anti-idiotypes against autoantibodies in pooled normal human polyspecific Ig. *J Immunol* 1989; 143:4104–4109.
75. Van Doorn PA, Rossi F, Brand A, et al: Treatment of chronic inflammatory demyelinating polyneuropathy with high-dose intravenous immunoglobulins. *J Neuroimmunol* 1990; 29:57–64.
76. Dietrich G, Pereira P, Algiman M, et al: A monoclonal anti-idiotypic antibody against the antigen-combining site of anti-factor VIII autoantibodies defines an idiotope that is recognized by normal human polyspecific immunoglobulins for therapeutic use (IVIg). *J Autoimmunity* 1990; 3:547–557.
77. Dietrich G, Kazatchkine MD: Normal immunoglobulin G (IgG) for therapeutic use (intravenous Ig) contain anti-idiotypic specificities against an immunodominant, disease-associated, cross-reactive idiotype of human anti-thyroglobulin autoantibodies. *J Clin Invest* 1990; 85:620–624.
78. Dietrich G, Piechaczyk M, Pau B, Kazatchkine MD. Evidence for restricted epitopic and idiotypic specificity of anti-thyroglobulin autoantibodies. *Eur J Immunol,* in press.
79. Bouanani M, Piechaczyk M, Pau B, et al: Significance of the recognition of certain antigenic regions on the thyroglobulin molecule by natural autoantibodies from healthy subjects. *J Immunol* 1989; 143:1129–1132.
80. Bresler HS, Lynne Burek C, Hoffman WH, et al: Autoantigenic determinants on human thyroglobulin: Determinants recognized by autoantibodies from patients with chronic autoimmune thyroiditis compared to auto-antibodies from healthy subjects. *Clin Immunol Immunopathol* 1990; 54:76–86.
81. Piechaczyk M, Bouanani M, Salhi SL, et al: Antigenic domains on the human thyroglobulin molecule recognized by autoantibodies in patients' sera and by natural autoantibodies isolated from sera of healthy subjects. *Clin Exp Immunol* 1987; 45:114–117.
82. Danz H, Takei M, Isenberg D, et al: Expression of interspecies idiotype in sera of SLE patients and their first-degree relatives. *Clin Exp Immunol* 1988; 71:445–450.
83. Takei M, Dang H, Wang RJ, et al: Characteristics of a human monoclonal anti-Sm antibody expressing an interspecies idiotype. *J Immunol* 1988; 140:3108–3113.
84. Zanetti M, Barton RW, Bigazzi PE: Anti-idiotypic immunity and autoimmunity. II. Idiotypic determinants of autoantibodies and lymphocytes in sponta-

neous and experimentally induced autoimmune thyroiditis. *Cell Immunol* 1983; 75:292–299.
85. Rossi F, Bellon B, Vial MC, et al: Effect of intravenous immunoglobulins on $HgCl_2$-induced autoimmunity in rats. *Clin Exp Immunol* 1991; 84:129–133.
86. Lefvert AK: Idiotypes and anti-idiotypes of human auto-antibodies to the acetylcholine receptor in myasthenia gravis. *Monogr Allergy* 1987; 22:57.
87. Zouali M, Eyquem A: Idiotypic-anti-idiotypic interactions in systemic lupus erythematosus: Demonstration of oscillating levels of anti-DNA antibodies and reciprocal anti-idiotypic activity in a single patient. *Ann Immunol* 1983; 134:377.
88. Sultan Y, Rossi F, Kazatchkine MD: Recovery from anti-VIIIc (anti-hemophilic factor) autoimmune disease is dependent on generation of anti-idiotypes against anti-VIIIc autoantibodies. *Proc Natl Acad Sci (USA)* 1987; 84:828–831.
89. Tiarks C, Pechet L, Huphreys RE: Development of anti-idiotypic antibodies in a patient with a factor VIII antibody. *Am J Hematol* 1989; 32:217–221.
90. Ruiz-Arguelles A: Spontaneous reversal of acquired autoimmune dysfibrinogenemia probably due to an anti-idiotypic antibody directed to an interspecies cross-reactive idiotype expressed on antifibrinogen antibodies. *J Clin Invest* 1988; 82:958–963.
91. Roux KH, Tankersley DL: A view of the human idiotypic repertoire: Electron microscopic and immunologic analyses of spontaneous idiotype-anti-idiotype dimers in pooled human IgG. *J Immunol* 1990; 144:1387–1392.
92. Tankersley DL, Preston MS, Finlayson JS: Immunoglobulin G dimer: An idiotype-anti-idiotype complex. *Mol Immunol* 1988; 25:41–48.
93. Gronski P, Bauer R, Bodenbender L, et al: On the nature of IgG dimers. *Behring Inst Mitt* 1988; 82:127–153.
94. Dietrich G, Algiman M, Sultan Y, et al: Origin of autoantibody-specific anti-idiotypic activity in normal polyspecific immunoglobulins for therapeutic use (IVIg). *Fed Proc,* in press.
95. Coutinho A: Beyond clonal selection and network. *Immunol Rev* 1989; 110:63–87.
96. Holmberg D, Forsgren S, Ivars F, et al: Reactions amongst IgM antibodies derived from normal neonatal mice. *Eur J Immunol* 1984; 14:435.
97. Portnoï D, Freitas A, Holmberg D, et al: Immunocompetent autoreactive B lymphocytes are activated cycling cells in normal mice. *J Exp Med* 1986; 164:25.
98. Kang C-Y, Kohler H: Immunoglobulin with complementary paratope and idiotope. *J Exp Med* 1986; 163:787–796.
99. Kaveri SV, Kang CY, Kohler H: Natural mouse and human antibodies bind to a peptide derived from a germline variable heavy chain: Evidence for evolutionary conserved sequence. *J Immunol* 1990; 145:4207–4213.
100. Rossi F, Guilbert B, Tonnelle C, et al: Idiotypic interactions between normal human polyspecific IgG and natural IgM antibodies. *Eur J Immunol* 1990; 20:2089–2094.
101. Kaveri SV, Halpern R, Kang CY, et al: Self-binding antibodies (autobodies) form specific complexes in solution. *J Immunol* 1990; 145:2533–2538.
102. Kaveri SV, Halpern R, Kang CY, et al: Antibodies of different specificities are self-binding: Implication for antibody diversity. *Mol Immunol* 1991; 28:773–778.
103. Rossi F, Dietrich G, Kazatchkine MD: Anti-idiotypes against autoantibodies in

normal immunoglobulins: Evidence for network regulation of human autoimmune responses. *Immunol Rev* 1989; 110:135–149.

104. Varela F, Anderson A, Dietrich G, et al: The population dynamics of antibodies in normal and autoimmune individuals. *Proc Natl Acad Sci (USA)* 1991; 88:5917–5921.

Treatment of Multiple Myeloma With Renal Involvement

Dominique Ganeval, M.D.
Department of Nephrology, Necker Hospital, Paris, France

Cécile Rabian, M.D.
Department of Nephrology, Necker Hospital, Paris, France

Violaine Guérin, M.D.
Department of Nephrology, Necker Hospital, Paris, France

Nathalie Pertuiset, M.D.
Department of Nephrology, Necker Hospital, Paris, France

Paul Landais, M.D.
Department of Nephrology, Necker Hospital, Paris, France

Paul Jungers, M.D.
Department of Nephrology, Necker Hospital, Paris, France

Renal failure is a common feature in myelomatosis, and more than 50% of patients with multiple myeloma have impaired renal function at presentation or during the course of the disease.[1, 2] Impaired renal function is generally reported as associated with poor prognosis. In observations before and around the 1970s, the median survival time of patients with myelomatosis and renal failure was very short, not exceeding 2 months in certain series.[3–5] However, in the past 2 decades the renal outlook has markedly improved in these patients due to better understanding and appropriate management of renal failure, and the use of hemodialysis when necessary. Consequently, deaths directly attributable to renal failure drastically decreased. Despite this improvement, the survival time of patients with myelomatosis and renal failure remains shorter than that usually reported in the general population of patients with myeloma. This prompted us to reexamine the literature concerning this problem and our own data.

Patients

Of the 85 patients with myelomatosis whom we observed between 1965 and 1990, only 5 had normal renal function. Since 5 cases were too few to form a control group, these patients were excluded from the study.

The main characteristics of the patients are summarized in Table 1. Fifty-

TABLE 1.
Main Characteristics at Presentation of 80 Patients With Multiple Myeloma and Renal Failure

Characteristic	Data
Sex, male/female	37/43
Age, yr	64 ± 13.4
M-protein	
IgG	26
IgA	15
IgD	2
BJ only	37
κ/λ	1.05
Stage (Durie and Salmon)	
I B	8
II B	14
III B	58
Plasma cell (%)	41.7 ± 32.8
Hemoglobin (g/dL)*	9.2 ± 1.9
Serum calcium (mmol/L)	2.6 ± 0.5
Serum creatinine (μmol/L)	700 ± 460
Bence Jones proteinuria (g/24 hr)	5.2 ± 5.5
Factors contributory to RF†	
Hypercalcemia	24
Dehydration	8
Use of contrast media	9
Nephrotoxic drugs	2
Infections	7
Other	2
Renal biopsy (30 patients)‡	
Myeloma kidney	19
Amyloidosis	2
LCDD†	8
Other	1

*Many patients had received blood transfusion before admission
†RF = renal failure; LCDD = light chain deposition disease.
‡During follow-up, LCDD developed in one patient with myeloma kidney, amyloidosis in two patients with myeloma kidney, and one patient with LCDD. Amyloidosis was also demonstrated in extrarenal localization in three patients who had not undergone renal biopsy.

six patients (70%) were admitted after 1977. Some of the 24 patients observed before 1977 were included in a preceding study.[6]

When patients observed after 1977 were compared to the subgroup previously seen, only few differences appeared. Classification of patients according to the type of immunoglobulin continuously showed a much higher incidence (46% for the whole series) of patients with myeloma cells excreting only Bence Jones protein (Bence Jones myeloma) compared to M-protein distribution in the general population of myeloma in which this group is under 20%. The percentage of Bence Jones myeloma in our series even increased in recent years (48% after and 40% before 1977). The percentage of patients at stage III of the study by Durie and Salmon[7] was high in both periods, with a mean of 73%. Renal insufficiency at presentation was severe, though slightly lower in the second subgroup (after 1977) than in the first. Finally, nearly half of the patients were referred to us from other hospitals, with already diagnosed myeloma and because of threatening renal failure and very poor status. Most of the patients with undiagnosed myeloma at admission had Bence Jones myeloma.

Survival analysis was performed with the product limit method. Comparisons between survival curves were tested by the log rank test. The proportional hazard model was used to define prognostic variables. The exponential of the regressive coefficient is considered as a relative risk in case of qualitative variable.

Renal Insufficiency

The association between light chain proteinuria and renal failure in myelomatosis has repeatedly been shown.[8, 9] The myeloma kidney is characterized by light-chain-derived tubular casts, surrounded by multinucleated giant cells.[9–11] It is generally thought that increased production of myeloma protein and emergence of light chains in tubules at high concentration, plus some contributing factors such as decreased tubular urine flow, lead to the precipitation of light chains, the formation of casts, tubular epithelial atrophy, interstitial fibrosis, and subsequent decreased renal function.[12, 13] Dehydration, hypercalcemia, infections, and nephrotoxic drugs may also be precipitating factors leading to acute renal failure or contributory factors to chronic renal deterioration.[14, 15] Besides typical lesions of the myeloma kidney, other lesions, also specifically related to light chains, can complicate multiple myeloma; i.e., renal amyloidosis[16] and light chain deposition disease (LCDD).[17, 18]

In our series, all patients had renal insufficiency (serum creatinine concentration >130 μmol/L) at admission and most of them suffered from severe renal failure (see Table 1). Overall mean serum creatinine concentration was 700 μmol/L. Thirty-eight patients had a serum creatinine concentration ≥700 μmol/L and one of them was already receiving dialysis. Only 12 patients had mild renal impairment with a serum creatinine concentration ≤200 μmol/L. In nearly half of the patients (47.5%), precipitating or factors contributory to renal failure were present. Hypercalcemia was most frequent. Dehydration appeared as the third factor, after the use of contrast media, but its frequency could have been underestimated, or it could have been corrected before transfer to our hospital. Seventy-six patients (95%) had Bence Jones proteinuria, among which 39 had IgG, IgA, or IgD myeloma with Bence Jones excretion, and 37 had only Bence Jones production. The mean level of Bence Jones proteinuria was 5 g/day (range, 0.10 to 55 g/day. Bence Jones protein, either in serum or in urine, was not measured with a direct technique. It was estimated from monoclonal pike intensity at electrophoresis, and values are only approximate). Of the 37 patients with Bence Jones myeloma, 11 had free Bence Jones protein in the serum, ranging from 0.5 to 15 g/L (mean, 6 g/L). It is particularly interesting that some of the patients with large amounts of free Bence Jones protein in their serum had moderate renal failure at that time (serum creatinine level ≤500 μmol/L), suggesting that the degree of renal failure was not the only factor responsible for the presence of Bence Jones protein in the serum.

Among clinical parameters that characterized the patients at presentation, the only association we found with creatinine was hemoglobin ($P <$ .005). However, this relationship was weaker than that observed in patients with renal insufficiency without myeloma. Although hypercalcemia was frequent at presentation, there was no association between its presence and serum creatinine level. Finally, there was no link, in our series, between creatinine level and stage of the disease.

Treatment of Renal Insufficiency

Since the presence of free light chains in renal tubules is the main factor responsible for the occurrence of renal failure in myeloma patients,[6, 8, 9] measures to reduce the concentration of light chains passing through the kidney are of major importance to prevent and treat renal insufficiency in such patients. The benefit of high urine flow, by maintenance of high fluid intake, has been well demonstrated.[6, 8, 19–21] The supplementary benefit of urine alkalinization to prevent precipitation of light chains in tubules is usually accepted, although it has been debated by some authors.[21] Dialysis, as long as necessary, is now a common measure in myeloma patients with end-stage renal disease (ESRD)[6, 12, 15, 22, 23] to allow administration of repeated courses of chemotherapy and remission of myeloma. Some authors have reported reversal of renal failure after a period of dialysis.[12, 15, 24, 25] Recently, plasmapheresis has been proposed as a means of rapidly reducing the plasma concentration of myeloma proteins and, as a consequence, avoiding the appearance of Bence Jones proteins in the tubular urine.[26–28] The exact benefit of this technique is still debated.[12]

In our series, the treatment of renal insufficiency has involved: (1) high fluid intake in all patients except a few with oliguria or congestive cardiac failure, who were fluid intolerant; (2) alkalinization of urine with oral or intravenous sodium bicarbonate in the amount necessary to maintain the pH of urine ≥7; (3) chemotherapy in all but 2 patients; (4) dialysis in 25 patients; and (5) plasmapheresis in 13 patients. This last treatment was not performed in a controlled study, and indications of plasmapheresis varied with time.

Results of Treatment of Renal Insufficiency

First Month

Patients could be classified into three groups according to their renal status 1 month after presentation (78 patients; 2 patients were excluded because of early death; Fig 1).

Group 1

Reversal of renal failure was observed in 38 patients (49%). Mean serum creatinine concentration at admission was 707 μmol/L and the mean decrease was 45% (standard deviation [SD], 18.3%; range, 20% to 86%). In 4 patients, serum creatinine reached normal values. In 2 in whom dialysis had been undertaken immediately after admission, renal function improved during the first month and dialysis could be stopped. Factors contributory to renal failure were present in many, but not in all, patients who improved during the first month.

Group 2

In 18 patients (23%), renal function stabilized. In this group mean serum creatinine concentration at admission was 255 μmol/L.

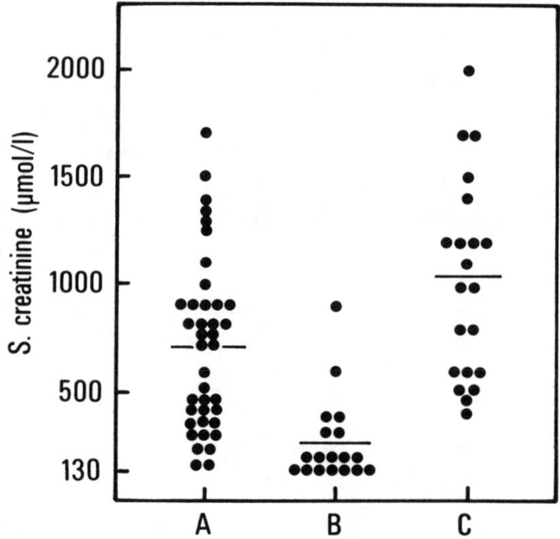

FIG 1.
Distribution of serum creatinine concentrations at presentation in groups defined according to evolution of renal function after 1 month: *A* = improved; *B* = stabilized; *C* = end-stage or worsened renal failure.

Group 3

At 1 month, 22 patients (28%) had either reached ESRD, or initial renal failure had worsened. The mean creatinine level at presentation was 1046 μmol/L.

Long-Term Results

For this analysis, we considered the minimal serum creatinine concentration obtained during evolution, or serum creatinine level observed at the end of follow-up, excluding creatinine values in the late terminal phase of relapsing myelomas; these values were considered more likely to be a consequence of hemodynamic or infectious complications than actual independent alteration of renal function. Nineteen patients were excluded because of early death (within the first 3 months) or absence of sufficient follow-up. Consequently, 59 patients could be analyzed. Table 2 shows a comparison of the evolution of renal function in the three groups defined at the end of the first month.

Group 1

Most patients who had improved renal function at 1 month had further improvement. Only 2 showed progressive renal failure and required dialysis after 36 and 65 months.

TABLE 2.
Long-Term Evolution of Renal Function in 59 Evaluable Patients With Multiple Myeloma and Renal Failure

			Long-Term Renal Function			
			Improved			
Renal Function After 1 Month	No. Patients	No. Evaluable	To Normal	Partially	Stabilized	ESRD
Group 1						
Normal renal function	4	4	4			
Partial recovery	34	25	4	10	9	2
Group 2						
Stabilized	18	17	5	5	4	3
Group 3						
Worsened	4	3		2		1
ESRD	18	10	—	—	—	10
Total	78	59	13	17	13	16

Group 2

In the 17 patients with unchanged renal function at 1 month, 10 improved (5 of them reaching normal creatinine values), and 3 had slowly progressed to ESRD and dialysis (time to hemodialysis: 8.53 to 64 months). The remaining 4 patients had stabilization of abnormal renal function at the level observed at admission up to the end of follow-up (mean duration, 32 months; range, 5 to 57 months).

Group 3

Only 2 of the 13 patients of this group had partially improved renal failure. All 9 patients who were receiving dialysis at 1 month continued dialysis until death (8 patients; mean duration, 10 months; range, 4 to 22 months) or until the end of the study (1 patient alive after 11 months). The eleventh patient progressively deteriorated and reached ESRD 3 months later.

Acute Renal Failure

Nine patients experienced acute deterioration of renal function during the follow-up. Reversal of renal failure was obtained in all but 1 patient. Renal failure was totally reversible in 5 patients and partially reversible in 3.

Renal and Extrarenal Histologic Studies

Renal biopsy was performed in 30 patients (among whom 6 patients underwent two, and 2 patients underwent three renal biopsies). The first biopsy specimen showed: myeloma kidney in 19 patients; amyloidosis in 2 patients; LCDD in 8 patients; and proliferative glomerulonephritis in 1. During the evolution, 1 patient with myeloma kidney developed renal and extrarenal LCDD, and 3 patients (2 with myeloma kidney, 1 with LCDD) developed amyloidosis. Extrarenal amyloidosis was also found in 3 patients who did not undergo renal biopsy. Thus, amyloidosis could be demonstrated in 9 patients with myeloma (11% of the whole series). However, we must stress that the prevalence of myeloma kidney observed in our series is probably underestimated, since only 37% of the 80 patients underwent renal histologic study, and since all patients with symptoms suggestive of LCDD or amyloidosis were systematically investigated.

Some interesting findings emerge from the analysis of renal failure in our patients with myeloma.

1. Improvement of renal failure may occur despite severe renal insufficiency at admission. More than half of the patients with serum creatinine concentration ≥800 μmol/L had improved after 1 month. However, taking all patients together, improvement appeared more frequent in patients with moderate or mild renal failure at admission than in those with severe

renal failure, and there was a positive correlation between serum creatinine levels at 1 month and at presentation (Fig 2). It is interesting that the 13 patients who regained normal renal function after 1 month or later had a mean serum creatinine concentration at admission of 256 μmol/L (range, 150 to 500 μmol/L).

2. Evolution of renal function after 1 month is a good indication of further evolution. Long-term improvement in renal function was found for 62% of the analyzable patients in group 1 (improvement after 1 month), for 58% in group 2 (stabilization after 1 month), and for only 15% in group 3 (worsened renal failure or ESRD after 1 month, see table 2). Thus, it appears that if the final outcome is to be favorable, improvement (or at least stabilization) must be obtained at 1 month.

3. Patterns of evolution of creatinine with time (Fig 3) in patients with improved renal function showed first a phase of rapid decrease in serum creatinine level within the first month, then a second phase of much slower improvement. The first phase of improvement was mostly independent of chemotherapy since it took place before the first signs of objective response and sometimes despite obviously uncontrolled growth of the tumor. The second phase is likely the result of both chemotherapy (in re-

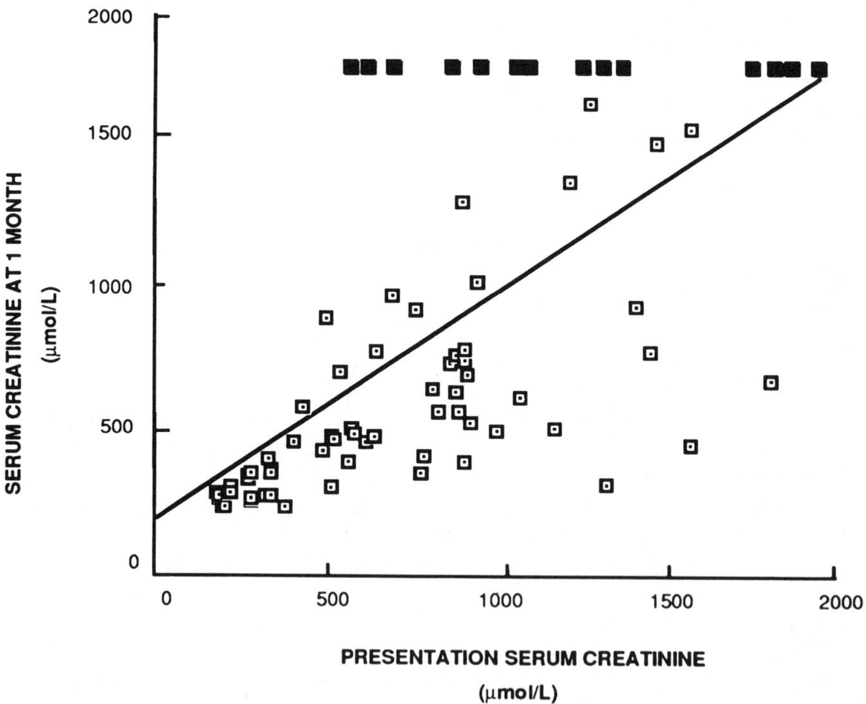

FIG 2.
Serum creatinine concentrations at presentation and after 1 month of 78 patients with multiple myeloma and renal failure. *Solid box* = patients receiving dialysis at the end of first month.

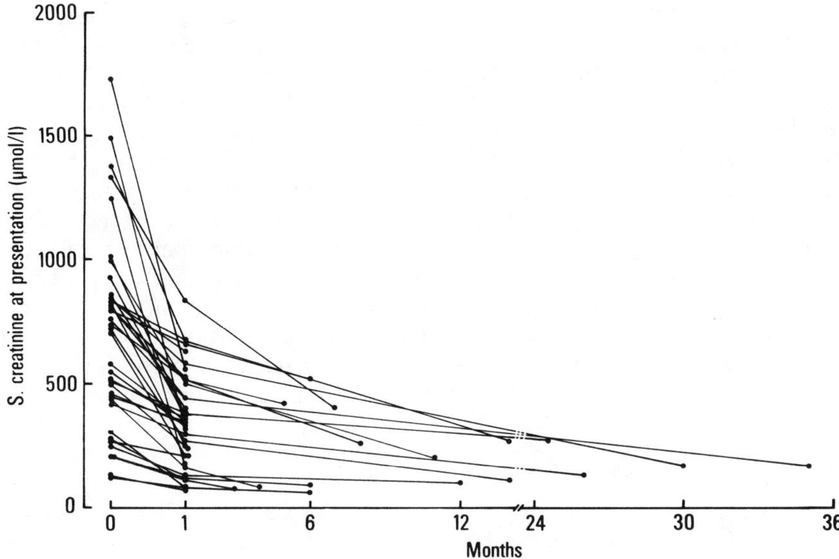

FIG 3.
Patterns of change in serum creatinine concentrations with time in 44 patients in whom renal function improved.

sponders) and continuation of measures undertaken to suppress the toxic renal effect of remnant light chains (i.e., maintenance of high urine flow and urine alkalinization). It must be emphasized that improvement can be very slow, as reported in some cases of acute renal failure[15, 29] and can last a very long time (see Fig 3) as shown by the interval before reaching the minimum value of serum creatinine concentration, up to 35 months (mean, 10.8 months).

4. Evolution to ESRD mostly occurs in the early phase of the follow-up, since of the 25 patients in our series who reached ESRD, 18 (72%) did so within the first month. Conversely, for patients who do not reach ESRD within the first month, a long interval before dialysis may be expected, as shown by the 7 patients who reached ESRD after 2 to 64 months (mean, 33 months).

5. When acute renal failure occurs during the course of the disease; i.e., in patients in whom risk factors are known and who are regularly followed up, recovery can be expected, as was the case for 8 of 9 patients. This observation is particularly interesting since this percentage is markedly higher than that reported for patients with myeloma presenting with acute renal failure.[8, 12, 15, 23, 29, 30]

Chemotherapy

Since the study was not prospective and entry of patients extended over a long period, chemotherapy regimens varied among patients. However, alkylating agents plus prednisone (± vincristine) were used as first-line chemotherapy (C1) in most patients (84%). In 32% of those (most observed before 1975), alkylating agents and prednisone were given daily. Treatment was administered to the other patients for 4 consecutive days every 4 weeks. Only 5 patients (6%) were given multidrug therapy, including doxorubicin (Adriamycin) and/or carmustine (BCNU) plus prednisone, as first-line treatment. Chemotherapy was administered according to tumor mass (Durie and Salmon staging) and age, and doses of alkylating agents were reduced according to serum creatinine values. Chemotherapy for relapses or refractory myeloma (C2) generally used a second type of alkylating agent in the early period, and doxorubicin and/or BCNU in the more recent period. Since, in our series, the type and method of treatment did not significantly influence the response rate or suvival time, the difference in protocols being used was not taken into account for further analyses.

Response to Chemotherapy

Four patients were excluded from the following analysis: 2 patients who did not receive chemotherapy because of age and obvious terminal phase of the disease, and 2 patients with myeloma and LCDD because they had such small traces of circulating light chains that detecting a response was hazardous. On the other hand, 15 patients died and we were unable to follow up 2 patients within the first 2 months. These 17 cases were studied as a separate group. Thus, 59 patients were analyzable for response to chemotherapy (Fig 4).

Response was defined as at least a 50% reduction in the initial M-protein concentration.[31] Response to C1 was completed in 34 patients (57.6% of the 59 evaluable patients or 44.7% of all treated patients). The exact time to response (calculated from the start of treatment until the first confirmed M-protein determination showing at least a 50% reduction) was known in 35 patients. It was short, with a mean of 4.8 months, due to the high number of rapid responders (time to response ≤2 months, 14 patients; time ≥3 months, 19 patients; mean time, 7.4 months; range, 3 to 18 months). Eleven patients had a partial response (20% to 50% reduction in M-protein) and 14 patients were refractory to C1.

C2 was given to 30 patients (14 of the 20 patients who had a relapse after a good initial response, 6 of the 11 patients who had only a partial response to C1, and 10 of the 14 patients with refractory myeloma). Response rate to C2 was different depending on the result of C1. Patients with partial initial response had the best response to C2 and 50% of them (3/6) achieved at least a 50% reduction in initial M-protein concentration. Similar results (≥50% reduction in M-protein) were observed in only 30% (3/10) of patients with refractory myeloma. Finally, patients who had a relapse after a good initial result of C1 had the worst response rate to C2 with only 21% of patients (3/14) achieving a 50% reduction in initial M-protein concentration.

In patients who did not respond to C2, it must be noted that 37% received

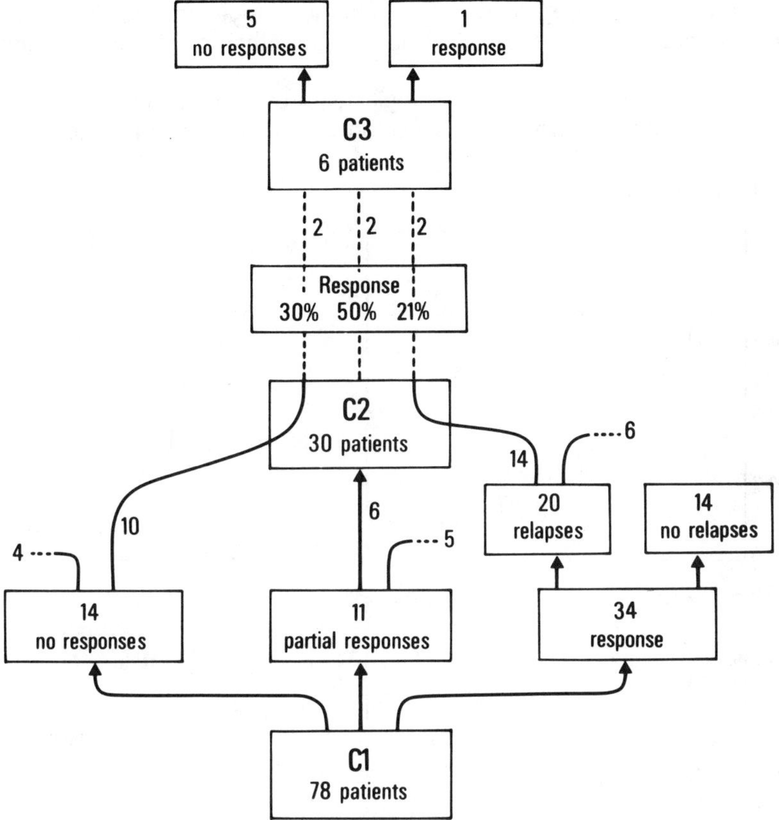

FIG 4.
Chemotherapy regimens and responses to therapy in 78 patients with multiple myeloma and renal failure. Numbers beside the *dotted line* indicate number of patients who did not receive a new treatment. Numbers beside the *dashed lines indicate number of treated patients.*

only one or two courses before death, suggesting either that they had a very aggressive form of disease, or that diagnosis of relapse and/or the decision to change drugs in refractory myeloma could have been difficult in these patients and the initiation of new treatment was subsequently delayed.

C3 was administered in only 6 patients and failed in most (5/6).

Survival Time

Median survival time for the 78 patients who received chemotherapy was 20 months (Fig 5). Seventeen patients died within the first 3 months. The median survival time in those patients alive and followed up after 3 months from presentation was 25 months. This median survival time is close to that of the general population of patients with myeloma receiving similar conventional chemotherapy (20 to 40 months),[32–35] though slightly shorter.

The analysis of clinical and biologic features at presentation (Table 3; see Fig 5) showed a positive association with prognosis for stage (see Fig

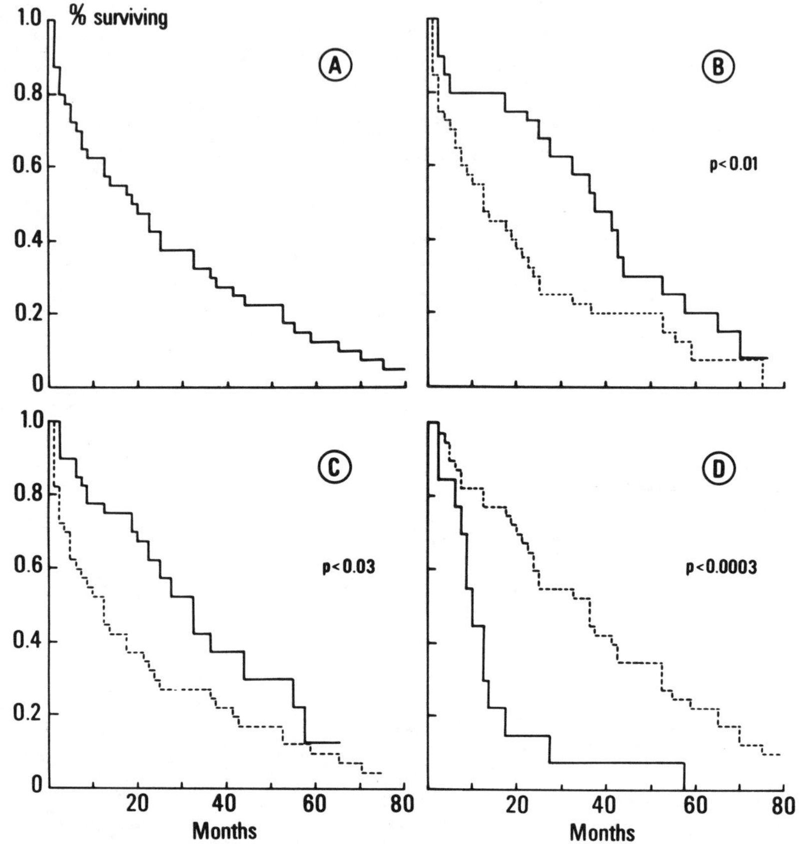

FIG 5.
A, survival curve of 78 patients with myeloma and renal failure who received chemotherapy. Median survival, 20 months. **B,** influence of staging (Durie and Salmon) on survival. *Solid line* = stages I + II; n = 21; median, 37 months. *Broken line* = stage III; n = 57; median, 12 months ($P < .01$). **C,** influence of evolution of renal function during first month on survival. *Solid line* = Serum creatinine returned to or remained at a value <300 μmol/L; n = 29; median, 32 months. *Broken line* = serum creatinine remained at or reached a value >300 μmol/L; n = 49; median, 12 months ($P < .03$). **D,** survival according to response to chemotherapy (early deaths excluded). *Broken line* = responsive patients; n = 45 (50% reduction of M-protein = 34 patients; partial response, 20% to 50% = 11 patients); median, 36 months. *Solid line* = unresponsive patients; n = 14; median, 10 months ($P < .0003$)

TABLE 3.
Effect of Certain Presentation and Follow-Up Disease Parameters on Survival in Patients With Multiple Myeloma and Renal Failure

Parameters Studied	No. Patients	*P*
Response to chemotherapy (C1)	59	<.0003
Stage (Durie and Salmon)	80	<.01
Renal function after 1 month	80	<.03
Age	80	
M-protein type (BJ > IgG > IgA > IgD)	80	
Lytic bone lesions*	80	
Hemoglobin*	80	<.05
Serum creatinine*	80	
Long-term evolution of renal function	59	
Sex	80	
Type of light chain	76	
Plasma cell count*	79	
Serum calcium*	80	
Serum albumin*	80	Not significant
Presence of amyloidosis	80	
Chemotherapy regimen (C1)	78	

*At presentation.

5); evolution of serum creatinine level at 1 month, with a discriminatory level of 300 μmol/L (see Fig 5); and above all for response to chemotherapy (see Fig 5) with a median survival time of 36 months for responders and 10 months for nonresponders ($P < .0003$). Of the remaining parameters investigated, type of M-protein, hemoglobin, lytic bone lesions, and long-term evolution of renal function also influenced survival time. In contrast, no such relationship was found for sex, age, κ vs. λ light chain, plasma cell count, albuminemia, calcemia, serum creatinine concentration at presentation, presence of amyloidosis, and nature or protocol of administration of C1.

When the individual influence on survival time of each variable was assessed with multivariate regression analysis (Cox model), response to chemotherapy was confirmed to be the dominant and independent feature for survival time.

Discussion

Improvements in the understanding of the disease and in techniques of treatment have drastically changed the prognosis of renal insufficiency associated with multiple myeloma. Overall prognosis (i.e., survival time), however, remains under that of patients with myeloma without renal involvement.

Several reasons could theoretically be responsible for this poorer prognosis of patients with myeloma and renal failure. We attempted to analyze them in our series and in the literature.

Period of Observation

Our study concerned patients observed between 1965 and 1990. In the first part of this period, renal involvement in myeloma was generally considered as associated with such a poor outcome that decision and choice of treatment was difficult. In particular, dialysis was usually considered as inappropriate in patients with myeloma, as in other malignant diseases. Thus, only supportive therapy was undertaken in several of our patients observed before 1970. Survival time was short in these patients and could influence the overall median survival time.

Severity of the Disease

It must be stressed that at admission the majority of our patients had several associated signs of serious disease, such as anemia, hypercalcemia, and advanced renal failure. The prognostic value of many clinical and biologic parameters has been widely analyzed in recent years.[5, 7, 36–34] Increasing tumor burden, which has been shown to be correlated with clinical parameters such as anemia, hypercalcemia, and (at least partially) renal insufficiency, is associated with a shorter survival time. Other variables have been investigated more recently.[45] Certain immunochemical types of tumor, myelomas with a large plasmablastic fraction, have a poor outcome.[4] The prognostic influence of parameters reflecting the whole tumor mass, in particular lactate dehydrogenase and serum β2 microglobulin (β2M),[46–50] or its proliferative part such as plasma cell labeling index or DNA content value,[46, 51–55] or factors associated with these parameters[51, 52, 56–61] have been analyzed, especially with regard to response rate, time to relapse, and survival time. Multivariate analysis indicates that the most important variables could be β2M level and labeling index.[46, 48, 50, 62] In our series, serum β2M was measured only in recent years, and results were in accordance with these conclusions.

Distribution of M-Protein Type

The distribution of M-protein type in our series showed a high frequency of patients with plasma cells excreting only Bence Jones proteins. These cases of Bence Jones myeloma represented 46% of our patients, compared to the 10% to 20% frequency generally found in myeloma without renal failure. Bence Jones myeloma has long been considered to be associated with poor prognosis. However, in our series, such poor prognosis was not confirmed and study of correlations between M-protein type and survival time showed that patients with myeloma and only Bence Jones proteinuria had a longer survival time than patients with intact Ig (survival of patients with Bence Jones myeloma > IgG > IgA > IgD, $P < .01$). A similar observation was reported by Alexanian et al.[36] who found that survival of patients with Bence Jones myeloma was better than that of patients with IgA, and was similar, but with a longer duration of remission, to that observed in patients with IgG peaks.[36] Since Bence Jones myelomas are highly associated with renal failure, an explanation of the observed differences in the influence of Bence Jones myeloma on prognosis could be the improved management and prognosis of renal failure itself. In the past, most patients with myeloma and renal failure died rapidly, while since the 1980s, renal failure is no longer a dominant problem, explaining the lesser influence of M-protein type on prognosis. The longer remission time was attributed by Alexanian et al. to the more rapid disappearance of Bence Jones proteins than intact Ig during remission, a fact we also observed in our series. In conclusion, the higher incidence of Bence Jones myeloma in our series compared to the series of myeloma without renal failure cannot directly account for the poorer survival time we observed.

Survival Time and Reversal of Renal Failure

The influence of reversal of renal failure on survival time has been diversely evaluated.[1, 8, 15, 25, 29] In our series, a high incidence of death was observed in patients with high serum creatinine levels at presentation (Table 4). However, improvement of renal function after 1 month (or more

TABLE 4.
Relationship of Serum Creatinine Value at Presentation to Frequency of Early Deaths* in 80 Patients With Multiple Myeloma

Serum Creatinine (μmol/L)	No. Patients	No. Deaths	Percent
≤200	12	1	8.3
200–800	35	6	17.1
≥800	33	12	36.3
Total	80	19	23.7

*Within the first 3 months.

precisely serum creatinine returning to or being maintained at a level <300 μmol/L) was associated with a longer survival time ($P < .05$). This favorable effect of renal failure reversal on overall prognosis has been reported in other series, especially for patients with acute renal failure.[13, 15] In our analysis, we also found an association between long-term improvement of renal function and survival time; however, it is more likely that it was the good response to chemotherapy and the reduction or disappearance of light chains that resulted in prolonged survival time and permitted subsequent long-term improvement of renal function, rather than the contrary.

If improvement of renal function, particularly in the first weeks, has a favorable effect on outcome, any measure that could contribute to such improvement should also influence survival. Plasmapheresis permitted a dramatic reduction in M-protein concentration in several studies, resulted in[12, 26, 30] and improved renal insufficiency in patients with myeloma with marked or end-stage renal failure.[12, 25, 30, 61] However, a beneficial effect of this technique on survival time has not yet been demonstrated.[12, 25]

Chemotherapy

We used only conventional chemotherapy, i.e., alkylating agents plus prednisone, in nearly all patients as first-line chemotherapy, with an administered/theoretical dose of 0.85 corresponding to the reduction of renal function. No difference in survival time was observed between patients who received either continuous or discontinuous regimens. With these protocols, the response rate was 45%, similar to that found in series with no or few patients with renal failure, suggesting that renal insufficiency does not alter the effect of chemotherapy on plasma cells. Therefore, the choice of initial chemotherapy in our patients did not explain the relatively short survival time we observed. In contrast, review of the second course of chemotherapy shows several findings that could be of interest for this analysis. Thirty percent of patients with a relapse and 29% of patients with refractory myeloma were not given a new regimen of chemotherapy. When given, courses before death were few, suggesting that very aggressive myeloma was present and/or that definite diagnosis of relapse was not easy to make in these patients especially in patients with Bence Jones myeloma, and that change of treatment could sometimes have been delayed. Furthermore, chemotherapy regimens for relapses and for patients refractory to C1 most often used a second alkylating agent, and unusually drugs such as doxorubicin and BCNU. In fact, no patient received aggressive multidrug therapy, widely used nowadays in the general population of patients with myeloma, which seems to induce a higher response rate and probably longer survival time than conventional treatment (Table 5).*

Early Deaths

Mean survival time in our patients was 20 months, better than the 13 months we found in an older series,[6] but shorter than that reported in pa-

*References 13, 15, 18, 20, 22, 23, 25, 26, 28, 33, 41, 42, 49, 54, 55, 62–65, 67–84.

TABLE 5.
Examples of Treatment Given for Multiple Myeloma

Treatment*	Percent Responses†	Median Survival (mo)‡	References
MP	30–60	20–40	26, 42, 64, 65
VMBCP (M2)			22, 55, 62, 67–71
VMCP-VCAP, VBAP			
VAD	45–87	20–50	15, 23, 54, 72, 73
M—h.d.	44–78	22–44	63, 74
Chemotherapy—h.d. + TBI + Allogeneic BMT	75	more than 36	41
Chemotherapy—h.d.			
+ TBI			49, 75–77
+ Autologous: BMT	75–80 (20–50 CR)	more than 36	18, 49, 76, 78
+ Blood stem cells autologous graft			58, 79, 80
Interferon α-2b + chemotherapy	75–80 (30–45 CR)		13, 25, 33, 81, 82
As maintenance treatment		52 since start of interferon	20, 28, 83

*M = melphalan; P = prednisone; V = vincristine; B = BCNU; C = cyclosphosphamide; A = adriamycin; D = dexamethasone; h.d. = high doses; TBI = total body irradiation; BMT = bone marrow transplantation; CR = complete response.
†Variations in percentages observed are in part due to variations in criteria. For the Myeloma Task Force,[31] ≥50% reduction, for the SWOG,[84] ≥75% reduction of M-protein is required.
‡Variations in percentages observed for survival are in part due to inhomogeneity of analyzed groups (number of patients, prognostic factors at presentation, chemotherapy given as first-line treatment or given for relapse or refractory myeloma).

tients with normal renal function, which is generally between 20 to 40 months with comparable treatment (see table 5).[32–35] We already noted that this shorter survival time was in part due to the very high percentage of patients who died within the first 3 months (6.8% per month, compared with the 3.8% per month during the next 3 months and the 2.9% in the next 6 months). This high frequency of early deaths in patients with myeloma and renal failure, which is not observed in patients with normal renal function, has been stressed by other authors, even in recent series.[20, 21] In the fourth Medical Research Council (MRC) myelomatosis trial (patients entered after 1980), 39% of the 80 patients with uremic myeloma had died within 100 days of entry.[21]

The risks of early death appear to be related to the degree of renal failure, as illustrated in our series, in which deaths within the first 3 months were more than four times as high in patients with serum creatinine ≥800 μmol/L at presentation than in those with serum creatinine ≤200 μmol/L (see Table 4). However, this is in part due to the fact that renal failure is more common in advanced myeloma disease.[20] Fifty-eight (73%) of our 80 patients were at stage III, a percentage markedly higher than that usually observed in the general population of patients with myeloma. MacLennan et al. found that in their patients with myeloma admitted to the fourth and fifth MRC myelomatosis trial,[20] the risk of early death attributable to progressive tumor growth was more than three times as high in patients presenting with serum creatinine >200 μmol/L than in those with normal renal function.

Another important cause of early death in patients with myeloma and renal failure is infectious complications.[2] In our series, sepsis was the second cause of early death. Perri et al.,[85] in a series of 60 patients with myeloma, found an overall incidence of infection of 1.46 per patient-year with the highest risk in the first 2 months after diagnosis and start of chemotherapy (4.68 infections per patient-year compared to 1.04 for subsequent months), and this risk of infection in the early time period was significantly increased in patients with renal failure,[85] an observation also recently reported by MacLennan et al.[20]

Conclusion

The role of renal failure in the prognosis of patients with multiple myeloma clearly emerges from our observations and from the literature. However, this influence appears extremely complex.

We and other authors have clearly stressed the prognostic significance of data such as: a high creatinine level at presentation (>800 μmol/L), leading to a low survival time (see Table 4); early deaths, not directly related to renal failure (at least presently) but to causes more frequently observed in multiple myeloma with than without renal failure. Renal function improvement at 1 month (serum creatinine decreasing or being maintained below 300 μmol/L), on the contrary, is a prognostic factor associated with a prolonged survival time.

Thus, all the factors influencing renal function within the first month are of capital importance: symptomatic measures such as alkaline diuresis, probably (and in some cases) plasmapheresis, and early chemotherapy. Even initially severe renal failure may regress to values below the critical level of 300 μmol/L. Certain features point to good evolution of renal failure: (1) normal or only slightly altered renal function in the weeks before; (2) the existence of precipitating factors, providing that (3) the interval between the appearance of renal failure and its treatment is short. In the absence of patient history, renal biopsy helps to distinguish those with mild lesions from those with diffuse and severe fibrosis (or extensive amyloidosis). Renal failure will mostly not or only slightly improve in this last group, in which plasmapheresis should probably be reserved for well-selected cases.

In the past, the poor prognosis associated with renal failure was unquestionable.[1, 43] At present, the importance attached to renal failure varies among authors. This may be explained by the heterogeneity of the population of patients with renal failure, including causes of renal deterioration, time, and type of treatments. The role of symptomatic measures, for example, has been stressed by the MRD myelomatosis trials.[20] The median survival time of patients with myeloma and with renal failure was 37 days in the third trial while it was 380 days in the fourth, in which high fluid intake and urine alkalinization were systematically added to previous treatment. Differences observed may also reflect a change in indications of dialysis and plasmapheresis. Finally, the differences in renal histologic lesions before treatment are rarely taken into account.

All this probably (at least partially) explains that when using multivariate analysis, the two dominant factors remain first the response to chemotherapy, and second the staging, and that creatinine values no longer emerge.

The management of chemotherapy is of capital importance for survival in patients in whom renal insufficiency is correctly treated and thus is no longer a major problem.

The important progress made in the past years in managing multiple myeloma could be of help in patients with myeloma and renal failure, provided it is adjusted to their particular problems. Conventional chemotherapy (i.e., alkylating agents plus prednisone) gives good results in patients with renal failure and could be maintained as first-line chemotherapy. More aggressive multidrug chemotherapy (see Table 5), especially the VAD protocol, could be beneficial in treatment of relapses and of refractory myelomas. Recombinant interferon α-2b (see Table 5) could be of interest as maintenance treatment, provided first results are confirmed in further studies. Finally, the effectiveness of a new strategy, high-dose chemotherapy with or without total body irradiation, supported by autologous marrow transplantation, should provide a new possibility of treatment in patients with myeloma and renal failure, after conventional therapy has allowed renal insufficiency to regain a level compatible with this technique.

References

1. Kyle RA, Elveback LR: Management and prognosis of multiple myeloma. *Mayo Clin Proc* 1976; 51:751–760.
2. Kyle RA: Multiple myeloma. Review of 869 cases. *Mayo Clin Proc* 1975; 50:29–40.
3. Medical research council's working party on leukaemia in adults: Report on

the second myelomatosis trial after five years of follow-up. *Br J Cancer* 1980; 42:813–822.

4. Report of the medical research council's working party for therapeutic trials in leukemia: Report on the first myelomatosis trial. Part I. Analysis of presenting features of prognostic importance. *Br J Haematol* 1973; 24:123–139.
5. Woodruff RK, Wadsworth J, Malpas JS, et al: Clinical staging in multiple myeloma. *Br J Haematol* 1979; 42:199–205.
6. Ganeval D, Jungers P, Noël LH, et al: La néphropathie du myélome, in Hamburger J, Crosnier J, Funck-Brentano JL (eds): *Actualités Néphrologiques de l'Hôpital Necker.* Paris, Flammarion Médecine-Sciences, 1977, pp 309–347.
7. Durie BGM, Salmon SE: A clinical staging system for multiple myeloma. Correlation of measured myeloma cell mass with presenting clinical features, response to treatment, and survival. *Cancer* 1975; 36:842–854.
8. Alexanian R, Barlogie B, Dixon D: Renal failure in multiple myeloma. Pathogenesis and prognostic implications. *Arch Intern Med* 1990; 150:1693–1695.
9. Verroust P, Morel-Maroger L, Preud'homme JL: Renal lesions in dysproteinemias. *Springer Semin Immunopathol* 1982; 5:333–356.
10. Hill GS, Morel-Maroger L, Méry JP, et al: Renal lesions in multiple myeloma: Their relationship to associated protein abnormalities. *Am J Kidney Dis* 1983; II:423–438.
11. Pirani CL, Silva F, D'Agati V, et al: Renal lesions in plasma cell dyscrasias: Ultrastructural observations. *Am J Kidney Dis* 1987; 10:208–221.
12. Johnson WJ, Kyle RA, Pineda AA, et al: Treatment of renal failure associated with multiple myeloma. Plasmapheresis, hemodialysis and chemotherapy. *Arch Intern Med* 1990; 150:863–869.
13. Pozzi C, Pasquali S, Donini U, et al: Prognostic factors and effectiveness of treatment in acute renal failure due to multiple myeloma: A review of 50 cases. *Clin Nephrol* 1987; 28:1–9.
14. Kyle RA: Monoclonal gammopathies and the kidney. *Ann Rev Med* 1989; 40:53–60.
15. Rota S, Mougenot B, Baudouin B, et al: Multiple myeloma and severe renal failure: A clinicopathologic study of outcome and prognosis in 34 patients. *Medicine* 1987; 66:126–137.
16. Kyle RA, Greipp PR: Amyloidosis (AL). Clinical and laboratory features in 229 cases. *Mayo Clin Proc* 1983; 58:665–683.
17. Ganeval D, Noël LH, Preud'homme JL, et al: Light-chain deposition disease: Its relation with AL-type amyloidosis. *Kidney Int* 1984; 26:1–9.
18. Randall RE, Williamson WC Jr, Mullinax F, et al: Manifestation of systemic light chain deposition. *Am J Med* 1976; 60:293–299.
19. Ganeval D, Cathomen M, Noël LH, et al: Kidney involvement in multiple myeloma and related disorders. *Contrib Nephrol* 1982; 33:210–222.
20. MacLennan ICM, Cooper EH, Chapman CE, et al: Renal failure in myelomatosis. *Eur J Haematol* 1989; 43:60–65.
21. Medical research council's working party on leukaemia in adults: Analysis and management of renal failure in fourth MRC myelomatosis trial. *Br Med J* 1984; 288:1411–1416.
22. Iggo N, Palmer ABD, Severn A, et al: Chronic dialysis in patients with multiple myeloma and renal failure: A worthwhile treatment. *Q J Med* 1989; 73:903–910.
23. Lazarus HM, Adelstein DJ, Herzig RH, et al: Long-term survival of patients with multiple myeloma and acute renal failure at presentation. *Am J Kidney Dis* 1983; 2:521–525.

24. Dahlberg PJ, Newcomer KL, Yutuc WR, et al: Myeloma kidney: Improved renal function following long-term chemotherapy and hemodialysis. *Am J Nephrol* 1983; 3:242–243.
25. Misiani R, Tiraboschi G, Mingardi G, et al: Management of myeloma kidney: An anti-light-chain approach. *Am J Kidney Dis* 1987; 10:28–33.
26. Sølling K, Sølling J: Clearances of Bence-Jones proteins during peritoneal dialysis or plasmapheresis in myelomatosis associated with renal failure. *Contrib Nephrol* 1988; 68:259–262.
27. Wahlin A, Grubb A, Holm J, et al: Effects of plasmapheresis on the plasma concentration of proteins used to monitor the disease process in multiple myeloma. *Acta Med Scand* 1988; 223:263–267.
28. Wahlin A, Löfvenberg E, Holm J: Improved survival in multiple myeloma with renal failure. *Acta Med Scand* 1987; 221:205–209.
29. Cohen DJ, Sherman WH, Osserman EF, et al: Acute renal failure in patients with multiple myeloma. *Am J Med* 1984; 76:247–256.
30. Zucchelli P, Pasquali S, Cagnoli L, et al: Controlled plasma exchange trial in acute renal failure due to multiple myeloma. *Kidney Int* 1988; 33:1175–1180.
31. Chronic leukemia—myeloma task force: National Cancer Institute Proposed guidelines for protocol studies—II Plasma cell myeloma. *Cancer Chemother Rep* 1973; 4:145–158.
32. Durie BGM, Salmon SE: The current status and future prospects of treatment for multiple myeloma. *Clin Haematol* 1982; 11:181–210.
33. Medical research council's working party on leukaemia in adults: Treatment comparisons in the third MRC myelomatosis trial. *Br J Cancer* 1980; 42:823–830.
34. Sporn JR, McIntyre OR: Chemotherapy of previously untreated multiple myeloma patients: An analysis of recent treatment results. *Semin Oncol* 1986; 13:318–325.
35. Woodruff K: Treatment of multiple myeloma. *Cancer Treat Rev* 1981; 8:220.
36. Alexanian R, Balcerzak S, Bonnet JD, et al: Prognostic factors in multiple myeloma. *Cancer* 1975; 36:1192–1201.
37. Alexanian R: Ten-Year survival in multiple myeloma. *Arch Intern Med* 1985; 145:2073–2075.
38. Buckman R, Cuzick J, Galton DAG: Long-term survival in myelomatosis. A report to the MRC working party on leukaemia in adults. *Br J Haematol* 1982; 52:589–599.
39. Cavo M, Galieni P, Grimaldi M, et al: Improvement of Durie & Salmon staging for multiple myeloma by adding platelet count as a stratifying variable: A multivariate regression analysis of 163 untreated patients. *Eur J Haematol* 1989; 43:99–104.
40. Cohen HJ, Bartolucci A: Age and the treatment of multiple myeloma. Southeastern cancer study group experience. *Am J Med* 1985; 79:316–324.
41. Fuzibet JG, Bataille R, Bagarry D, et al: Survie prolongée au cours du myélome multiple. Caractéristiques de présentation et de réponse au traitement de 73 malades ayant vécu 5 ans ou plus. *Presse Med* 1986; 15:1913–1916.
42. Medical research council's working party on leukaemia in adults: Results of the MRC myelomatosis trials for patients entered since 1980. *Hematol Oncol* 1988; 6:145–158.
43. Merlini G, Gobbi PG, Ascari E: The Merlini, Waldenström, Jayakar staging system revisited. *Eur J Haematol* 1989; 51:105–110.
44. Merlini G, Waldenström JG, Jayakar SD: A new improved clinical staging sys-

tem for multiple myeloma based on analysis of 123 treated patients. *Blood* 1980; 55:1011–1019.
45. Barlogie B, Epstein J, Selvanayagam P, et al: Plasma cell myeloma—New biological insights and advances in therapy. *Blood* 1989; 73:865–879.
46. Barlogie B, Alexanian R: Prognostic factors in multiple myeloma: The MD Anderson experience. *Eur J Haematol* 1989; 43:84–87.
47. Bartl R, Frisch B, Diem H, et al: Bone marrow histology and serum beta 2 microglobulin in multiple myeloma—a new prognostic strategy. *Eur J Haematol* 1989; 43:88–98.
48. Bataille R, Durie BGM, Grenier J, et al: Prognostic factors and staging in multiple myeloma: A reappraisal. *J Clin Oncol* 1986; 4:80–87.
49. Garewal H, Durie BGM, Kyle RA, et al: Serum $beta_2$-microglobulin in the initial staging and subsequent monitoring of monoclonal plasma cell disorders. *J Clin Oncol* 1984; 2:51–54.
50. Greipp PR, Katzmann JA, O'Fallon WF, et al: Value of β_2-microglobulin level and plasma cell labeling indices as prognostic factors in patients with newly diagnosed myeloma. *Blood* 1988; 72:219–223.
51. Barlogie B, Alexanian R, Dixon D, et al: Prognostic implications of tumor cell DNA and RNA content in multiple myeloma. *Blood* 1985; 66:338–341.
52. Barlogie B, Smallwood L, Smith T, et al: High serum levels of lactic dehydrogenase identify a high-grade lymphoma-like myeloma. *Ann Intern Med* 1989; 110:521–525.
53. Durie BGM, Salmon SE, Moon TE: Pretreatment tumor mass, cell kinetics, and prognosis in multiple myeloma. *Blood* 1980; 55:364–372.
54. Greipp PR, Kyle RA: Clinical, morphological, and cell kinetic differences among multiple myeloma, monoclonal gammopathy of undetermined significance, and smoldering multiple myeloma. *Blood* 1983; 62:166–171.
55. Greipp PR, Witzig TE, Gonchoroff NJ, et al: Immunofluorescence labeling indices in myeloma and related monoclonal gammopathies. *Mayo Clin Proc* 1987; 62:969–977.
56. Cozzolino F, Torcia M, Aldinucci D, et al: Production of interleukin-1 by bone marrow myeloma cells: Its role in the pathogenesis of lytic bone lesions. *Blood* 1989; 74:380–387.
57. Dewald GW, Kyle RA, Hicks GA, et al: The clinical significance of cytogenetic studies in 100 patients with multiple myeloma, plasma cell leukemia, or amyloidosis. *Blood* 1985; 66:380–390.
58. Epstein J, Barlogie B, Katzmann J, et al: Phenotypic heterogeneity in aneuploid multiple myeloma indicates pre-B cell involvement. *Blood* 1988; 71:861–865.
59. Garrett IR, Durie BG, Nedwin GE, et al: Production of lymphotoxin, a bone-resorbing cytokine, by cultured human myeloma cells. *N Engl J Med* 1987; 317:526–532.
60. Latreille J, Barlogie B, Johnston D, et al: Ploidy and proliferative characteristics in monoclonal gammopathies. *Blood* 1982; 59:43–51.
61. Zhang XG, Klein B, Bataille R: Interleukin-6 is a potent myeloma-cell growth factor in patients with aggressive multiple myeloma. *Blood* 1989; 74:11–13.
62. Durie BGM, Bataille R: Therapeutic implications of myeloma staging. *Eur J Haematol* 1989; 43:111–116.
63. Samson D, Newland A, Kearney J, et al: Infusion of vincristine and doxorubicin with oral dexamethasone as first-line therapy for multiple myeloma. *Lancet* 1989; ii:882–885.

64. Medical research council's working party on leukaemia in adults: Prognostic features in the third MRC myelomatosis trial. *Br J Cancer* 1980; 42:831–840.
65. Westin J: Interferon alpha-2b therapy during the plateau phase of multiple myeloma. V Hannover Interferon Workshop, Feb 21–23, 1990, p 50.
66. Alexanian R, Dreicer R: Chemotherapy for multiple myeloma. *Cancer* 1984; 53:583–588.
67. Case DC, Lee BJ, Clarkson BD: Improved survival times in multiple myeloma treated with melphalan, prednisone, cyclophosphamide, vincristine and BCNU: M2 protocol. *Am J Med* 1977; 63:897–903.
68. Cooper MR, McIntyre OR, Propert KJ, et al: Single, sequential, and multiple alkylating agent therapy for multiple myeloma: A CALGB study. *J Clin Oncol* 1986; 4:1331–1339.
69. Harousseau JL, Milpied N, Guilhot F, et al: Traitement de première intention des myélomes graves du sujet jeune par melphalan à haute dose. *Presse Med* 1988; 17:1471–1474.
70. Oken MM, Kyle RA, Greipp PR: Alternative cycles of VBMCP with interferon (r IFN alpha-2) in the treatment of multiple myeloma. *Proc Am Soc Clin Oncol* 1988; 7:225.
71. Oken MM, Tsaltis A, Abramson N: Evaluation of intensive (VBMCP) vs standard (MP) therapy for multiple myeloma (abstract). *Proc Am Soc Clin Oncol* 1987; 6:203.
72. Alexanian R, Barlogie B, Dixon D: High-dose glucocorticoid treatment of resistant myeloma. *Ann Intern Med* 1986; 105:8–11.
73. Barlogie B, Smith L, Alexanian R: Effective treatment of advanced multiple myeloma refractory to alkylating agents. *New Engl J Med* 1984; 310:1353–1356.
74. Barlogie B, Alexanian R, Smallwood L, et al: Prognostic factors with high-dose melphalan for refractory multiple myeloma. *Blood* 1988; 72:2015–2019.
75. Barlogie B, Alexanian A, Dicke KA, et al: High dose chemoradiotherapy and autologous bone marrow transplantation for resistant multiple myeloma. *Blood* 1987; 70:869–872.
76. Groupe d'Études et de Recherches sur le Myélome (GERM): Traitement des myélomes multiples résistant aux alkylants par vincristine-adriamycine en perfusion continue et dexaméthasone. *Presse Med* 1986; 15:2001–2004.
77. Hansen OP, Clausen NT, Drivsholm A, et al: Phase III study of intermittent 5-drug regimen (VBCMP) versus intermittent 3-drug regimen (VMP) versus intermittent melphalan and prednisone (MP) in myelomatosis. *Scand J Haematol* 1985; 35:518–524.
78. Anderson K, Barut B, Takvorian T: Monoclonal antibody purged autologous bone marrow transplantation for multiple myeloma (abstract). *Blood* 1989; 74:202.
79. Benbunan M, Adam M, Fermand JP, et al: Collection, cryopreservation and autologous transplantation with circulating hemopoietic stem cells in patients with multiple myeloma and lymphoma. *Bone Marrow Transplantation* 1990; 5:33–34.
80. Mandelli F, Avvisati G, Amadori S, et al: Maintenance treatment with recombinant interferon alfa-2b in patients with multiple myeloma responding to conventional induction chemotherapy. *New Engl J Med* 1990; 322:1430–1434.
81. Cooper MR, Fefer A, Thompson J, et al: Alpha-2-interferon/melphalan/prednisone in previously untreated patients with multiple myeloma: A phase I-II trial. *Cancer Treat Rep* 1986; 4:473–476.

82. Lokhorst HM, Meuwissen OJATh, Bast EJEG, et al: VAD chemotherapy for refractory multiple myeloma. *Br J Haemat* 1989; 71:25–30.
83. Peest D, Deicher H, Coldewey R, et al: Induction and maintenance therapy in multiple myeloma: A multicenter trial of MP versus VCMP. *Eur J Cancer Clin Oncol* 1988; 24:1061–1067.
84. Alexanian R, Bonnet J, Gehan E, et al: Combination chemotherapy for multiple myeloma. *Cancer* 1972; 30:382–389.
85. Perri RT, Hebbel RP, Oken MM: Influence of treatment and response status on infection risk in multiple myeloma. *Am J Med* 1981; 71:935–940.

Part IV

Kidney Transplantation

Bioreagents in Allograft Immunosuppression

J.P. Soulillou, M.D.

University Hospital, INSERM U211, Nantes, France

Bioreagents, defined earlier as antilymphocyte polyclonal gammaglobulins used for immunosuppression of graft recipients, now comprise a growing family of monoclonal antibodies (MoAb), modified MoAb (chimeric or humanized), or artificial molecules aimed at target immunocompetent cells.

Since, so far, these compounds are—for at least some of their parts—of nonself molecules, they invariably elicit a recipient immune response and are therefore restricted in their indications to short-term treatment, i.e., prophylaxis of early rejection or treatment of ongoing rejection episodes.

To date, only a few types of bioreagents have been used clinically on a large scale: rabbit or horse antilymphocyte globulins and, more recently, ortho pan OKT3, a mouse IgG1 MoAb directed against the epsilon component of the CD3 complex.[1] However, many other monoclonal antibodies or fusion proteins have been tested in pilot randomized studies and will probably add some diversity to the immunosuppression arsenal for the treatment of allograft recipients.

Antilymphocyte Polyclonal Globulins

Sir W. Wooldruff first showed that anti-rat lymphocyte polyclonal sera could prolong the life of an allograft.[2] In humans, antilymphocyte globulin (ALG) was introduced in 1967 by Monaco et al.,[3] and various kinds of polyclonal globulins have been used since, comprising antibodies directed at thymocytes (ATG),[4] thoracic duct lymphocytes,[5] B-cell[6] or T-cell immortalized cell lines,[7] and more recently, a normal alloreactive T-cell clone.[8]

Almost all reports have been concordant in describing ALG as a very efficient means of treating steroid-resistant rejection episodes before the use of cyclosporine A (CsA) as maintenance treatment. Although they also seem active in patients receiving CsA,[9, 10] their use in this context has been reported to increase the incidence of lymphoma.[11] ALG can also be given immediately after grafting—and for the following 1 to 3 weeks—to prevent early rejection. This approach has become popular in the era of CsA due to the early toxicity of the drug. Early randomized studies showed a decreased incidence of rejection and an increase of graft function at 6 and 12 months in patients receiving prophylactic ALG, although graft survival rates were almost identical at 2 years.[12, 13] In these studies, patients receiving ALG also had a lower incidence of primary graft nonfunction, shorter hospitalization times, and less need for dialysis. The choice of the best strategy (i.e., sequential therapy or CsA immediately after grafting) has become less evident when lower initial doses of CsA were recommended, with only few differences after 1 year in almost all parameters recorded in a controlled randomized study.[13] Again, experience of the medical groups with one or the other strategy is an important factor in success. In addition, many centers have chosen to restrict the use of ALG to primary nonfunctioning grafts only.

Optimal use of ALG requires the monitoring of some lymphocyte markers. Among various unexplored possibilities (for instance monitoring of $CD2^+$, or $CD3^+$ circulating cells), monitoring of sheep red blood cell rosetting T cells[14] has been proposed.[15] Since 1982, we have adapted ALG doses in all patients to maintain rosetting T cells below 10% (test performed on ficoll hypaque purified mononucleated cells). Such a procedure was associated with an extremely low incidence of rejection during treatment (2%),[16] achieved with daily doses much lower (0.77 to 1.4 mg/kg[16] for instance for Merieux rabbit ATG) than those recommended (2.5 to 5 mg/kg), with much lower doses often observed in the elderly or in women. However, children seem to require somewhat higher doses (2.23 ± 84 mg/kg) for the same ATG as compared to adults (C. Guyot, personal communication). In addition, this monitoring also helps in detecting recipient-blocking anti-ALG antibodies whose appearance is contemporary to an elevation of rosetting T cell levels above 20%, mimicking what was described for monitoring of $CD3^+$ circulating T cells during anti-CD3 treatment.[17]

In contrast, monitoring of circulating ALG levels appears hopeless due to the fact that only a portion of the rabbit Ig corresponds to anti-lymphocyte antibodies. However, interestingly, the monitoring of ALG circulating levels has shown prolonged persistence of detectable rabbit Ig in recipients. This observation, combined with the finding that rosetting T cell levels are significantly depressed for at least 60 days after 2 weeks of ALG treatment,[16] indicates that the suppressive action of such bioreagents far exceeds its period of administration, which may contribute to explaining the increased rate of infection reported in patients treated with ALG. The monitoring of the recipient anti-ALG immune response, which cannot distinguish antibodies directed against antilymphocyte antibodies and against rabbit Ig, seems to be of poor predictive value as compared with the measurement of rosetting T-cell levels. Finally, comparison of the respective advantages of rabbit or horse ALG remains hazardous because of the significant batch-to-batch variations that are a common feature of these reagents.

The precise description of the molecules functionally active at the lymphocyte surface and which could be recognized by antibodies present in ALG has raised the possibility that some discrete specificities could have a dominant role in the suppressive ALG effect. We were unable to detect significant levels of antibodies against CD25, CD2, CD3, or CD4 in a rabbit ALG raised against a $CD4^+$ alloreactive clone[8, 18, 19] in competition experiments with labeled MoAb specific to the corresponding CDs.[8] Although these experiments (using flow cytometry) did not allow us to work at concentrations above 2 mg/mL (which is already extremely high) and since in vitro observation cannot predict what will happen during long-term in vivo treatment, the complement-fixing capacity of ALG and the resultant leukopenia (lasting throughout the treatment) suggest a major role for lymphocyte deprivation, rather than for more restricted and specific targeting in ALG effectiveness. However it is possible that the surface determinants of the immunizing cells confer some additional specific capacities to ALG prepared against blast cells. For instance, we have recently prepared an ALG by immunizing rabbits against a normal (i.e., untransformed) allostimulated T-cell clone.[8, 20] This clone has been derived from graft infiltrating cells and expanded by coculture with the corresponding graft donor Epstein-Barr virus (EBV)-transformed B-cell line.[18] ALGs raised against this clone ($CD4^+$ and specific for HLA-DRW8) have been used successfully in a pilot prophylactic study. However, only a study with a larger cohort of patients could provide evidence of its potential advantages (more antibodies against activation determinants, more stereotyped antigens, etc.) compared to other available ALG.

In conclusion, although ALGs have been commonly used for the past two decades and remain among the most powerful immunosuppressive agents available to date, their mechanisms of action are not clarified. However, they may still be useful in the future in protocols aimed to induce specific tolerance in recipients against donor antigen. Indeed, like TLI,[21] ALG seems to be able to induce, in some cases, a graft tolerance state when injected with donor bone marrow.[22] Additionally, in some way, they are still a paradigm of possible antilymphocyte MoAb cocktails that would mediate complement cytotoxicity.

Although clearly efficient in preventing or reversing rejection, ALGs are nevertheless associated with various side effects, including early fever and sometimes symptoms reminiscent of what is usually observed after OKT3 therapy and which are probably due, as for OKT3,[23] to cytokine release.[24] Severe and frequent serum sickness, probably related to the presence of large amounts of circulating xenoantigens, is also observed in recipients producing anti-ALG antibodies. More threatening is the possibility of a high incidence of severe opportunistic infections or lymphoma after ALG treatment, although this has only been clearly demonstrated when ALG was associated with other major immunosuppressive drugs.[11]

Monoclonal Antibodies

The availability of monoclonal antibodies and a better knowledge of interactive surface membrane molecules have opened new possibilities of targeted immunosuppression. Among the various theoretical advantages of a MoAb vs. a polyclonal antibody is its specificity and, therefore, the opportunity for precise monitoring of reagent effectiveness and for intelligent targeting. However, unmodified antibodies exhibit strong immunogenicity, forbidding long-term and often even sequential treatment, and usually act as poor effectors in terms of complement binding and opsonization.

So far, no MoAb other than ortho pan OKT3 has been used on a large scale in humans, and the clinical experience available for the MoAbs that have reached clinical trials is still limited. Basically, two kinds of MoAbs are under study. First, there are those that interact with determinants present on all lymphocytes or on a large proportion of T cells and second, there are those that interact with discrete subsets of lymphocytes. In addition, a third category consists of MoAbs that interact both with effectors (mostly lymphocytes) and with target tissues (anti-ICAM 1 for instance). We will first review the effects of MoAbs that have been tested in the past, then those that are currently under study, and finally those of potential interest. However, we will restrict this review to MoAbs that have reached clinical studies.

Anti-T12

This MoAb, directed at a surface membrane determinant present on all mature lymphocytes, was one of the very first to be tested in a clinical trial.[25] Recipients treated with anti-T12 did not appear to present less rejection compared to a historical control group,[25] although the number of patients reported has remained too small to allow a definitive conclusion. Nevertheless, this first trial suggested that, except for MoAbs able to destroy the targeted lymphocyte by complement-mediated toxicity such as campath 1M,[26] a MoAb directed at an antigen not involved in the function of the cell was likely to be ineffective.

Anti-CD3

MoAb directed against the epsilon component of the CD3 complex flanking the T cell receptor for antigens is so far the only one extensively studied and used in human allograft recipients.[1] This MoAb (ortho pan OKT3) can modulate the CD3-TCR complex at the surface of T cells and therefore makes it impossible for the lymphocytes of treated patients to interact with the antigen. Accordingly, the effectiveness of the MoAb in vivo can be monitored by the disappearance of CD3 markers at the surface membrane of lymphocytes whereas other T-cell CD (such as CD2) remain unmodified,[27] although graft infiltrating lymphocytes may not modulate CD3 as well.[28] Ortho pan CD3 has been shown to be a powerful agent for reversing rejections and, more recently, it has been shown to have a preventive effect in prophylactic protocols.[29] Although anti-CD3 MoAbs target all mature T cells, including resting ones, they are more specific than ATG since monocytes and natural killer (NK) and B cells lacking the CD3 marker are not targeted. However, the use of ortho pan OKT3 MoAb in the clinic has been tempered by adverse side effects present in a majority of treated patients including flu-like syndrome, pseudomeningitis, high-grade fever, chills, vomiting, and diarrhea and increased vascular permeability.[1] This syndrome has been shown to be related to acute T cell activation preceding CD3 modulation and to result in release of lymphokines such as interleukin (IL)2 or IL6.[23] In addition, TNF-α (but not IL1-β or interferon [IFN]-α)[23] is also over-produced, probably reflecting the involvement of the anti-CD3 Fc fragments with monocytes, bridging these cells with T cells.[30, 31] Recently, the involvement of TNF in this syndrome has been directly confirmed by the effect of an anti-TNF that has been shown to decrease the mentioned side effects when injected in conjunction with anti-CD3.[32] This syndrome, usually limited to the first 3 days of treatment, requires careful surveillance for detection of hyperhydration when given to patients with renal failure.

Several other anti-CD3 or antibodies directed against a monomorphic epitope of the alpha-beta heterodimeric T-cell receptor (TCR) have been recently tested in short series of graft recipients.[33] Preliminary data suggest that some of these MoAbs may result in lower T cell activation (principally anti-TCR) while still remaining able to modulate the CD3-TCR complex at the T cell surface.[33] When available, such reagents may represent an attractive alternative to ATG or classic anti-CD3 treatment; however, we will still be interfering with all lymphocytes and still lack the specificity for antigen-committed cells.

Anti-CD7

CD7 is present on all T cells, including thymocytes. Although the function of this molecule is unknown, the fact that accessory signals can be delivered by some anti-CD7 to costimulated lymphocytes suggests that this molecule might be involved in some activation pathways. A chimeric form of CD7 in which Fc constant fragments from human IgG1 have been tested in primates has been shown to decrease the T cell counts and to modulate CD7 at the T-cell surface membrane.[34] Recently, this chimeric antibody has been tried in a pilot study in humans and seems to be devoid of important side effects.[35] This prophylactic study does not yet allow any conclusion as to the possible efficacy of anti-CD7 in preventing rejection, because of the small number of cases reported. However, the authors report no rejection episode during the time of anti-CD7 treatment ($n = 11$)[35] (P. Sweny, personal communication). More promising is the fact that this chimeric MoAb appeared to have elicited no anti-MoAb antibodies in this first report.

Anti-CD4

Anti-CD4 MoAb comprise a heterogeneous cluster in terms of in vivo efficacy as suggested in the mouse model.[36, 37] In this species, an anti-CD4 (anti-L3T4) was able to prolong skin or cardiac allografts and to induce in the recipient a state of tolerance for the nonidiotypic determinants of the

MoAb itself as well as for those of other xenogeneic antigens (aggregated Ig for instance) when given simultaneously to the animals.[39] Moreover, anti-CD4 MoAb can induce graft tolerance when injected in large doses at grafting. How anti-CD4 operates remains mysterious because some MoAbs deplete the $CD4^+$ lymphocyte subset while others do not. It is, however, probable that the T helper signals delivered to the B cell are attenuated. Actions through inhibition of the interaction between CD4 and class II molecules or through direct regulatory signals (CD4 is linked to P56 LKC, a kinase that can be activated during CD4-class II interaction) are also possible. Recently, an anti-CD4 (a mouse IgG2a: BL4) has been used immediately after transplantation and until day 3 to day 14 in a short series of human kidney graft recipients.[40] This pilot study was too limited to make conclusions concerning the potential BL4 effect on early rejection incidence (four episodes occurred in the 12 patients treated), but quite remarkable was the observation that only one patient developed anti-BL4 antibodies,[40] suggesting that some blocking effect of this MoAb could occur in the recipient anti-MoAb immune response, as reported with some anti-CD4 in the mouse.[39]

Anti-LFA1 and ICAM 1

Adhesion molecules (interaction CD8/class I, CD4 class II, LFA1 ICAM 1 and 2, CD2/LFA3) are required for optimal T cell activation by alloantigens. They operate by delivering accessory activation signals, as restriction elements, and by increasing the physical interactions between attacking and target cells.[41] Antibodies directed at the CD11a determinant of the LFA1 heterodimeric molecules or at ICAM 1 (one of the known ligands of LFA1), have been shown to inhibit various immune reactions ranging from the initial recognition steps to effector functions.[41] A rat anti-CD11a MoAb (Ig2a, MoAb 25-3) has been used with success for the first time in humans to prevent rejection in pediatric patients with mismatched bone marrow grafts.[42] Moreover, the MoAb appeared to have only few and minor side effects. Although similar results were not obtained with an anti-CD18[43] or with the same MoAb in another pilot study in adult bone marrow recipients,[44] the results did appear sufficiently promising for us to try this antibody in organ transplantation. However, preliminary results (seven patients) obtained in a protocol of treatment of first ongoing acute cellular rejection episodes did not suggest that MoAb 25-3 can reverse rejection according to clinical and histologic criteria, even when high circulating levels are maintained (~6 μg/mL; nb: Kd of 25-3:2nM) by increasing the administered dose.[44a] Interestingly, monitoring of recipient anti-MoAb 23-5 immune response showed an extremely low level of immunization. Only one patient developed a low level of anti-MoAb 25-3. For comparison, in similar conditions, injection of an anti-IL2 receptor (also a rat Ig) led to 100% immunization[45] and, according to the literature, treatment with ortho pan OKT3 leads to 50% to 80% of immunization.[46, 47] Although these results are as yet preliminary (due to the small number of patients analyzed), these differences are nevertheless important and are reminiscent of what was observed by Benjamin et al. in the mouse[39] and noted above with treatment with the BL4 anti-CD4.[40] However, as we decided that it was not ethically acceptable to pursue this study in ongoing rejections (because of its apparent inefficacy), no further data will be available from our center for this clinical situation. Nevertheless, a new protocol in which the same MoAb will be given prophylactically for early rejection episodes should help to clarify this situation. Interestingly, almost no recipient anti-LFA1 response has either been noted in bone marrow recipients who do, however, mount some responses against another rat Ig (M. Hirn, personal communication). Again, these results are not yet conclusive since these bone marrow recipients underwent strong immunosuppression with aggressive chemotherapy. However, the differences are notable and should prompt further studies.

Although ICAM 1 is the only specific ligand of LFA1 and the only anti-LFA1 tested seems to be ineffective in reversing rejection, an anti-ICAM 1[48] has been shown to be very efficient in monkeys.[49] In addition, this anti-ICAM 1 prevented early kidney rejection.[49] That a MoAb targeting only one of the LFA1 ligands was strongly efficient whereas an anti-LFA1 itself was not was not expected since even in the presence of an anti-ICAM I, LFA1 should still be able to combine with another ligand in patients receiving anti-ICAM I MoAb. Although the difference could be in the epitopes involved (LFA1 can have two conformations associated with different levels of affinity for ICAM),[50] the fact that ICAM 1, in addition to lymphocytes, is expressed on target kidney and endothelial cells may play an important role in understanding its effectiveness. Extremely interesting is the fact that graft endothelial cells of treated animals exhibited a normal aspect even though they were covered by rat Ig for several days. These results suggest that a non-complement fixing MoAb directed at graft endothelial cell determinants may have no harmful effect but may instead protect these cells from recipient effectors.[51] However, the high level of expression of this ubiquitous molecule (which should absorb large quantities of MoAb) may cause some problems in obtaining optimal circulating concentrations of the MoAb in humans. Further results are expected from a recently initiated study in humans (B. Cosimi, personal communication). Interestingly, anti-ICAM 1 triggered a normal immune response in primate recipients.[49]

Activated T Cell Targeting

Anti-IL2 Receptor MoAb

Besides the use of agents interacting with all or with large subsets of lymphocytes, another approach to immunointervention in allograft recipients arose from the characterization of surface membrane molecules expressed almost exclusively on T cells upon antigen stimulation. Immediately after transplantation, such activation molecules would therefore be expressed only on the alloreactive lymphocytes genetically devoted to the recognition of donor class I or class II MHC antigens. Although the immunologic process leading to rejection is extremely complex and involves multiple interactions between immunocompetent cells and various mediators, the initial events are nevertheless apparently restricted to the recipient immune repertoire and are therefore under the control of a minority (~1:1000) of anti-donor committed recipient lymphocytes.[47]

The α chain (P55 or Tac chain) of the IL2-R, which is virtually not expressed on resting T cells but specifically expressed on antigenic stimulation, has been previously recognized to represent an almost perfect candidate for such a strategy of targeting activated cells. Theoretically, other lymphokine receptors such as IL4 could also be used. Kirkman et al. first showed that an anti-P55 MoAb could prevent or reverse rejection of heart allografts in mice.[51a] This in vivo capacity, almost completely restricted to MoAbs directed at the IL2 binding epitope of P55, has been reproduced in various species and models including skin, heart, and kidney grafting,[52, 53, 54, 55] DTH reaction,[58] and autoimmune diseases.[47] In 1987,[59] we reported the first study in the human with a rat IgG2a anti-human IL2 receptor MoAb produced by D. Olive et al.[60] This MoAb belongs to a cluster that can inhibit the binding of IL2 on both isolated P55 and IL2-receptor in its high affinity conformation and blocks IL2-induced growth on IL2-dependent clones.[61] This study indicated that this MoAb was devoid of side effects and, when used at 10 mg/day for 14 days starting immediately after transplantation, led to a rejection incidence comparable to that observed in an ALG-treated historical group.[59]

These preliminary results were recently confirmed in a randomized trial in which 33B3.1 has been respectively compared to anti-thymocyte globulins in a prophylactic protocol.[16] In this study, the incidence of rejection during MoAb treatment was slightly increased compared to an ATG group (12% vs. 2% of rejection within the first 2 weeks), but was almost similar at 1 or 3 months. In addition, patients treated with the anti-P55 MoAb had fewer infections than those receiving ATG. Other anti-P55 MoAb are currently being tested by several groups and, although all the studies are not yet complete and still include a small number of patients, various results have been reported. While some antibodies can significantly decrease the incidence of rejection and delay its occurrence in kidney[62] and liver[63] graft recipients, others cannot.[64] More information has to be accumulated to allow some conclusion on the possibility of various other parameters that may affect the MoAb effectiveness; for example, the role of the epitope recognized or the isotype of the MoAb (for instance, the two IgG2a MoAbs of rat origin could be more potent). The use of new genetically[65] or chemically[66] engineered chimeric anti-IL2-R preparations may circumvent the strong recipient antibody response elicited by 33B3.1 MoAb.

Finally, there has been only one study on the effect of an anti-IL2-R in the treatment of ongoing rejection; only partial and inconsistent recovery was noted in a series of ten acute rejection episodes and the study was interrupted.[45] These preliminary results suggest that IL2-R$^+$ cells are not directly involved in the rejection process at the time of ongoing rejection when the majority of the infiltrating cells are monocyte/macrophage cells[67] and when clonal expansion of T cells has already taken place. Alternatively, one cannot rule out other mechanisms of escape, such as high ligand concentration in the microenvironment of the graft and difficulties of access of the MoAb molecules to the graft infiltrating cells. Other related IL2-receptor-targeting agents, such as IL2-diphterlatoxin able to kill the target cells may be even more active. Additionally, it has been recently reported that a synergistic effect exists between some anti-β chain (P75) MoAb (TU27 for instance) and 33B3.1.[68] A combination of these two MoAbs in vitro results in a strong diminution in the levels of 33B3.1 required to achieve a profound inhibition of either IL2 binding on its high affinity receptor or on IL2-dependent growth of CTLL2 cell lines, two assays in which TU27 is ineffective alone.[68] Although targeting the β chain of IL2-R may result in the loss of the strict specificity of activated cell targeting (some β chains are present on resting lymphocytes), the combination of the two MoAbs may be more effective on high affinity IL2-R positive cells and therefore may be of some interest in the future.

Other Means of IL2-R Targeting

Some preliminary reports in humans, as well as the concordant results obtained in animals,[47] have sustained the concept that the IL2 receptor P55 chain and the high affinity receptor complex are important targets in transplantation. There is, therefore, a need for reagents that, in contrast to MoAb, would be cytotoxic for IL2R$^+$ cells in the human body environment and/or that would not elicit a rapid immune response in recipients.

The work of J. Murphy and T.B. Strom has initiated a family of original artificial molecules obtained by transfection of two fused genes, one being the cytokine corresponding to the receptor to target (IL2[69, 70] but also IL4[71]) and the second a toxin derived from several microorganisms (the first construct used diphtheria toxin).[69] IL2 diphtheria toxin fusion molecules[69, 71] that have an apparent affinity intermediate between the national ligand and a MoAb (~80 pM) are internalized after binding to activated lymphocytes and, after an initial and transient activation phase,[72] the cells are killed. Such a reagent has been shown to be extremely potent in inhibiting DTH reactions[70] and in prolonging graft survival in rodents. However, more information is required for primates about its possible toxicity and effectiveness in allograft models. In addition, there is as yet no information about recipient immunization against the toxin part of the molecule, particularly in diphtheria vaccinated patients, although in the fusion protein, the receptor binding part of the toxin, which seems also to be the dominant epitope, has been deleted. Obviously, there is an important therapeutic potential for these reagents that could be adapted to a variety of ligands. Other fusion molecules composed of only human components and theoretically unable to elicit a recipient immune response are under study in our laboratory.

Recently, another promising approach to inhibition of the cytokine-mediated cascade has consisted of the use of soluble truncated forms of cytokine receptors corresponding to the extracellular part of the molecule. In two instances, IL1[74] and IL4 receptors[75] (both with one chain receptor structure), the ligand binding affinity was maintained. S-IL1 and S-IL4 receptors can slightly prolong heart allograft survival (5[74] and 4[75] days, respectively) in mice but completely inhibited the response to a local injection of allogenic cells.[74]

At the end of this review, we hope that it is apparent to the reader that the immunosuppressive properties offered by bioreagents are promising and are far from being completely explored. There are many other membrane molecules involved in the development of the allogenic immune response that are potential candidates for targeting. This first step of exploration, which is virtually awaiting only the availability of monoclonal antibodies, is further complicated by the important role of the epitope recognized by these antibodies and by their degree of effector function, which is related to MoAb isotypes. Ultimately, the first merit of these reagents will be the contribution they make in indicating the best targets for interaction with the lymphocyte surface membrane. It is, however, likely that the future tools we will use to interact with these targets will be either engineered humanized MoAb or artificial antagonist molecules, more resembling classical drugs than MoAbs.

References

1. Ortho Multicenter Transplant Study Group: A randomized clinical trial of OKT3 monoclonal antibody for acute rejection of cadaveric renal transplant. *N Engl J Med* 1985; 313:337–341.
2. Wooldruff MFA, Anderson MF: Effect of lymphocyte depletion by thoracic duct fistula and administration of antilymphocyte serum on the survival of skin homografts in rats. *Nature* 1963; 200:702–704.
3. Monaco AP, Wood ML, Russel PS: Some effects of purified heterologous antihuman lymphocyte serum in man. *Transplantation* 1967; 5:1106–1111.
4. Wechter WJ, Brodie JA, Morrell RM, et al: Anti-thymocyte globulin (ATGAM) in renal allograft recipients. *Transplantation* 1979; 28:294–299.
5. Traeger J, Carraz M, Fries D, et al: Studies of antilymphocyte globulins made from thoracic duct lymphocytes. *Transplant Proc* 1969; 1:455–458.
6. Howard RJ, Condie RM, Sutherland DER, et al: The use of antilymphoblast globulin in the treatment of renal allograft rejection. *Transplant Proc* 1981; 13:473–476.
7. Laufer G, Miholic J, Laczkovics A, et al: Independent risk factors predicting acute graft rejection in cardiac transplant recipients treated by triple drug immunosuppression. *J Thorac Cardiovasc Surg* 1989; 98:1113–1121.
8. Bonneville M, Carcagne J, Vie H, et al: Polyclonal rabbit gamma globulins against a human cytotoxic $CD4^+$ T cell clone. I. Clone characteristics and antiblast globulin preparation. *Transplantation* 1989; 48:253–260.

9. Filo RS, Smith EJ, Leapman SB: Therapy of acute cadaveric renal allograft rejection with adjunctive antithymocyte globulin. *Transplantation* 1980; 30:445–451.
10. Hoitsma AJ, Van Lier HJJ, Reekers P, et al: Improved patient and graft survival after treatment of acute rejections of cadaveric renal allograft with rabbit antithymocyte globulin. *Transplantation* 1985; 39:274–280.
11. Touraine JL, Bozi E, El Yafi S: Infectious lymphoproliferative syndrome in transplant patients under immunosuppressive treatment. *Transplant Proc* 1985; 17:96–98.
12. Kupin WL, Venkatachalam KK, Oh HK, et al: Sequential use of Minnesota antilymphoblast globulin and cyclosprine in cadaveric renal transplantation. *Transplantation* 1985; 40:601–604.
13. Hourmant M, Soulillou JP, Guenel J: Comparison of three immunosuppressive strategies in kidney transplantation: Antithymocyte globulin and conventional treatment, antithymocyte globulin and cyclosporine. A one-center randomized study. *Transplant Proc* 1985; 17:1158–1161.
14. Madsen M, Johnsen HE: Methodological study of E rosette formation using AET treated sheep red blood cells. *J Immunol Method* 1979; 27:61–65.
15. Soulillou JP, Peyrat MA, Guenel J: Association between treatment resistant kidney allograft rejection and post-transplant appearance of antibodies to be lymphocytes alloantigen. *Lancet* 1978; 1:354–356.
16. Soulillou JP, Cantarorich D, Le Mauff B, et al: Randomized trial of an anti-interleukin 2 receptor monoclonal antibody (33B3.1) versus rabbit antithymocyte globulin (ATG) in prophylaxis of early rejection in human renal transplantation. *N Engl J Med* 1990; 322:1175–1182.
17. Debure A, Chkoff N, Chatenoud L, et al: One-month prophylactic use of OKT3 in cadaver kidney recipients. *Transplantation* 1988; 45:546–552.
18. Moreau JF, Bonneville M, Peyrat MA, et al: T-lymphocyte cloning from rejected human kidney allografts. Growth frequency and functional/phenotypic analysis. *J Clin Invest* 1986; 78:874–879.
19. Bonneville M, Moreau JF, Blokland E, et al: T-lymphocyte cloning from rejected human kidney allograft. Recognition repertoire of alloreactive T-cell clones. *J Immunol* 1988; 141:4187–4195.
20. Hourmant M, Babinet F, Cantarovich D, et al: Polyclonal rabbit gammaglobulins against a human cytotoxic $CD4^+$ T cell clone. II. Use in prevention of rejection in kidney transplantation: A pilot study. *Transplantation* 1989; 48:260–263.
21. Stroberg S, Slavin D, Gottlieb M, et al: Allograft tolerance after total lymphoid irradiation (TLI). *Immunol Rev* 1979; 46:87–112.
22. Barber WH: Induction of tolerance to human renal allografts with bone marrow and antilymphocyte globulin. *Transplant Rev* 1990; 4:68–78.
23. Chatenou L, Ferran C, Legendre C, et al: Clinical use of OKT3: The role of cytokine release and xenosensitization. *J Autoimmunity* 1988; 1:631–641.
24. Debets JMH, Leunissen KML, Van Hooff HJ, et al: Evidence of involvement of tumor necrosis factor in adverse reactions during treatment of kidney allograft rejection with antithymocyte globulin. *Transplantation* 1989; 47:487–492.
25. Kirkman RL, Aranjo JL, Brusch GJ, et al: Treatment of acute allograft rejection with monoclonal anti-T12 antibodies. *Transplantation* 1983; 36:620–626.
26. Hale G, Waldman H, Friend P, et al: Pilot study of Campath-1, a rat mono-

clonal antibody that fixes human complement, as an immunosuppressant in organ transplantation. *Transplantation* 1980; 42:308–310.
27. Chatenoud L, Baudrihaye MF, Kreis H, et al: Human in vivo antigenic modulation induced by the anti T-cell OKT3 monoclonal antibody. *Eur J Immunol* 1982; 12:919–984.
28. Kerr PG, Atkins RC: The effects of OKT3 therapy on infiltrating lymphocytes in rejecting renal allografts. *Transplantation* 1989; 48:33–36.
29. Vigeral P, Chkoff N, Chatenoud L, et al: Prophylactic use of OKT3 monoclonal antibody in cadaver kidney recipients. *Transplantation* 1986; 41:730–733.
30. Frenken L, Koene R, Tax W: Role of isotype in anti CD3 induced interferon gamma synthesis. *Transplantation* 1991; 51:881–886.
31. Woodle E, Thislethwaite J, Stuart F, et al: T lymphocyte activation and lymphokine production induced by anti human CD3 monoclonal antibodies is dependent on antibody isotype and epitope specificity. *Transplant Proc* 1991; 23:81–82.
32. Ferran C, Sheehan K, Schreiber R, et al: Anti-TNF monoclonal antibody significantly abrogates the anti CD3 induced reaction. *Transplant Proc* 1991; 23:849–850.
33. Land W, Hillebrand G, Illner WD, et al: First clinical experience with a new TCR/CD3-monoclonal antibody (BMA 031) in kidney transplant patients. *Transplant Int* 1988; 1:116–117.
34. Heimich G, Gram H, Kocher HP, et al: Characterization of a human T cell specific chimeric antibody (CD7) with human constant and mouse variable regions. *J Immunol* 1989; 143:3589–3597.
35. Sweny P, Amlot P, Fernando O, et al: Pilot study of chimeric human/mouse CD7 monoclonal antibody (SD2 CMH 380) in renal transplantation (abstract). Presented at the meeting of the Transplantation Society, August, 1990.
36. Alters SE, Sakai K, Steinman L, et al: Mechanisms of anti CD4-mediated depletion and immunotherapy. A study using a set of chimeric anti CD4 antibodies. *J Immunol* 1990; 144:4587–4592.
37. Waldor MK, Mitchell P, Kipps TJ, et al: Importance of immunoglobulin isotype in therapy of experimental autoimmune encephalomyelitis with monoclonal anti CD4 antibody. *J Immunol* 1987; 139:3660–3664.
38. Deleted in proofs.
39. Benjamin RJ, Qin S, Wise MP, et al: Mechanisms of monoclonal antibody-facilitated tolerance induction: A possible role for the CD4 (L3T4) and CD11a (LFA1) molecules in self-non-self discrimination. *Eur J Immunol* 1988; 18:1079–1088.
40. Morel P, Vincent C, Cordier G, et al: Anti CD4 monoclonal antibody administration in renal transplanted patients. *Clin Immunol Immunopathol,* in press.
41. Springer TA, Dustin ML, Kishimoto TK, et al: The lymphocyte function associated LFA1, CD2 and LFA3 molecules: Cell adhesion receptors of the immune system. *Ann Rev Immunol* 1987; 5:223–252.
42. Fisher A, Griscelli C, Blanche S, et al: Prevention of graft failure by an anti-LFA1 monoclonal antibody in HLA-mismatched bone marrow transplantation. *Lancet* 1986; ii:1058–1061.
43. Baume D, Kuentz M, Pico JL, et al: Failure of a CD18/anti-LFA1. Monoclonal antibody infusion to prevent graft rejection in leukemic patients receiving T depleted allogeneic bone marrow transplantation. *Transplantation* 1989; 47:472–474.

44. Maraninchi D, Mawas C, Stoppa AM, et al: Anti-LFA1, monoclonal antibody for the prevention of graft rejection after T cell depleted HLA-matched bone marrow transplantation for leukemia in adult. *Bone Marrow Transplant* 1989; 4:147–150.
44a. Le Mauff B, Hohrmant M, Rohgier JP, et al: *Transplantation* 1991; in press.
45. Cantarovich D, Le Mauff B, Hourmant M, et al: Anti-interleukin 2 receptor monoclonal antibody in the treatment of on-going acute rejection episodes of human kidney graft. A pilot study. *Transplantation* 1989; 47:454–457.
46. Goldstein G, Fuccello AJ, Norman DJ, et al: OKT3 monoclonal antibody plasma levels during therapy and the subsequent development of host antibodies to OKT3. *Transplantation* 1986; 42:507–510.
47. Le Mauff B, Cantarovich D, Jacques Y, et al: Monoclonal antibodies against interleukin-2 receptors in the immunosuppressive management of kidney graft recipients. *Transplant Rev* 1990; 4:79–92.
48. Stannton DE, Martin SD, Stratowa C, et al: Primary structure of ICAM-I demonstrates interaction between members of the immunoglobulin and integrin supergene families. *Cell* 1988; 52:925–933.
49. Cosimi AB, Geoffrion C, Anderson T, et al: Immunosuppression of cynomolgus recipients of renal allografts by R6.5, a monoclonal antibody to intercellular adhesion molecule-1, in Springer TA, Anderson DC, Rosenthal AS, et al: (eds): *Leukocyte Adhesion Molecules.* New York, Springer-Verlag, 1988, pp 274–281.
50. Arnaout MA: Structure and function of the leukocyte adhesion molecules CD11/CD18. *Blood* 1990; 75:1037–1050.
51. Cosimi AB, Conti D, Delmonico FL, et al: In vivo effects of monoclonals antibody to ICAM-1 (CD54) in non human primates with renal allografts. *J Immunol* 1990; 144:4604–4612.
51a. Kirkman RL, Barrett LV, Koltun WA, et al: Prolongation of murine cardiac allograft survival by anti-interleukin 2 receptor monoclonal antibody AMT-13. *Transplant Proc* 1987; 14:618–619.
52. Burkhardt K, Loughnan MS, Diamantstein T, et al: Immunosuppressive effect of the anti-IL2 receptor monoclonal antibody, AMT-13, on organ-cultured fetal pancreas allograft survival. *Transplantation* 1988; 46:726–731.
53. Granstein RD, Goulston C, Gaulton GN: Prolongation of murine skin allograft survival by immunologic manipulation with anti-interleukin 2 receptor antibody. *J Immunol* 1986; 136:898–902.
54. Tighe H, Friend PJ, Collier SJ, et al: Delayed allograft rejection in primates treated with anti-IL2 receptor monoclonal antibody Campath-6. *Transplantation* 1987; 45:226–228.
55. Tellides G, Dallman MJ, Morris PJ: Mechanism of action of interleukin-2 receptor (IL-2R) monoclonal antibody (Mab) therapy: Target cell depletion or inhibition of function? *Transplant Proc* 1989; 21:997–998.
56. Deleted in proofs.
57. Deleted in proofs.
58. Dantal J, Jacques Y, Soulillou JP: Cluster-function relationship of rat-anti mouse P55 112-receptor monoclonal antibodies. In vitro studies on the CTL-L2 mouse cell line and in vivo studies in a delayed type hypersensitivity model in mice. *Transplantation,* in press.
59. Soulillou JP, Peyronnet P, Le Mauff B, et al: Prevention of rejection of kidney transplants by monoclonal antibody directed against interleukin 2 receptor. *Lancet* 1987; 1:1339–1342.

60. Olive D, Raymond J, Dubreuil P, et al: Anti-interleukin 2 receptor monoclonal antibodies. Respective role of epitope mapping and monoclonal antibody-receptor interactions in their antagonist effects on interleukin 2-dependent T cell growth. *Eur J Immunol* 1986; 16:611–616.
61. Le Mauff B, Olive D, Moreau JF, et al: Epitopic analysis of the human interleukin 2 receptors by the use of monoclonal antibodies: Epitope-function relationship. *Transplant Proc* 1987; 19:281–284.
62. Reed MH, Shapiro ME, Milford EL, et al: Interleukin 2 receptor expression on peripheral blood lymphocytes in association with renal allograft rejection. *Transplantation* 1989; 48:361–366.
63. Otto G, Thies J, Kabelitz D, et al: Anti CD25 monoclonal antibody inhibits early rejection in liver transplantation. A controlled pilot study. *Transplant Proc* 1991; 23:1387–1389.
64. Friend P, Woldman H, Cobhold S, et al: Prophylactic use of the anti IL2 receptor monoclonal antibody YTH-906 after liver transplantation. A randomized controled trial. *Transplant Proc* 1991; 23:1390–1392.
65. Queen C, Schneider WP, Selick HE, et al: A humanized antibody that binds to the interleukin 2 receptor. *Proc Natl Acad Sci USA* 1989; 86:10029–10033.
66. Carosella ED, Latour M, Jacques Y, et al: Anti human IL2 receptor monoclonal antibody isotypic switching: chimeric rat-human antibodies. *Hum Immunol* 1990; 29:233–246.
67. Bouchot O, Anegon I, Romaniuk A, et al: Interleukin 2 receptor in rat allograft rejection. *Transplant Proc* 1990; 22:1995–1997.
68. Audrain M, Boeffard F, Soulillou JP, et al: Synergistic action of Mabs directed at p55 and p75 chains of the human IL2-receptor. *J Immunol* 1991; 146:884–892.
69. Bacha P, Williams DP, Waters C, et al: Interleukin 2 receptor-targeted cytotoxicity. Interleukin 2 receptor-mediated action of a diphtheria toxin-related interleukin 2 fusion protein. *J Exp Med* 1988; 167:612–622.
70. Kelley VE, Bacha P, Pankewycz O, et al: Interleukin 2-diphtheria toxin can abolish cell-mediated immunity in vivo. *Proc Natl Acad Sci USA* 1988; 85:3980–3984.
71. Ogata M, Chaudray VK, Fitzgerald DJ, et al: Cytotoxic activity of a recombinant fusion protein between IL4 and pseudomonas exotoxin. *Proc Natl Acad Sci USA* 1989; 86:4215–4219.
72. Walz G, Zanker B, Brand K, et al: Sequential effects of interleukin 2-diphtheria toxin fusion protein on T-cell activation. *Proc Natl Acad Sci USA* 1989; 86:9485–9488.
73. Deleted in proofs.
74. Fanslow WL, Sims JE, Sassenfeld H, et al: Regulation of alloreactivity in vivo by a soluble form of IL1 receptor. *Science* 1990; 248:739–742.
75. Fanslow W, Clifford K, Beckman M, et al: Regulation of in vivo alloreactivities by IL4 and the soluble IL4 receptor (abstract). Presented at the Meeting of the Transplantation Society, San Francisco, August, 1990.

Xenografting: A New Hope for Organ Transplantation

Claus Hammer, M.D., Ph.D.

Professor, Institute for Surgical Research, University of Munich, Klinikum Grosshadern, Munich, Germany

The shortage of human organs is a persistent and increasing problem in transplantation. According to German statistics for 1989, 1,918 kidneys were transplanted, more than 5,849 patients were on the waiting list, and the number of patients on dialysis exceeded 20,937. This need has stimulated studies aimed at the use of organs from outside the human species for grafting; i.e., xenotransplants. The use of animal organs would have many advantages, including:

1. no shortage of organs, because one could select the appropriate species (e.g., pig, sheep, or monkey). They could be bred in large and sufficient numbers.
2. no logistic problems, because the breeding stations or sterile animal facilities could be located close to transplant centers.
3. fewer ethical problems, because the donor situation, with all its crucial questions, would be solved.
4. fewer financial problems because, at least in the future, the production of specific pathogen-free (SPF) animals would not be too expensive.

Xenotransplantation must be looked at in terms of evolutionary considerations and under different physiologic conditions and immunologic aspects than allogeneic transplantation. Xenogeneic immunologic problems, especially preformed natural antibodies, are important in widely divergent species. Transplantation of organs of more closely related species; i.e., concordant systems in which cellular mechanisms dominate rejection, has to be distinguished from that in widely divergent or discordant systems in which organs are destroyed by humoral mechanisms.

Evolutionary Considerations in Xenotransplantation

The classification of phylogenetic relationships and their impact on histocompatibility of organs or cells of the various animal species and man is possibly the most challenging question in xenogeneic transplantation. In the early days of allogeneic and xenogeneic transplantation at the beginning of this century, the evolutionary aspects were not taken into consideration. Organs from animals unselected for their genetic background were transferred to human beings with poor results. Today it is understood that organs taken from closely related species survive much better than those harvested from species that are phylogenetically widely divergent. Such evolutionary considerations and their impact in terms of zoological relationships are obviously of extreme importance with regard to the highly restrictive criteria involved in the choice of a suitable xenograft for man.[1] These criteria include not only the availability of appropriate species, organ size, blood group compatibility, and protein histocompatibility, but also the fact that certain characteristics of these parameters have undergone specific evolutionary changes. Such changes occur to a different extent in different species, and might therefore be quite disparate even in zoologically similar species. The rates of morphologic change in animal species appear to shift tremendously in a short time, simply under the pressure of the environment, for example during domestication.[2]

Chromosome analyses have opened new avenues for the study of genetic diversity and relationship in xenogeneic transplantation. The genetic relationship between species is determined on the basis of similar structural and organizational development of the DNA. In reassociation experiments and DNA-DNA hybridization, it was shown that 98% of human DNA can be found in the genes of chimpanzees, 92% in other Old World monkeys, and 85% in Asiatic primates.[3–5] The major histocompatibility (MHC) locus has been highly conserved throughout vertebrate evolution, and much of the MHC polymorphism is passed on from species to species.[6]

Another aspect of the analysis of evolutionary development is the numerous analogous enzymes that occur in animal cells. They possess similar substrate specificities but show considerable immunologic variation among different species. Comparisons between mammalian hemoglobins have shown that the α and β chains are derived from one common ancestor. However, they have undergone different degrees of mutational changes and the speed of mutation has also changed.[7–9] Blood perfusion of the graft and its clotting mechanisms are the main problems in xenogeneic transplantation. Blood viscosity in domestic animals is very similar. This constant factor relates to various blood components, including total protein, and red blood cells and white cells, the numbers of which change significantly.

Immunologic Aspects

Preformed natural antibodies (PNAb) are believed to be the primary reason for triggering hyperacute xenogeneic rejection. Sera from 111 animals representing seven zoological orders and 45 species showed considerable dependence on zoology; i.e., evolutionary system, in more than 8,000 individual tests. The more distantly related the species, the higher the titers of PNAb. Only primates and ungulates appear to produce isohemagglutinins. Closely related mammals within a zoologic family have no PNAbs. Many environmental factors influence the production of these PNAbs, including age, domestication, biorhythm, disease, and radiation. These PNAbs can be specific as shown by absorption experiments.[10, 11] A close correlation between the formation of PNAbs has been shown in two related species, the fox and dog. When erythrocytes from each species were used for absorption, the cross-reacting specificity was absorbed to a major degree, leaving some highly specific antibodies behind. The success of absorption of such antibodies decreases with the divergency of species. Given the above observations, it would seem that only closely related species within zoologic families; e.g., hare-rabbit, mouse-rat, the canines or primates, are suitable combinations for xenotransplantation. Transplant survival times (SVT) of some significance can be achieved within these combinations. Other combinations of widely divergent species with high titers of antibodies show very short SVTs without laborious modulations.[12, 13] The use of animal donors smaller than the recipient (most primates are smaller than human beings) poses additional problems. It is not known if, for example, baboon hearts or kidneys are able to exceed their genetically predetermined size to match that of the larger recipient. It is also unknown whether the various growth factors or other peptide hormones, such as erythropoietin or anti-diuretic hormone, can function properly in widely divergent species.

Transplantation in Closely Related Systems

The rate and pattern of rejection of xenografts depends mainly on the genetic disparity of the species involved. As long as the animals subjected to xenografting belong to the same zoologic family, rejection episodes are observed that are primarily of cellular character. The survival time reaches intervals close to that of allogeneic transplant models. They are therefore called concordant.

Modern, highly potent immunosuppressive drugs and new immunomodulating methods have recently pushed xenogeneic transplantation into a clinically interesting position. To elucidate the various participating mechanisms during xenogeneic rejection in concordant and discordant systems, we have used animal species of varying phylogenetic relationships. The zoologic family of canines of the order Carnivora was found to be appropriate. Skin, hearts, and mainly kidneys from wolves *(Canis lupus)*, dingos *(Canis dingo)*, and foxes *(Vulpes vulpes)* were transplanted into inbred beagles and mongrel dogs to mimic a concordant system comparable to that of primates.[12]

The discordant situation was studied by hemoperfusing pig or sheep kidneys with blood from dogs; i.e., from a species of a different zoologic order.[14] The most important approach was to determine genetic and immunogenetic markers in this experimental model to demonstrate the phylogenetic relationship of the species used.

Kidney Transplantation

Beagles, weighing 12 to 15 kg and mongrel dogs of the same size received closely related xenogeneic fox kidneys. In the fox-dog model, both kidneys were removed en bloc, perfused, and cooled. Foxes of 3 to 4 kg body weight served as kidney donors. The animals were raised on farms. The kidneys were connected to the iliac vessels and the ureters were implanted into the bladder.[15] Wolf kidneys, originating from animals of 30 to 40 kg body weight, had to be transplanted into dogs of larger size (25 ± 4.5 kg). The donors had been injured in hierarchy fights but were basically healthy adults. Renal transplants from wolves and dingos were performed between matched donors and recipients. One kidney was implanted heterotopically into a nephrectomized recipient, with anastomosis to the iliac vessels.[16] Dingos were bred for scientific reasons. Dingos, the wild dogs of Australia, are believed to have been imported into New Guinea and Australia 10,000 years ago by the aborigines. They have developed from stone-age dogs into a naturally highly inbred strain. Before transplantation, the following immunogenetic markers were tested: karyotypes,[17] DLA histocompatibility,[18] mixed lymphocyte (MLR),[19] canine erythrocyte antigens,[20] red blood cell enzymes, haptoglobin electorphoresis, and other immunoelectrophoretic patterns (Fig 1).

Skin Transplantation

Thirty mongrel dogs of 8.5 ± 1.2 kg body weight were used as recipients of fox, wolf, and dingo skin. One animal of each species was selected as the only donor for all recipients. A skin flap of 2 × 3 cm was transplanted to the left thoracic wall under sterile conditions with atraumatic sutures at the four edges, while the remainder of the xenogeneic skin was attached with a tissue adhesive. The grafts were protected from destruction by a plastic cast with a wire mesh placed over the graft. The window allowed daily examination. Rejection was defined as 50% graft destruction.[12, 16]

	DOG	DINGO	WOLF	FOX
KARYOTYPE	2n= 78	2n= 78	2n= 78	2n= 38
DL - A	ORIGINAL	SIMILAR	SIMILAR	DETECTABLE IN FEW CASES
CEA	ORIGINAL	SIMILAR	SIMILAR	DETECTABLE IN MANY CASES
RBC-ISO-ENZYMES	ORIGINAL	DIFFERENT	DIFFERENT	DIFFERENT
SERUM-PROTEIN	ORIGINAL	SIMILAR	SIMILAR	DIFFERENT

FIG 1.
Markers tested in canine species.

Immunosuppressive Therapy

Recipients of dingo kidneys were not immunosuppressed. Wolf kidneys were transplanted to untreated dogs or dogs receiving horse anti-dog lymphocyte globulin (ALG). The ALG was raised in horses with thoracic duct lymphocytes of dogs as antigen. After absorption, the cytotoxic antibodies against lymphocytes showed a titer of 1:2,048; ALG was given in doses of 20 mg/kg body weight. To prevent antibody formation against ALG, the recipients were pretreated with deaggregated normal horse IgG on days −9 and −6 before transplantation. ALG was started on day −3, together with 1 mg/kg prednisolone, and was subsequently continued. ALG was also deaggregated before intravenous injection.[21] Fox kidneys were transplanted to dogs receiving:

1. ALG treatment as applied in the wolf-dog group;
2. anti-macrophage serum (AMS) with a titer of 1:4 after exhaustive absorption, applied at 0.3 mL/kg body weight 3 days prior to and 6 days after surgery;[15]
3. cyclosporin (CSA), given 1 day prior to transplantation (9 mg/kg body weight) intravenously (IV) dissolved in 20% Intralipid (5 mg/mL). Methylprednisolone (MP) was also given IV.[22] From the second postoperative day, 4 mg/kg CSA was given and tapered by 1 mg/kg body weight every third day.
4. 15-Deoxyspergualin, given at day 0 with a loading dose of 2.5 mg/kg body weight IV and 1.5 mg/kg daily from day 1 until the end of the experiment.

Results

Wolf Kidneys

Survival time (SVT) of 12 wolf kidneys ranged between 11 and 32 days in animals without surgical or other accidental failure. The mean SVT was 19.4 ± 2.8 days and was significantly longer ($P < .002$) than the survival time of allogeneic dog kidneys (11.4 ± 3.0) that served as controls. Treatment of the recipient with ALG prolonged SVT in four animals to 24, 27, 34, and 35 days, with a mean of 30.4 ± 2 days. Wolf skin transplanted onto mongrel dogs survived 12.5 ± 2.6 days with a range between 7 and 33 days. This was not significantly longer than the survival time of allogeneic dog skin, 8.6 ± 2.4 days. Daily treatment with ALG resulted in a prolongation up to 218 days with a mean SVT of 85.6 ± 20.6 days. Around 40 days after transplantation, fur was growing on the grafts.[16]

DLA Typing

All graft combinations between wolf and dog showed two or more mismatches in SD antigens. Like other immunogenetic markers, DLA antigens were scarcely different between dog and wolf. All wolves were proven to be an outbred population according to the SD antigens. With the sera used, the wild canines showed more blanks than the dogs.[12]

Mixed Lymphocyte Reaction

On the basis of the MLR, bidirectional stimulation could be established in all cases. A marked response between wolf and dog lymphocytes and vice versa was found. The rate of stimulation was comparable to that of an allogeneic system.[12]

Histologic Findings

The histologic picture of rejected wolf kidneys and skin was of cellular type, similar to that in allogeneic transplants. Signs of humoral involvement were detected in only three kidneys surviving longer than 25 days.

Dingo Kidneys

The semi-allogeneic kidneys were rejected after 11.5 ± 3.0 days in an allogeneic fashion. Creatinine and urea showed increasing values on day 6 after transplantation. The immunologic monitoring revealed no differences as compared to the allogeneic system. DLA typing and MLRs confirmed the allogeneic situation.[12]

Fox Kidneys

The xenogeneic renal grafts without treatment reached survival times of 6.5 ± 1.2 days. Prolongation achieved with the different immunosuppressive regimens is shown on Figure 2. The following mean survival times were measured: ALG 13.4 ± 1.0; AMS, 15.8 ± 0.7; ALG + AMS, 17.7 ± 0.9; CSA + MP, 10.9 ± 3.0 (see Fig 1).[22, 23] The cellular fluctuations in the peripheral blood as measured with fine-needle aspiration cytology reached maximum values of inflammation on day 7 after transplantation. The most common cells were lymphocytes and monocytes and their activated forms. No lymphoblasts, plasma cells, or macrophages were detected in the peripheral blood.[23]

Histologic investigations indicated massive infiltration of lymphocytes and lymphoblast-like cells in the transplanted fox kidneys. Immunofluorescence studies of renal biopsy specimens did not show any gamma globulin or complement deposits in the vessels of the rejected kidneys. These results along with the unchanged complement activities in the serum favor a predominantly cellular mechanism of rejection comparable to that of an allograft.[23] Xenogeneic skin from foxes survived 5.9 ± 1.4 days. The rejection was characterized by edema, hemorrhages, and induration. The interval between the first signs of rejection and 50%

ORGAN	IMMUNOSUPPRESSION	SVT (d)	N
KIDNEY	CONTROL	6.5 ± 1.2	8
KIDNEY	XENO BT	5.6 ± 0.9	6
KIDNEY	ALLO BT	6.3 ± 2.1	6
KIDNEY	ALG	13.4 ± 1.0	9
KIDNEY	AMS	15.8 ± 0.7	5
KIDNEY	ALG + AMS	17.7 ± 0.9	7
KIDNEY	CSA + MP	10.9 ± 3.0	7
KIDNEY	DEOXYSP.	13.0 ± 3.4	6
HEART	CONTROL	8.4 ± 1.9	6
HEART	CSA + MP	20.2 ± 4.1	6

FIG 2.
Survival times of fox kidney and heart grafts under various immunosuppressive regimens.

necrosis of the graft was 1 to 2 days. A correlation between the survival time of skin transplants and the histocompatibility results from dog and fox lymphocytes could not be established. The differences between genetic markers in this closely related xenogeneic transplantation system are shown in Figure 1.[12, 15] Heterotopic fox hearts transplanted to the recipient's neck functioned for 8.4 ± 1.9 days, slightly longer than that for fox kidneys. Immunosuppressive treatment with CSA and MP resulted in a survival time of 20.2 ± 4.1 days. The rejection was of the cellular type and comparable to mechanisms seen in kidneys (see Fig 2).

Pig Kidneys

Organs from widely divergent species hemoperfused with dog blood never showed typical function. The hyperacute xenogeneic rejection was of the pure humoral type. Factors such as preformed natural antibodies, complement, leukocytes, and platelets were eliminated from the perfusing blood (Figs 3–5). Manipulations including hemodilution, lymph drainage, or enhancing antibodies had no long-lasting effect (Fig 6).[14] The literature on this field has been compiled in an extensive review.[24]

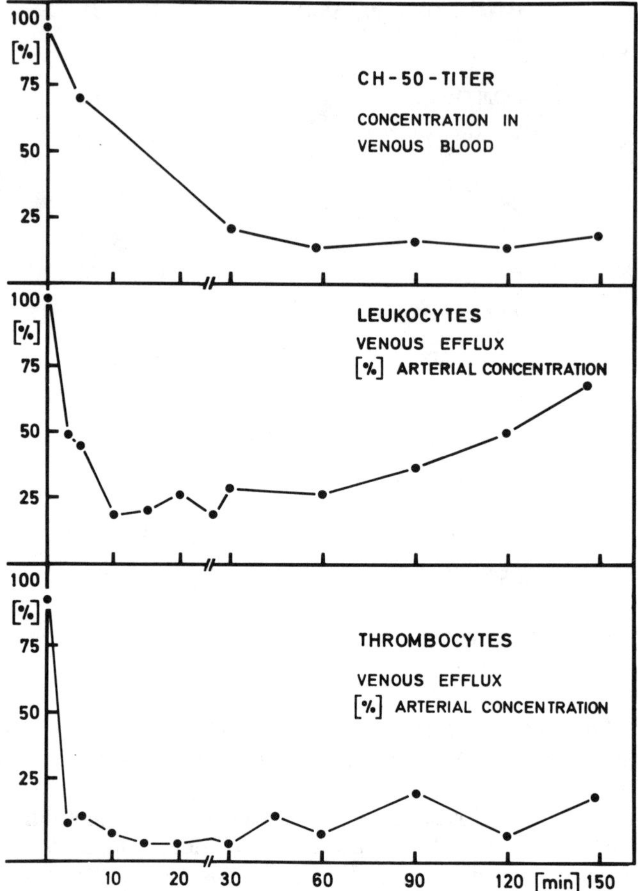

FIG 3.
Decrease in complement activity and cellular components in dog blood perfusing pig kidneys.

Discussion

Systematic evaluation of xenogeneic graft rejection is only possible by using donor-recipient combinations of different zoologic relationships. For clinical investigations, few animal species of appropriate body size are available. Closely related or so-called concordant species are even rarer. Primates have been widely used for such studies. We had access to various species of canines such as the wolf, dingo, and fox, all of different evolutionary distance from the domestic dog. On the basis of their genetic backgrounds, the domestic dog, the dingo, wolf, and jackal are closely related. They all produce fertile hybrids. The chromosome number (78) and the karyotype are identical or very similar. They are totally different from

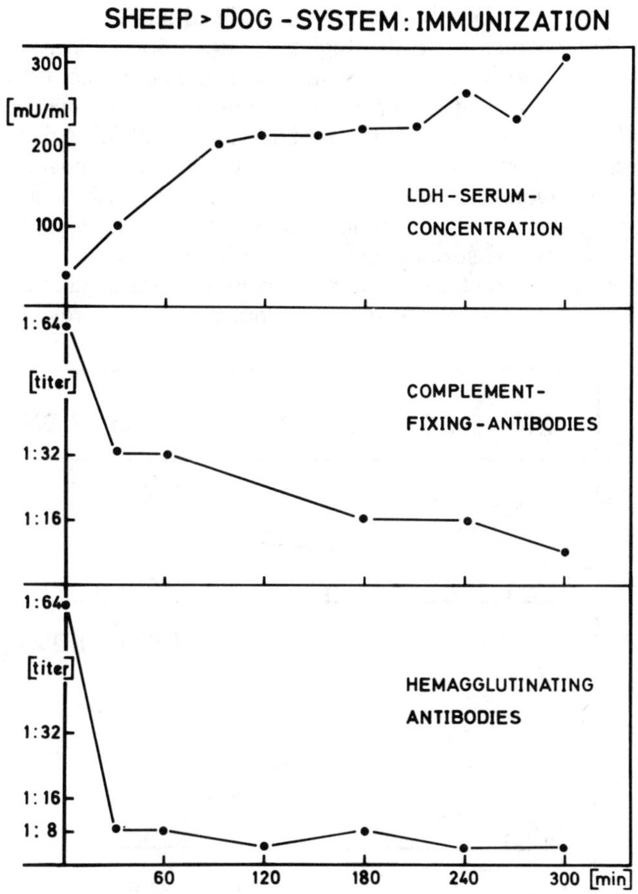

SHEEP > DOG - SYSTEM: IMMUNIZATION

FIG 4.
Decrease in humoral factors in dog blood perfusing pig kidneys.

foxes, which have 38 chromosomes and do not hybridize with dogs. Using DLA typing sera we found, however, more blanks in the wolves tested and could detect only some weak antigens on fox lymphocytes.

Posttransplant sera showing strong activity against fox transplantation antigens revealed only a few DLA specificities. It was difficult to type foxes with DLA sera. However, the recipients of fox organs produced antibodies that showed strong cross-reactions, not only with the dog lymphocytes, but also with their own red blood cells. Some of the recipients died from anemia, probably due to the high titers (1:64) of hemolytic antibodies induced by long-surviving fox kidney grafts at the time of rejection. Canine erythrocyte antigens, serum proteins, and erythrocyte isoenzymes showed similar behavior in our three dog species, but were completely different in the foxes.

With the use of serum albumin amino acid sequences as markers, it was calculated that coyotes have the highest genetic correlation with the domestic dog, followed by wolves, jackals, and, finally, foxes. MLR, used to test the evolutionary relationship between the species, showed no correlation at all. It would, however, seem that stimulation of MLR decreases with evolutionary divergency, with the exception of wolves. Between donor and recipient in the wolf-dog system, we found a statistically insignificant increase in ratios despite the exceptionally long survival time. This consistent finding of a prolonged survival time of wolf kidneys and skin in dogs, but not in the opposite direction, remains to be investigated. All rejections were primarily a cellular type. Dingo and wolf kidneys showed rejection mecha-

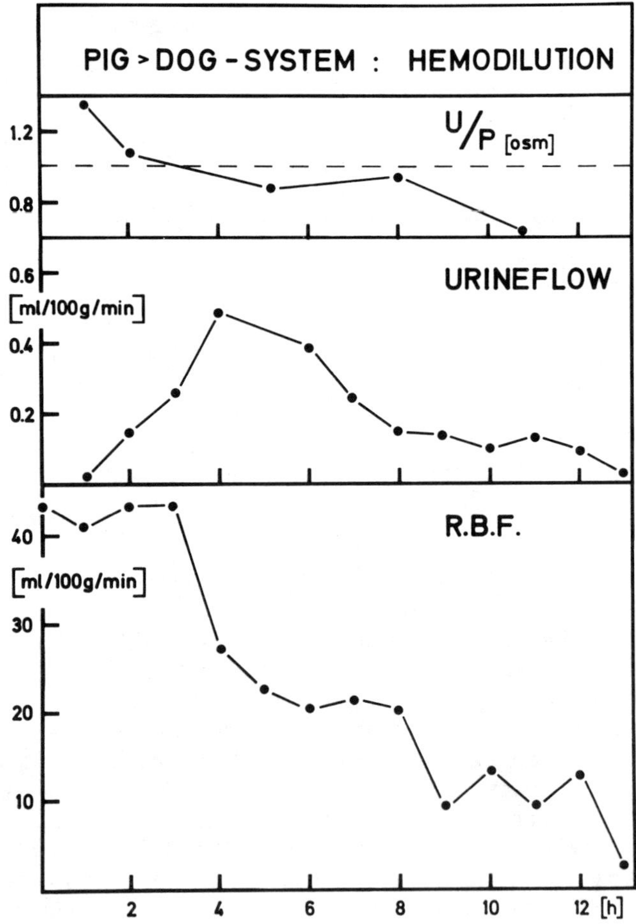

FIG 5.
Decrease in function (concentration, flow, and urine production) in xenogeneic kidneys under isovolemic hemodilution.

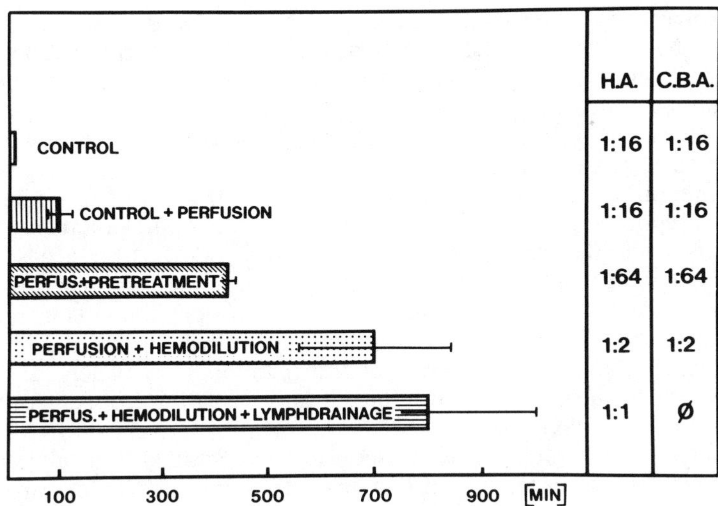

FIG 6.
Survival time of pig kidneys perfused with dog blood (control: no treatment; control + perfusion [Euro-collins solution]; perfusion + pretreatment [second set serum]); perfusion + hemodilution; perfusion + hemodilution + lymph drainage). Note difference in titer of PNab. *H.A.* = hemagglutinating antibody; *C.B.A.* = complement binding antibody.

nisms not distinguishable from those of allogeneic dogs. Fox organs were rejected in a more vigorous fashion.

The initial cellular mechanisms switched to humoral rejection shortly before the loss of graft function. Powerful immunosuppressive antibodies, CSA and deoxyspergualin, were able to prolong the survival time and to modify the rejection process. The surprisingly strong effect of antimacrophage serum (AMS) in dogs could be explained by new aspects of expression of class II antigens on canine mononuclear cells.[25, 26] Xenografts of widely divergent species like pig and sheep and even cats are rejected in a hyperacute fashion. It seems to us that the canines reject such discordant organs even more vigorously than primates. The mechanisms are of pure humoral character. However, depletion of antibodies by various methods, as reported by many authors,[24] did not lead to clinically important survival times. Thus, the xenogeneic canine model reflects known results from experiments performed in primates and even humans, and therefore proves its applicability as a clinically relevant model. What is the future direction of xenotransplantation?

In discordant systems, it appears that depletion of performed natural antibodies would be of major importance. Absorption columns, lymph drainage, and hemodilution are able to reduce the blood components, including preformed natural antibodies, to almost zero values. However, after a few days, most of the serum factors return to normal levels or show rebound effects. Clonal depletion of cells producing antibody directed against the xenogeneic antigen has been proposed, a procedure as difficult as the induction of antiidiotypic antibodies against PNAbs. Chemical destruction of preformed antibodies could be feasible. Dithiothreitol has been used to split sulphur bonds of IgM antibodies in patients who are highly sensitized. In patients in whom these antibodies disappeared, no rejection episodes developed after transplantation. Manipulation of the blood clotting system with antagonists to platelet-activating factor (PAF) and drugs inhibiting Ca^{2+}-transport have been suggested. Depletion of complement or inhibition of one specific part of the complement cascade has been described. The protection of cells or cultured cells against the immune response with membranes like alginate seems to be feasible. Our experiments with rat islets in a Goretex double membrane graft have been functional in dogs. However, it appears that discordant transplantation in widely divergent species remains a dream of the future. If and when it becomes feasible, it will revolutionize medicine.

Total lymphoid irradiation was used quite successfully in a primate and rat-hamster models (concordant systems). Together with potent immunosuppression, this could be a reasonable approach. Induction of transplant tolerance or transplantation of bone marrow to produce xenogeneic mixed chimeras has been successfully carried out in rats and mice. Transplantation of cultured cells depleted of passenger cells or class II antigens has been possible in histoincompatible allogeneic systems. Thus, concordant transplantation has an immediate therapeutic future. With our most powerful immunosuppressive strategies, xenotransplantation is ready to bridge desperate situations for a time that is ethically justifiable.

References

1. Reemtsma K, McCracken BH, Schlegel JU, et al: Renal heterotransplantation in man. *Ann Surg* 1964; 160:384–405.
2. Herre W, Röhrs M: *Haustiere Zoologisch Gesehen.* Stuttgart, Gustav Fischer Verlag, 1973.
3. Rake AC: DNA reassociation kinetics of closely related species. *Biochem Genet* 1974; 11:261–277.
4. Walker PMB: How different are the DNAs from related animals? *Nature* 1968; 219:228–232.
5. Wilson AC, Sarich VM, Maxson LR: The importance of gene rearrangement in evolution: Evidence from studies on rates of chromosomal, protein, and anatomical evolution. *Proc Natl Acad Sci USA* 1974; 71:3028–3030.
6. Figueroa F, Günther E, Klein J: MHC polymorphism pre-dating speciation. *Nature* 1988; 335:265–267.
7. Dolittle RF, Blombäck B: Amino-acid sequence investigations of fibrinopeptides from various mammals: Evolutionary implications. *Nature* 1964; 202:147–152.
8. Sarich VM, Wilson AC: Rates of albumin evolution in primates. *Proc Natl Acad Sci USA* 1967; 58:142–148.
9. Smith LF: Species variation in the amino acid sequence of insulin. *Am J Med* 1966; 40:662–666.

10. Hammer C: Isohemagglutinins and preformed natural antibodies in xenogeneic organ transplantation. *Transplant Proc* 1987; XIX:4443–4447.
11. Hammer C, Chaussy C, Brendel W: Preformed natural antibodies in animals and man. *Eur Surg Res* 1972; 5:162–166.
12. Hammer C, Chaussy C, von Scheel J, et al: Survival times of skin and kidney grafts within different canine species in relation to their genetic markers. *Transplant Proc* 1975; VII:439–447.
13. Schilling A, Land W, Pielsticker K: Experimental xenografting in widely divergent species; interaction of humoral factors in hyperacute xenograft rejection in the rat-dog system. *Res Exp Med* 1975; 165:79–92.
14. Messmer K, Hammer C, Land W, et al: Modification of hyperacute xenogeneic kidney rejection. *Transplant Proc* 1971; III:542–544.
15. Chaussy C, Hammer C, von Scheel J, et al: Xenogeneic skin and kidney transplants in a closely related canine system fox-dog. *Transplantation* 1975; 20:150–154.
16. Hammer C, Chaussy C, Welter H, et al: Exceptionally long survival time in xenogeneic organ transplantation. *Transplant Proc* 1981; XIII:881–884.
17. Lin CC, Johnston DH, Ramsden RO: Polymorphism and quirincrine fluorescence karyotypes of red foxes *(V. vulpes)*. Can J Genet Cytol 1972; 14:573–580.
18. Vriessendorp HM, Albert ED, Templeton JW, et al: Joint report of the second international workshop on canine immunogenetics. *Transplant Proc* 1976; VIII:289–314.
19. Grosse-Wilde H, Baumann P, Netzel B, et al: One way nonstimulation in MLC to DL-A homozygocity. *Transplant Proc* 1973; 5:1567–1571.
20. Swicher SN, Yang LE: The blood grouping system of dogs. *Physiol Rev* 1961; 41:495–503.
21. Brendel W, Duswald KH, von Scheel J, et al: Prolonged survival time of canine xenografts using a new schedule of horse-anti-dog lymphocytic globulin. *Transplant Proc* 1977; IX:379–381.
22. Krombach F, Hammer C, Gebhard F, et al: The effect of cyclosporine on wolf to dog kidney xenografts. *Transplant Proc* 1985; XVII:1436–1437.
23. Böhm D, Krombach F, Hammer C, et al: Fine needle aspiration cytology in cyclosporine treated xenogeneic kidney rejection. *Transplant Proc* 1985; XVII:2128–2129.
24. Auchincloss H: Xenogeneic transplantation. *Transplantation* 1988; 46:1–20.
25. Doxiadis I, Krumbacher K, Neefjes JJ, et al: Biochemical evidence that the DLA-B locus for class II determinants is expressed on all canine peripheral blood lymphocytes. *Exp Clin Immunogenet* 1989; 6:219–224.
26. Krumbacher K, van der Feltz JM, Happel M, et al: Revised classification of the DLA loci by serological studies. *Tissue Antigens* 1986; 27:262–268.

Subject Index

A

B

L

M

N

O